EASY REFERENCE TABLE

PACKAGED SIDES, MEALS & MEAL HELPERS

CONDIMENTS, SAUCES & DRESSINGS

Symbols Defined

gf = gluten-free

⚇   **Gluten-Free** lines, equipment, environment or facilities.

⚇   **Gluten Testing** is done on products, ingredients and/or equipment.

( )   **Cross-Contamination** is a possibility; or

       Shared Facility, Equipment or Line, as noted by the company; or,

       The product is made with "gluten-free ingredients" (with no mention of overall status by the company).

    Gluten-Free based on Triumph's independent review of ingredient label. Manufacturer has indicated that any gluten would be identified clearly on labels, but has not provided a GF list.

see p 17 for more tips! >>

INTRODUCTION

2nd edition

This guide is about making gluten-free grocery shopping safe, easy and full of choices. And, if you're keeping score at home, this new 2nd edition has 50% more listings than last year's, featuring over 30,000 gluten-free products.

I remember when gluten-free products were almost exclusively available at health food stores. Not only were these stores not as convenient or ubiquitous as local supermarkets, but their prices were often very expensive. Today, even mainstream supermarkets like Wal-Mart, Kroger and Trader Joe's are jumping on the gluten-free bandwagon with expanded gluten-free aisles, lists and product labeling. Talk about progress!

While a lot has changed for gluten-free shoppers in the last five years, gluten-free grocery shopping still remains a challenge. Despite advances in labeling, very few products are clearly labeled "gluten-free." And, a typical grocery store caries over 40,000 products. Where do you even start? As individual consumers searching for gluten-free products, we're often left guessing in grocery store aisles or calling dozens of manufacturers on a regular basis. This guide gives us a better way. It's designed to help you save valuable time and money anywhere you shop.

We've pulled together information about tens of thousands of gluten-free products from hundreds of manufacturers, and compiled it all in one convenient, easy-to-use grocery guide. Our goal is for you to use this guide as a starting point to find the right products, so that you can quickly hone in on items that are likely to suit your needs.

I've also seen some of our customers use the 1st edition of this guide to drastically reduce their monthly food bills. They did it by finding lower priced stores, focusing on private label products, and cleverly rationing the more expensive specialty items they were buying in the past. I choose to support companies that go the extra mile to test and label for gluten, and I hope you will, too. But, for those on a limited budget, you don't always have to pay a lot more to eat gluten-free.

Speaking of tough economic times, the last few months have been marked by rising commodity prices, affecting the price you pay at the gas pump and grocery store. Equally worrisome for a publishing company, paper and ink prices have also skyrocketed. Despite increased printing costs (and a 2nd edition that has 50% more listings than the first), we've gone to great lengths to keep the price of this guide stable. This year, we added advertising from some of the best and most exciting gluten-free products out there. The generous support of our advertisers has helped us keep this guide affordable. Please consider rewarding their generosity with your support.

On a final note, many of you have been with us since the beginning, when we launched our dining cards as a passion project in 2005. With your incredible support and encouragement, we've grown into a full-fledged publishing company. As we continue this evolution, our goal remains the same: to bring you world-class products that make gluten-free living safe, easy and fun. We have some exciting products in the pipeline, but if there are additional things you'd like to see from us, please don't hesitate to contact me. As always, I would love to hear your comments, thoughts, or questions.

Wishing you a peaceful, prosperous and gluten-free year,

Ross

Ross Cohen
President
Triumph Dining
ross@triumphdining.com

Everyone knows how to grocery shop – we've all been doing it most of our adult lives. The interesting thing is that each person approaches shopping slightly differently. Some people spend hours methodically comparing prices in search of the best deal, and others race through the store as quickly as possible so they can move on to other things. There's no right or wrong way to shop, but what follows are a few basic tips and ideas to help make your gluten-free shopping trips a little more successful – no matter what your personal shopping style is.

Choosing a Grocery Store

Some grocery stores are simply better for the gluten-free shopper than others. Generally, I prefer to do my shopping in stores that cater to gluten-free clientele in some way – it makes my shopping easier, and I prefer to support the businesses that focus on my needs.

A store's focus on gluten-free customers can manifest itself in several ways:

1. Grouping gluten-free goods in one section, like Kroger does;

2. Stocking an extensive selection of gluten-free products – many smaller, specialty stores like Martindale's in Springfield, PA, Against the Grain in Salt Lake City, UT, and Gluten-Free Trading Company in Milwaukee, WI pride themselves on carrying hundreds or thousands of specialty, gluten-free items;

3. Labeling gluten-free foods – either in the grocery aisle like Whole Foods, or on packaging itself; Wegman's in New York marks their gluten-free, private label foods with a little "G";

4. Publishing a list of gluten-free items that can be found in their stores, like the Trader Joe's chains (though sometimes they run out of their printed lists, which is why their list is incorporated in this guide).

Stores that fit into these categories will tend to have more options for gluten-free customers, resulting in a better shopping experience. Try to frequent these types of stores when you can.

But, we understand that not everyone lives near a Trader Joe's, or can afford to buy all their groceries from premium and specialty stores. That's why this guide is designed to help you find gluten-free options in any grocery store – whether or not it specifically caters to gluten-free customers.

Common Pitfalls to Avoid

One ongoing concern for people on the gluten-free diet is cross-contamination. It can happen anywhere, there's no way to know whether it's happened to a product, and it's rarely ever flagged for us. Also, the Food Allergen Labeling and Consumer Protection Act does not set specific standards for using cross-contamination advisory statements or require manufacturers to identify the possibility of inadvertent cross-contamination. (See the next chapter for a more in-depth discussion of the FALCPA.)

And, concerns about cross-contamination extend beyond grocery store shelves, to bulk bins, deli/meat counters, and the prepared foods sections.

Bulk Bins

Bulk bins are largely left unattended by grocery store personnel. There's often no way to tell that other customers haven't inadvertently shared serving scoops across products, potentially contaminating anything that otherwise would have been gluten-free. And, there's no indication whether products rotate through the bins or, if they do, whether the bins are thoroughly cleaned before transitions. In other words, the bin that holds a seemingly gluten-free product today could have been full of wheat flour last week. For these reasons, we recommend avoiding bulk bins and buying packaged items, instead.

The Deli Counter

Deli counters and prepared food sections present a different challenge. Here, store personnel directly handle food products meant for your consumption. The easiest way to navigate these challenges is to think of the deli counter and prepared food section like "mini restaurants." (For more information about issues to consider in gluten-free restaurant dining, please refer to *The Essential Gluten-Free Restaurant Guide*, also available from Triumph Dining.)

Before you make a purchase, you need to understand both the ingredients in the food and the preparation methods used to create it. There are many issues to consider in making a decision about these foods. Some examples include: Do gluten-containing meats go in the deli slicer?

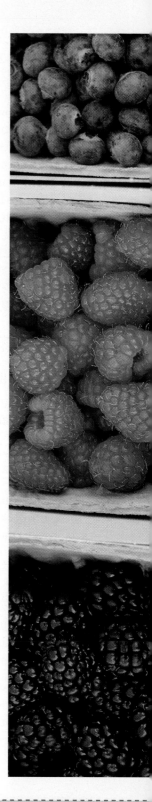

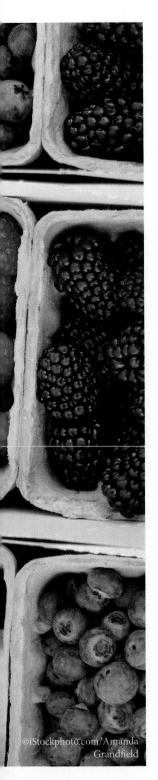

What, if any, precautions are taken in the prep area to avoid cross-contamination? Are there ingredient labels on the prepared foods? How accurate are those labels?

Often times, however, it's challenging to interface with the employees who prepared these foods. At some grocery stores we've seen, the prepared foods are made off-site or by an early morning crew that's long since cleared out by the time the typical person shops, making it hard to get questions answered about dish contents and preparation methods. For these reasons, we recommend frequenting deli counters and prepared food sections only when you've done sufficient due diligence to confirm the products you're purchasing truly are gluten-free.

Selecting Your Groceries

Despite a restricted diet, there are still many wonderful foods for gluten-free shoppers to choose from. When given a choice, I prefer to support the companies that cater to the needs of gluten-free customers. Some of these companies produce specialty products for the gluten-free market. Others have dedicated manufacturing lines and/or carefully test their products for gluten. Please consider buying their products and calling or writing in to let them know you appreciate their efforts. The more we support these businesses, the more products we'll have to choose from in the future.

Consider Your Information Source

When thinking about which products to purchase and evaluating information available to you, please keep in mind that primary source information, like ingredient statements on packages and manufacturer statements, is always better and more reliable than secondary source information, like postings on message boards and compilation lists (this guide included). Think of it like a game of telephone – the more people who handle information before you receive it, or the older that information gets, the greater chance there is of it having inaccuracies or other problems.

Always Read Labels

The goal of this guide is to drastically cut your label-reading time, but the reality is that no product obviates the need for label-reading entirely. Product formulations can change without notice, companies can make mistakes on their gluten-free list, and people compiling information can make mistakes, as well. That's why you need to read labels every time you make a purchase, and regularly contact the company to confirm the gluten-free status of the products you consume. Visit www.triumphdining. com for a free online database with contact information for over a thousand companies. Please take advantage of this resource.

Never Make Assumptions

When contacting companies, please keep in mind that the FDA has yet to issue a rule defining the term "gluten-free." Meanwhile, there's a lot of conflicting information on the gluten-free diet, even among dieticians, support groups and the many other experts in the field. Some believe that blue cheese is gluten-free, others do not. And, the emerging question about the suitability of oats in the gluten-free diet adds even more confusion. So, don't expect a company to guess what your definition of gluten-free is. Always ask questions to make sure you understand what their particular definition of gluten-free is.

GLUTEN FREE OATS?

Ask your doctor to see if "gluten-free" oats may be right for you. Recent research suggests that moderate consumption of oats can be safe for most Celiacs. However, there's a catch . . . it's only pure, uncontaminated oats.

In contrast, normal oats and oat products, like the ones found at your local grocer, are usually cross-contaminated with wheat during harvest, transport, or processing. Consequently, they are unsafe for the gluten-free diet.

However, pure, uncontaminated oats are available. They have to be specially grown and processed to avoid cross-contamination, so they are harder to find and more expensive than traditional oats. But if you're hankering for oatmeal-raisin cookies or a crunchy bowl of granola, you may finally have a safe option!

BOB'S RED MILL
(800) 553-2258

CREAM HILL ESTATES
(866) 727-3628

GLUTEN FREE OATS
(307) 754-2058

Where to Find More Information

This guide pre-supposes that you are already familiar with the gluten-free diet. But for those just starting out, there are some excellent resources available to help you understand the gluten-free diet and to make informed choices. For example, there are a host of helpful resources available from local and national support groups, widely available books and online materials. Doctors and nutritionists are also an excellent source of information. In short, please be proactive about educating yourself. When it comes to the gluten-free diet, an educated shopper is really a healthy shopper!

Effective January 1, 2006, the Food Allergen Labeling and Consumer Protection Act of 2004 (FALCPA), set requirements for the labeling of eight major allergens on packaged foods. This is a quick overview of the elements of the FALCPA that are likely to be relevant to consumers on a gluten-free diet.[1]

Allergens Covered

The FALCPA covers eight major allergens that are credited with causing 90% of all food allergies. Those allergens include: milk, eggs, fish, crustacean shellfish, tree nuts, peanuts, soybeans and, most importantly, wheat. The FDA notes that, for the purposes of the FALCPA, wheat includes common wheat, durum wheat, club wheat, spelt, semolina, Einkorn, emmer, kamut and triticale.

Allergens Not Covered

It's important to note that the FALCPA does **not** cover barley or rye. Nor does it cover oats, which is likely to be cross-contaminated with wheat.

Labeling: What's Required

The FALCPA requires food manufacturers to identify allergens in ingredient lists in one of two ways:

1. In the ingredient listing, the common or usual name of the major food allergen must be followed in parenthesis by the name of the food source from which the major allergen is derived. For example: "Enriched flour (wheat flour…)," or

2. Immediately following the ingredient listing, a "Contains" statement must indicate the name of the food source from which the major food allergen is derived. For example: "Contains: milk, wheat, and eggs."

Allergens present in flavorings, coloring and additives must also be identified in one of the two ways listed above.

Labeling: What's Not Required

It is important to note that the FALCPA does not apply to major food allergens that are unintentionally added to food as a result of cross-contamination. Cross-contamination can result during the growing and harvesting of crops, or from the use of shared storage, transportation, or production equipment.

---

[1]Please note this brief overview is not meant to be comprehensive, nor is it intended as medical or legal advice. If you have questions about food labeling laws or their impact on your dietary choices and decision making, please consult a legal professional, dietician or doctor, as appropriate.

The FALCPA also does not address the use of advisory labeling, including statements designed to identify the possibility of cross-contamination. The FALCPA does not require the use of such statements, nor does it specifically articulate standards of use for advisory statements.

Application

The FALCPA applies to all packaged foods sold in the U.S. that are regulated by the FDA and that are required to have ingredient statements.

It's important to note that the FALCPA does not apply to meat products, poultry products and egg products that fall under the authority of the USDA.

The Big Picture

What does this all mean for people following the gluten-free diet? There are three important limitations of the FALCPA to keep in mind:

1. As far as gluten is concerned, the FALCPA does not cover it. The FALCPA covers wheat, but not rye, barley, or other potentially troublesome grains.

2. The FALCPA covers only products regulated by the FDA that require ingredient lists. For any product that does not require an ingredient list (such as raw fruits), or that falls outside the FDA's jurisdiction (such as meat, poultry and egg products that fall under the authority of the USDA), the FALCPA does not require manufacturers to identify major allergens.

3. The FALCPA does not require manufacturers to identify the possibility of inadvertent cross-contamination, nor does it set specific standards for using advisory statements warning of potential cross-contamination.

The important thing to remember is that, despite improved labeling laws, hidden gluten in grocery items is still a very real possibility. Gluten can come from non-wheat sources, result from cross-contamination, or can occur in products not covered by the FALCPA. For those reasons, it's important to remain vigilant and carefully scrutinize the products you buy. It's not enough to just read labels; contacting manufacturers directly is often necessary.

What is Gluten-Free Anyway?

One final note on the FALCPA: The FALCPA required the FDA to issue a rule to define and permit the use of the term "gluten-free" on food labels by August 2008 (this ruling has been delayed). We expect that ruling in the near future, but when it comes, it will not require food companies to label gluten-free products as such. Rather, the the FDA will establish a uniform standard definition of the term "gluten-free" to be used voluntarily by food manufacturers, likely after some period of notice to allow companies time to comply. For more information, please visit the FDA at www.fda.gov.

While we hope that this guide makes gluten-free shopping easier, we do recognize that there are some limitations, which we would like to call out so that you can make informed shopping decisions.

Gluten-Free Lists

As mentioned in previous chapters, there is currently no FDA rule defining gluten-free and generally no consensus in the community as to an exact definition. (Consider the controversies surrounding blue cheese and oats, just to name a few.) So when a company reports that its products are gluten-free, there is the possibility that their definition of gluten-free may differ from yours. We provide the contact information for over a thousand companies in our free online database, which can be found at www.triumphdining.com, to make it easier to contact companies.

In addition, the information published in this guide for each food item has been obtained directly from that item's manufacturer, the entity that licensed the manufacturing, or an affiliate, unless otherwise noted. The accuracy of the information provided by these sources has not been verified.

Always Read Labels

It's important to keep in mind that product formulations and ingredient sourcing can and do change without notice, companies can make mistakes on their gluten-free list, and people compiling and categorizing large volumes of information (like the content for this guide) can make mistakes, as well. For these reasons, Triumph Dining cannot assume any liability for the correctness or accuracy of any information presented in this guide. You should read labels every time you make a purchase and regularly contact companies to confirm the gluten-free status of the products you consume.

Contact the Company with Questions

Our online brands database (www.triumphdining.com) contains the contact information for over a thousand companies, including those whose products are listed in this guide. Please contact them directly with any questions or for updates. Any information provided in this guide was obtained from the company (unless otherwise noted), and they will always be your best source of information on their products.

A Question of Semantics

Since there is still no FDA regulation defining the term "gluten-free" and no requirement that companies report the possibility of cross-contamination, as consumers, we're very much still on our own. A company may claim its products are "gluten-free" and free of "cross-contamination," but since there's no universally accepted definition of either term, you may still not be getting the whole story. Therefore, a product's appearance in this guide does not mean that the product is entirely free of gluten (besides, that would likely be an impossible standard, as the most sensitive, sophisticated commercially-available tests for gluten do not measure to 0 ppm).

This guide is largely a compilation of the information over 1,000 companies provide when consumers reach out to them asking about the gluten-free status of their products.

Common Sense is Your Best Guide

A guide like this should never be a replacement for your own knowledge, common sense, and diligence. This guide is intended as a starting point only, and not a final determination that a listed product is gluten-free, suitable for the gluten-free diet, or safe for you personally to consume. It is not a substitute for reading labels and contacting companies. Rather, this guide is designed to help you hone in on the products most likely to be suitable for the gluten-free diet, so that you can focus your label-reading and company-contacting efforts on the most promising products, without wasting dozens and dozens of hours chasing dead ends. Always exercise caution when using any lists, even this one or ones directly from a brand. People make mistakes, so if something doesn't feel right, it probably isn't.

Some Final Notes

The information published in this guide is intended for use in the United States and with products manufactured with the intent to be sold in the United States, only. Products sold or intended to be sold outside the United States may have completely different ingredients than their U.S. counterparts, and may not be gluten-free.

This guide is for limited educational purposes only and is not medical advice. If you have questions about the gluten-free diet, what ingredients are appropriate to consume, whether or not particular items are appropriate for your consumption, etc. please consult with your physician.

For the foregoing reasons, Triumph Dining cannot assume any liability for any losses or damages resulting from your use of this product listing. It's up to you to determine whether a product is appropriate based on your individual dietary needs. For more information about a particular company's testing practices, standards and thresholds, please contact that company directly.

Use of this guide indicates your acknowledgement of and agreement to these terms.

Section 2:
Gluten-Free Product List

Symbols Defined

gf = gluten-free

Gluten-Free lines, equipment, environment or facilities.

Gluten Testing is done on products, ingredients and/or equipment.

( ) **Cross-Contamination** is a possibility; or

Shared Facility, Equipment or Line, as noted by the company; or,

The product is made with "gluten-free ingredients" (with no mention of overall status by the company).

Gluten-Free based on Triumph's independent review of ingredient label. Manufacturer has indicated that any gluten would be identified clearly on labels, but has not provided a GF list.

more information >>

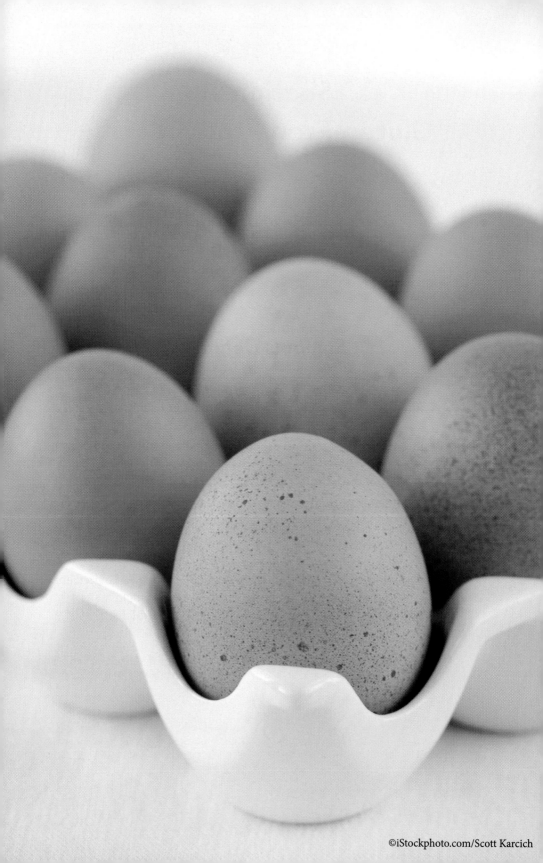

USING THIS PRODUCT LIST
A Quick Tutorial

Our goal is for this guide to make your shopping trips easier, safer, and full of choices. There are a few things you need to know about this guide's content and organization to help us fulfill on that goal.

PRODUCTS FEATURED

Our guide covers over 30,000 products from hundreds of different brands. The products listed are groceries likely to be found in typical American grocery stores like Safeway, Kroger, Albertson's, etc. They include brand names, as well as private label brands from some of the larger grocery chains. In cases where the grocery chain's name is different from their private label brand, we've also put the chain's name in parentheses next to the private label brand name.

Some brands publish a list enumerating each gluten-free item, while others chose to simply say all foods in a particular category are gluten-free. In the latter case, we list the brand name in the appropriate category and sub-category, followed by a description of the products covered and the word "All," where applicable. For example, if a company, let's call it "Brand X," tells us that all its cheeses are gluten-free, it will be listed under "Brand X," followed by "Cheeses (All)." Alternatively, sometimes the brand communicated that all of their products were gluten-free, in which case, they will be noted in the guide as "Brand X (All)."

Sometimes, the brand communicated that all but a few of its products were gluten-free. In those cases, they're listed as "Brand X (All BUT ...)." That qualifier will always appear with Brand X across all categories to cut down on the need to cross-reference multiple sub-categories as you shop.

DON'T SEE YOUR LOCAL STORE IN THE GUIDE?

Even if you don't see your local store's private label products in this guide, that doesn't mean they're not in here!

Some grocery stores operate under several names and indicate that their gluten-free lists are applicable to multiple stores brands. For example, Safeway's gluten-free list also applies to Genuardi's and Von's brands. Here is a list of overlapping stores and store brands:

SAFEWAY: Dominick's, Genuardi's, Randalls, Tom Thumb & Vons

KROGER: Buena Comida, City Market, Dillons, First Choice, Food 4 Less, Fred Meyer, Fry's, King Soopers, Naturally Preferred, Private Selection, QFC, Ralphs, Smith's & Value

ALBERTSON'S: Acme, Equaline Good Day & Jewel

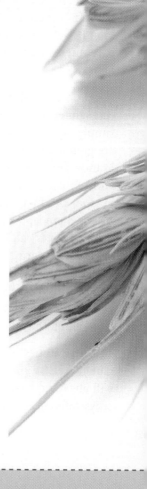

Products Not Featured

You will not find "boutique" gluten-free brands in this guide, unless those brands are likely to be found in typical grocery stores. This list is also far from comprehensive; there are smaller brands and new items popping up all the time. Just because a product isn't listed in these pages, doesn't mean it's not gluten-free. If there's something you're interested in that's not listed in this guide, call the company directly or let us know, and we'll look into adding it for the next edition.

There are some brands missing from the product listings because they simply do not provide or maintain lists of their gluten-free products.

We haven't listed some items that are generally accepted and widely known to be gluten-free. For example, plain dairy milk is not listed. However, we have listed flavored milk, sour cream and other items that contain ingredients (e.g., thickeners or other additives) that may be a concern to some shoppers. Of course, what is "generally accepted" and "widely known" to be gluten-free is subjective. So while one person may find an entire sub-category of items we cover in the guide to be obviously gluten-free, some will not. We try to be as inclusive as possible for the sake of the latter audience.

Finally, for the sake of simplicity, this guide only lists items on a company's gluten-free list. We have excluded items that were reported to contain gluten.

GENERAL OVERVIEW OF ORGANIZATION

The product list is organized into a three tier system: first by category, then by subcategory, then by product name.

TIP!

The Easy Reference Table of Contents on the inside front cover is a quick visual reference for the different categories and sub-categories.

Organization by Category

The products listed in this guide are arranged like a typical grocery store. The list is organized first by master categories that align with aisles in a grocery store, like those for Dairy and Eggs, Snacks, and Frozen Foods.

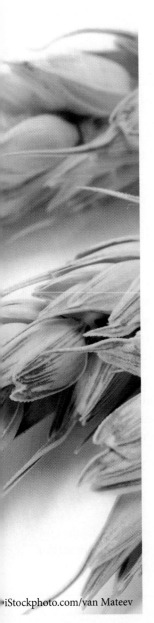

Our belief is that organizing the guide by grocery aisle will make your trip through the store quicker – you can follow along in the guide as your shop through the store.

There are a few exceptions to the link between master category and grocery aisle: in some cases our consumer research found it more helpful to organize items by general category as opposed to aisle. For example, while refrigerated orange juice is often found in the Dairy and Eggs aisle, you'll find it listed here in the Beverages category.

Organization by Sub-Category

Each master category is further sub-divided by sub-categories that align with the particular types of food products found in the master category aisle. For example, sub-categories within the Snacks master category include: Chips, Cookies, Crackers, etc. Sub-categories are organized alphabetically within the master category.

Organization by Brand & Product

Within these subcategories, you'll find individual products listed alphabetically by brand name (in bold), then product name (not in bold). While we've done our best to organize the products into the "correct" category and sub-category, we hope you'll understand it was a subjective process and there will be some variances.

Symbols

Information on all items listed in this section 2, except the items in gray (more about these later) is obtained directly from the brand, manufacturer or brand representative (we refer to these as just the "company" for short). Occasionally, they also send along additional information, ranging from legal disclaimers to in-depth notes on manufacturing procedures.

In order to make this guide portable and convenient, it's not practical to reprint all these notes provided by a company. But, there are a few exceptions. We know that you want to know which items may pose cross-contamination concerns and conversely, when companies go the extra mile by having dedicated production lines or gluten testing, for example. Therefore, those and other relevant situations are marked with special symbols. Check out the beginning of this section for a symbol key.

Placement of Symbols

If a symbol applies to a brand as a whole, we placed the symbol next to the brand name. If it only applies to a particular product, the symbol will only appear next to the specific product. For example, if Brand X's entire line comes with a cross-contamination warning, the disclaimer icon will appear next to the Brand X name. If the warning only applies to its Chocolate Chip flavor, we place the symbol next to the Chocolate Chip flavor listing only.

Limitation of Symbols

Another thing to keep in mind is that any information, including disclaimers like cross-contamination warnings, are provided by companies at their discretion. Unfortunately, companies are not required by law to warn shoppers of cross-contamination, so just because a company does not have a cross-contamination warning does not mean it's not an issue! We sincerely hope that the FDA will resolve this issue in the near future.

Going the Extra Mile

Some prominent brands do not maintain or share gluten-free lists. When you're gluten-free, your choices are naturally limited. The goal of this book is to open up more choices, not limit them.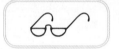

Therefore, in cases where these brands do not have a gluten-free list, but DO have a policy of accurately labeling for gluten, no matter how small the amount, Triumph independently reviewed each product's ingredients (based solely on reviewing the product labeling at the time of review) to determine which are gluten-free.

The information for these particular product listings did not come directly from the brand or manufacturer, as with the other products in this guide, so we have distinguished them with a special reading-glass symbol and gray text color.

This feature is new for the 2nd edition, and we hope you enjoy the new expanded, in-depth coverage it allows us to provide.

Where to Go for More Information

For additional information, please visit our free Brands Information database on our website (www.triumphdining.com). It contains company contact information so you can easily contact companies with questions or for updated lists.

Happy shopping!

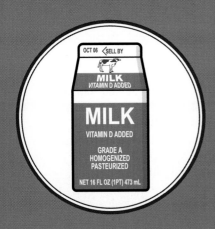

DAIRY & EGGS

BUTTER

Challenge
Retail Butter Items (All)

Crystal Farms
60/40 Butter Blend
Butter and Unsalted Butter

Giant
Salted Butter Quarters
Unsalted Butter Quarters

Hy-Vee
Sweet Cream Butter Quarters
Sweet Cream Butter Solid
Sweet Cream Whipped Butter
Unsalted Sweet Butter Quarters

Kroger ()
Butter

Laura Lynn (Ingle's)
Butter

Lucerne (Safeway)
Butter

Lurpak
Lurpak (All)

Meijer
Butter AA Qtrs

Meyenberg
Meyenberg Goat Milk Products (All)

Nature's Promise (Giant)
Organic Butter

Nature's Promise (Stop & Shop)
Organic Butter

Publix ()
Butter - Salted
Butter - Unsalted

Butter - Whipped, Salted
Butter - Whipped, Unsalted
Sweet Cream Butter

Stop & Shop
Salted Butter Quarters
Unsalted Butter Quarters

Tillamook
Butter (All)

Trader Joe's ()
Butter (All)

Vermont Butter & Cheese Company
Vermont Butter & Cheese Company (All)

BUTTERMILK

Giant
1% Buttermilk

Hood
Buttermilk

Lucerne (Safeway)
Buttermilk - Fat Free
Buttermilk - Low Fat
Buttermilk - Regular

CHEESE & CHEESE SPREADS

A & E Cheese
Pre-Sliced American Cheese
Pre-Sliced Colby Jack Cheese
Pre-Sliced Havarti Cheese
Pre-Sliced Mild Cheddar Cheese
Pre-Sliced Mozzarella Cheese
Pre-Sliced Muenster Cheese
Pre-Sliced Pepper Jack Cheese

Pre-Sliced Provolone Cheese
Pre-Sliced Swiss Cheese
Shredded Colby Jack Cheese
Shredded Mexican Mix Cheese
Shredded Mild Cheddar Cheese
Shredded Mozzarella Cheese
Shredded Sharp Cheddar

Albertsons
Cottage Cheeses
Ricotto Cheese

Alouette
Baby Brie - Herb
Baby Brie - Plain
Chive & Spring Onion
Cilantro Lime
Creamy Onion & Shallots
Crème de Brie - Herb
Crème de Brie - Original
Crème de Cheddar
Crème de Havarti Garlic & Herb
Crème de Parmesan
Crème de Swiss
Crème Fraîche
Elégante Roasted Garlic/Pesto
Elégante Roasted Sweet Pepper/Olive
Elégante Sundried Tomato & Garlic
Garlic & Herbs
Garlic Supreme
Goat Spreadable - Plain
Light Cucumber Dill
Light Garlic & Herbs
Peppercorn Parmesan
Petit Baby Brie Original
Reserve Plain Brie
Savory Vegetable
Spinach Artichoke
Sundried Tomato & Basil

Alpine Lace ()
Cheeses (All)

Andrew & Everett
Cheese (All)

Apetina
Apetina Products (All)

Applegate Farms
Applegate Farms (All BUT Chicken
Nuggets, Chicken Pot Pie, & Chicken
Strips)

Athenos ᐴ
Blue Cheese Crumbled Natural
Chunk Mild
Chunk with Basil & Tomato
Chunk with Black Peppercorn
Chunk with Garlic & Herb
Crumbled Mild
Crumbled Reduced Fat
Crumbled Traditional
Crumbled Traditional Value Size
Crumbled with Basil & Tomato
Crumbled with Basil & Tomato
Reduced Fat
Crumbled with Black Peppercorn
Crumbled with Garlic & Herb
Crumbled with Lemon Garlic &
Oregano
Crumbled with Roasted Bell Peppers &
Garlic
Feta Crumbled Reduced Fat
Feta Crumbled with Basil & Tomato
Natural
Feta Crumbled with Garlic & Herb
Natural
Feta Traditional Chunk Packed in Brine
Natural
Gorgonzola Crumbled Natural
Traditional Feta Crumbled Natural

BelGioioso Cheese
American Grana
Asiago
Auribella
Blue Cheese
Burrata
CreamyGorg
Crèma Di Mascarpone
Crescenza-Stracchino
Crumbly Gorgonzola
Fontina
Fresh Mozzarella - Water-Packed, Curd
& Thermoform
Italico
Kasseri
Manteche
Mascarpone
Parmesan
Parmesan For Vegetarians

Pepato
Peperoncino
Provolone - Medium
Provolone - Mild
Provolone - Sharp
Ricotta con Latte 73
Ricotta con Latte 75
Ricotta con Latte 75 Smooth
Romano
Tiramisu Mascarpone
Toscanello

Bett's ()
Bett's Food Products (All)

Boar's Head
Cheeses (All)

Borden
Borden Cheese Products (All)

Boursin
Boursin Cheese (All Flavors)

Breakstone's
Whipped Temp Tee

Cabot Creamery
Cabot's Products (All)

Chavrie
Plain
Plain Log with Basil/Roasted Garlic

Country Crossing (Save-A-Lot) ()
Country Crossing Cheeses ()

Cracker Barrel
Cheese Sticks - Extra Sharp Cheddar
2% Milk Reduced Fat Cheese
Cheese Sticks - Natural Extra Sharp
Cheddar White Cheese
Cheese Sticks - Natural Sharp Cheddar
Cheese
Cracker Cuts - Extra Sharp
Cracker Cuts - Extra Sharp Cheddar 2%
Milk Reduced Fat
Cracker Cuts - Vermont Sharp-White
Emmentaler Swiss
Extra Sharp
Extra Sharp Cheddar 2% Milk Reduced
Fat Shredded
Extra Sharp White
Fontina
Havarti

Natural Baby Swiss
Natural Cheddar Vermont Sharp-White
Natural Extra Sharp Cheddar
Natural Extra Sharp Cheddar 2% Milk
Reduced Fat
Natural Extra Sharp White Cheddar
Reduced Fat
Natural Sharp Cheddar
Natural Sharp Cheddar 2 Stacks Slices
Natural Sharp Cheddar 2% Milk
Reduced Fat
Natural Sharp Cheddar Slices
Natural Sharp White Cheddar Reduced
Fat
Natural Vermont's Sharp White Cheddar
2% Milk Reduced Fat
White Colby

Crystal Farms
2% and Fat Free IWS
72 & 120 Sliced American Cheese (All)
Aerosol Cheese (All Flavors)
American Deluxe Sliced
American IWS
Blue Cheese & Gorgonzola
Cheese Spread Loaf
Cold Packs
Jar Cheese (All Flavors)
Natural Cheeses - Chunks & Shreds
(All Varieties and Flavors)
Parmesan and Romano - Shaker &
Shredded
Ricotta (All Varieties)
Salami Cheese
String Cheese & Stick Cheeses
Swiss, Sharp, Pepper Jack IWS

Deliano's (Save-A-Lot)
Deliano's Grated Parmesan Cheese

Denmark's Finest
Denmark's Finest (All)

Dofino
Dofino (All)

Ekte Gjetost
Ekte Gjetost (All)

Finlandia Cheese
Finlandia Cheese (All)

Friendship Dairies
Friendship Products (All BUT Toasted Onion Flavored Sour Cream)

Giant
Colby and Monterey Blend (All Varieties) ()
Colby Half Moon Single Slices ()
Fat Free White Cheese Singles ()
Feta (All Varieties) ()
Havarti (All Varieties) ()
Horseradish Cheddar Cheese ()
Mexican Cheese Blend ()
Mild Cheddar (All Varieties) ()
Mild Longhorn Style Cheddar (All Varieties) ()
Monterey Jack (All Varieties) ()
Mozzarella (All Varieties) ()
Muenster (All Varieties) ()
Neufchatel Cheese ()
NY Extra Sharp Cheddar (All Varieties) ()
NY Sharp Cheddar (All Varieties) ()
Parmesan Cheese (All Varieties) ()
Port Wine Cheddar Cheese ()
Provolone (All Varieties) ()
Ricotta (All Varieties) ()
Sharp Cheddar (All Varieties) ()
Sharp Cheddar Cold Pack Cheese Food ()
String Cheese ()
Swiss Cheese (All Varieties) ()
Taco Cheese Blend ()
Vermont Sharp Cheddar (All Varieties) ()
Wisconsin Sharp (All Varieties) ()

Heini's
Amish Farm Milk Cheeses (All)

Heluva Good
All Solid Block Style Cheese

Hy-Vee
American Cheese Food
American Singles
American Singles 2% Milk
Cheeze-Eze
Colby 1/2 Moon Longhorn Cheese
Colby Cheese
Colby Hunk Cheese
Colby Jack 1/2 Moon Longhorn Cheese
Colby Jack Cheese
Colby Jack Cheese Cubes
Colby Jack Hunk Cheese
Colby Jack Slices
Colby Longhorn Cheese
Colby Slice Singles
Extra Sharp Cheddar Cheese
Fancy Shredded 4 Italian Cheese
Fancy Shredded Cheddar Jack Cheese
Fancy Shredded Colby Jack Cheese
Fancy Shredded Mild Cheddar 2% Cheese
Fancy Shredded Mild Cheddar Cheese
Fancy Shredded Mozzarella 2% Milk
Fancy Shredded Mozzarella Cheese
Fat Free Singles
Fat Free Swiss Cheese Slices
Finely Shredded Colby Jack Cheese
Finely Shredded Mild Cheddar Cheese
Grated Parmesan Cheese
Hot Pepper Cheese
Lil' Hunk Colby Jack Cheese
Lil' Hunk Mild Cheddar Cheese
Low Fat Ricotta Cheese
Medium Cheddar Cheese
Medium Cheddar Longhorn Cheese
Mild Cheddar Cheese
Mild Cheddar Cheese Cubes
Mild Cheddar Hunk Cheese
Mild Cheddar Slices
Monterey Jack Cheese
Monterey Jack Hunk Cheese
Mozzarella Cheese
Mozzarella Hunk Cheese
Muenster Cheese
Muenster Cheese Slices
Part Skim Ricotta Cheese
Pepper Jack Cheese
Pepper Jack Cheese Cubes
Pepper Jack Hunk Cheese
Pepper Jack Singles
Pepper Jack Slices
Provolone Cheese
Provolone Cheese Slices
Sharp Cheddar Cheese

Sharp Cheddar Hunk Cheese
Sharp Cheddar Longhorn Cheese
Shredded Colby Jack Cheese
Shredded Mexican Blend Cheese
Shredded Mild Cheddar Cheese
Shredded Mozzarella Cheese
Shredded Parmesan Cheese
Shredded Pizza Cheese
Shredded Sharp Cheddar Cheese
Shredded Taco Cheese
Sliced Low-Moisture Part-Skim
   Mozzarella
Swiss Cheese
Swiss Singles
Swiss Slices

Isaly's
Cheese Items (All)

Jarlsberg
Jarlsberg (All)

Kraft Cracker Cuts
Colby & Monterey Jack Natural
   Marbled Cheese Cuts
Natural Baby Swiss Cheese Cuts
Natural Mild Cheddar Cheese Cuts
Sharp Cheddar Cheese Cuts

Kraft Deli Deluxe
American 2% Milk Slices Cheese
American Slices Cheese
American White Slices Cheese
Colby Jack Slices Cheese
Mild Cheddar Slices Cheese
Mozzarella Slices - Low Moisture
   Cheese
Natural Swiss Slices Cheese
Pepper Jack Spicy Slices Cheese
Provolone Slices Cheese
Sharp Cheddar 2% Milk Slices Cheese
Sharp Cheddar Slices Cheese
Swiss 2% Milk Reduced Fat Slices
   Cheese
Swiss Slices Cheese

Kraft Easy Cheese
American
Cheddar
Sharp Cheddar

Kraft Grated Cheese
Parmesan & Romano Medium 100%
   Grated
Parmesan 100% Grated
Parmesan Original
Parmesan Reduced Fat
Parmesan Shredded
Parmesan, Romano & Asiago Shredded
Romano 100% Grated

Kraft Natural Cheese
2% Cubes - Cheddar & Monterey Jack
2% Cubes - Cheddar Sharp
2% Cubes - Colby & Monterey Jack
Cheddar & Monterey Jack Marbled
Cheddar Bacon
Cheddar Extra Sharp
Cheddar Mild
Cheddar Mild 2% Milk Reduced Fat
Cheddar Sharp
Colby
Colby & Monterey Jack
Colby & Monterey Jack Marbled
Colby 2% Milk Reduced Fat
Extra Sharp Cheddar
Extra Sharp Cheddar Cheese
Medium Cheddar
Mild Cheddar
Mild Cheddar Cheese
Mild Cheddar Longhorn Style 2% Milk
Monterey Jack
Monterey Jack 2% Milk Reduced Fat
Mozzarella Low-Moisture Part-Skim
Organic Cheddar
Pepper Jack
Roasted Garlic Cheddar
Sharp Cheddar
Sharp Cheddar 2% Milk Reduced Fat
Smoky Swiss & Cheddar

Kraft Natural Crumbles
Blue Cheese
Feta Cheese
Italian Style Cheese
Mediterranean Style Cheese
Mexican Style 2% Milk Reduced Fat
   Cheese
Mozzarella Cheese
Reduced Fat-Colby & Monterey Jack

Cheese
Sharp Cheddar Cheese
Three Cheese-Monterey Jack/Colby &
  Cheddar Cheese

Kraft Natural Shredded Cheese ᐭ
Cheddar Fat Free
Cheddar Mild 2% Milk Finely Shredded
  Reduced Fat
Cheddar Mild 2% Milk Reduced Fat
Colby & Monterey Jack
Colby & Monterey Jack 2% Milk
  Shredded
Colby & Monterey Jack Finely
  Shredded
Colby & Monterey Jack Shredded
Italian Style Five Cheese
Mexican Cheddar Jack
Mexican Cheddar Jack with Jalapeno
  Peppers
Mexican Four Cheese
Mexican Four Cheese 2% Milk
Mild Cheddar Finely Shredded
Monterey Jack
Mozzarella
Mozzarella 2% Milk Reduced Fat
Mozzarella Fat Free
Mozzarella Low Moisture
Mozzarella Low-Moisture Finely
  Shredded
Mozzarella Low-Moisture Part-Skim
Organic Cheddar
Organic Mozzarella
Pizza Mozzarella & Cheddar
Sharp Cheddar 2% Milk Reduced Fat
Sharp Cheddar Finely Shredded
Sharp Cheddar Finely Shredded 2%
  Milk
Swiss

Kraft Singles ᐭ
Aged Swiss
American 2% Milk Slices
American Fat Free Slices
American Slices
American White
Organic American Slices
Pepperjack 2% Milk Slices
Select American Slices

Sharp Cheddar
Sharp Cheddar 2% Milk Slices
Sharp Cheddar Fat Free Slices
Swiss 2% Milk
Swiss Fat Free Slices
Swiss Slices
White American
White American 2% Milk Slices
White American Fat Free Slices
White American Slices

Kraft String-Ums ᐭ
Mozzarella String Cheese

Kraft Twist-Ums & String-Ums ᐭ
Mozzarella & Cheddar
Mozzarella & Cheddar Super Long

Kroger ()
Bar Cheeses
Cubed Cheeses
Shredded Cheeses
Sliced Cheeses

Laughing Cow ⅋
Laughing Cow Cheese (All)

Laura Lynn (Ingle's)
Cheese Chunks (All Sizes)
Parmesan & Romano Cheese
Parmesan Cheese
Ricotta Cheese

Lifeway
Lifeway (All)

Lucerne (Safeway)
Cheese (All Varieties)
Ricotta Cheese
String Cheese

Maggio
Ricotta

Meijer
2% Individual Wrap American
2% Individual Wrap Sharp
American Cheese Spray Aerosol
Cheddar - Fancy Shred
Cheddar - Jack Fancy Shred Zip Pouch
Cheddar - Medium Bar
Cheddar - Midget Horn
Cheddar - Mild Bar
Cheddar - Mild Chunk
Cheddar - Sharp Bar
Cheddar - Sharp Chunk

Cheddar - Shred
Cheddar - Shred Sharp Zipper Pouch
Cheddar - Shred Zipper Pouch
Cheddar - Sliced Longhorn Half Moon
Cheddar - X-Sharp Bar
Cheddar - Mont Jack Bar
Cheddar - Sharp Fancy Shred
Cheddar - Sharp Shredded
Cheese - Individual Wrap Slice Pepper
Cheese - Mexican Blend Shredded
Cheese Cheddar Aerosol
Cheese Individually Wrapped
Cheese Sharp Cheddar Aerosol
Cheese Swiss Individually Wrap
Cheezy Does It - Jalapeno
Cheezy Does It - Processes Spread Loaf
Cheezy Does It - Spread Loaf
Colby - Jack Longhorn Half Moon
Colby Bar
Colby Chunk
Colby Jack - Fancy Shred
Colby Jack Bar
Colby Jack Sliced Shingle
Colby Longhorn Full Moon
Colby Longhorn Half Moon (Sliced)
Colby Midget Horn
Colby Shred Fancy
Fancy Italian Blend Shred
Fancy Mexican Blend Shred
Fancy Shred Colby Jack
Fancy Shred Mild Cheddar
Fancy Shred Mozzarella
Fancy Shred Nacho/Taco
Hot Pepper Jack Chunk
L.M. Part Skim Mozzarella Bar
L.M. Part Skim Mozzarella Shred
L.M. Part Skim Mozzarella Square
L.M. Part Skim String Cheese
Low Moisture Part Skim Mozz. Shred
Marble Cheddar (C&W Cheddar)
Mexican Shred
Monterey Jack Chunk
Mozz Slice Chunk L/M Part Skim
Mozzarella Chunk L/M Part Skim
Mozzarella Single Slice
Mozzarella Shred
Muenster Slice Single
Parmesan & Romano Cheese (Grated)

Parmesan Cheese (Grated)
Parmesan Cheese - 1/3 Less Fat
Pepper Jack Bar
Pepperjack Sliced Stack Pack
Pizza Shrd Mozzarella/Cheddar
Processed American Cheese
Processed F.F. Sharp Individ. Slices
Provolone Stacked Slice
Ricotta Cheese - Part Skim
Ricotta Cheese - Whole Milk
String Cheese
Swiss Chunk
Swiss Slice Single
Swiss Sliced Sandwich/Cut

Meyenberg
Meyenberg Goat Milk Products (All)

Midwest Country Fare (Hy-Vee)
American Sandwich Slices
Shredded Cheddar Cheese
Shredded Mozzarella Cheese

Mini Babybel 🏅
Mini Babybel Cheese (All)

Montrachet
Chives
Herbs
Original Flavor

Old Chatham Sheepherding Company
Cheeses (All)

Polly-O Cheese ⤻
Fat Free Ricotta
Lite Ricotta
Mozzarella / Parmesan Finely Shredded
Mozzarella Fat Free
Mozzarella Part Skim
Mozzarella Shredded - Fat Free
Mozzarella Shredded - Lite
Mozzarella Shredded - Part Skim
Mozzarella Shredded - Whole Milk
Original Ricotta
Parmesan - Grated
Part Skim Ricotta

Primo Taglio (Safeway)
American Cheddar
Caesar Jack Cheese
Crumbled Danish Blue
Danish Havarti
Hot Pepper Jack

Imported Ages White Cheddar
Lacy Swiss Cheese
Muenster
Provolone
Regular Jack Cheese
Shredded Asiago
Smoked Fontina Cheese

Publix ()

Asiago Wedge (Specialty Cheeses)
Blue Crumbled (Specialty Cheeses)
Cheddar - Extra Sharp (All Forms: Block, Chunk & Shreds)
Cheddar - Medium (All Forms: Block, Chunk & Shreds)
Cheddar - Mild (All Forms: Block, Chunk & Shreds)
Cheddar - Sharp (All Forms: Block, Chunk & Shreds)
Cheese Spread (Processed Cheese)
Colby (All Forms: Block, Chunk & Shreds)
Colby Jack (All Forms: Block, Chunk & Shreds)
Creative Classic Queso Blanco (Specialty Cheeses)
Creative Classic Queso de Freir (Specialty Cheeses)
Crumbled Feta (Specialty Cheeses)
Crumbled Goat (Specialty Cheeses)
Crumbled Reduced Fat Feta (Specialty Cheeses)
Deluxe American Cheese Slices (Processed Cheese)
Feta Chunk (Specialty Cheeses)
Garden Jack Stick (Specialty Cheeses)
Garlic and Herb Cheese Spread (Specialty Cheeses)
Gorgonzola Crumbled (Specialty Cheeses)
Grated Parmesan (Specialty Cheeses)
Horseradish Jack Stick (Specialty Cheeses)
Hot Pepper Cheese Spread (Specialty Cheeses)
Italian 6-Cheese Blend - Shredded
Mexican 4-Cheese Blend - Shredded
Monterey Jack (All Forms: Block, Chunk & Shreds)
Monterey Jack & Cheddar - Shredded
Monterey Jack with Jalapeño Peppers (All Forms: Block, Chunk & Shreds)
Mozzarella (All Forms: Block, Chunk & Shreds)
Muenster (All Forms: Block, Chunk & Shreds)
Parmesan Wedge (Specialty Cheeses)
Parmesan, Grated (Specialty Cheeses)
Provolone (All Forms: Block, Chunk & Shreds)
Reduced Fat Feta Chunk (Specialty Cheeses)
Reduced Fat Pepper Jack (Specialty Cheeses)
Ricotta (All Forms: Block, Chunk & Shreds)
Salsa Jack Stick (Specialty Cheeses)
Shredded Parmesan (Specialty Cheeses)
Singles - Pasteurized Process American Cheese Food
Singles - Pasteurized Process American Cheese Food (Thick Slice)
Singles - Pasteurized Process Swiss Cheese Food
Swiss (All Forms: Block, Chunk & Shreds)

Raley's ()

Baby Swiss Sliced Cheese
Cheddar Mild Cheese
Colby Jack Sliced Cheese
Danish Havarti Sliced Cheese
Fresh Deli Horseradish Cheese (Processed)
Fresh Deli Jalapeno Jack Cheese
Fresh Deli Mild Cheddar Cheese
Fresh Deli Monterey Jack Cheese
Fresh Deli Provolone Cheese
Fresh Deli Swiss Cheese
Gouda Smoked Sliced
Horseradish Processed Sliced
Hot Pepper Jack Sliced (Processed)
Jarlsburg Sliced
Mild Cheddar - Sliced
Monterey Jack
Monterey Jack - Sliced

Muenster Cheese
Provolone
Sliced Muenster
Sliced Provolone
Sliced Swiss
Swiss Cheese

Redwood Hill Farm
Redwood Hill Farm & Creamery (All)

Rosenborg
Rosenborg (All)

Safeway
Grated Parmesan Cheese
Quick Cheese - Sharp Cheddar

Saga
Saga (All)

Saladena
Blue Cheese Crumbles
Feta Crumbles - Mediterranean
Feta Crumbles - Plain
Goat Crumbles - Plain
Goat Crumbles - Provencal
Gorgonzola

Select Brand (Safeway)
Cheese Fondue
Shredded Parmesan

Ski Queen Gjetost
Ski Queen Gjetost (All)

Snøfrisk
Snøfrisk (All)

Stop & Shop
Colby and Monterey Blend (All
    Varieties) ()
Colby Half Moon Single Slices ()
Fat Free White Cheese Singles ()
Feta (All Varieties) ()
Havarti (All Varieties) ()
Horseradish Cheddar Cheese ()
Mexican Cheese Blend ()
Mild Cheddar (All Varieties) ()
Mild Longhorn Style Cheddar (All
    Varieties) ()
Monterey Jack (All Varieties) ()
Mozzarella (All Varieties) ()
Muenster (All Varieties) ()

NY Extra Sharp Cheddar (All Varieties) ()
NY Sharp Cheddar (All Varieties) ()
Parmesan Cheese (All Varieties) ()
Port Wine Cheddar Cheese ()
Provolone (All Varieties) ()
Ricotta (All Varieties) ()
Sharp Cheddar (All Varieties) ()
Sharp Cheddar Cold Pack Cheese Food ()
String Cheese ()
Swiss Cheese (All Varieties) ()
Taco Cheese Blend ()
Vermont Sharp Cheddar (All Varieties) ()
Vermont White Cheddar Cheese ()
Wisconsin Sharp (All Varieties) ()

Tillamook
Cheese (All)

Trader Joe's ()
Cheese (All Shredded, Blocks &
    Wedges BUT Blue Cheese)
Parmesan and Romano Cheese Blend
Sun Dried Tomato Pesto Torta
    (Refrigerated)

Ukrop's
Dips/Spreads/Sauces - Pimento Cheese
    Spread

Velveeta ᗧ
2% Milk Cheese
Cheese Slices
Cheese Slices Extra Thick
Mexican Mild Cheese
Pepper Jack Cheese
Regular Cheese

Vermont Butter & Cheese Company
Vermont Butter & Cheese Company
    (All)

CHEESE, VEGAN

Lisanatti
Cheese Alternatives (All)

Publix ()
Imitation Mozzarella Cheese - Shredded

Rice
Rice (All)

Rice Vegan
Rice Vegan (All)

Sunergia Soyfoods
Organic Lemon Oregano Soy Feta
Organic Mediterranean Soy Feta
Organic Soy Bleu
Organic Tomato Garlic Soy Feta

Trader Joe's ()
Soy Cheese Slices (Deli)

Vegan
Vegan (All)

Vegan Gourmet
Cheddar
Monterey Jack
Mozzarella Cheese Alternative
Nacho

Veggie
Veggie (All)

Veggy
Veggy (All)

COTTAGE CHEESE

Axelrod
Cottage Cheese

Breakstone's 〰
Cottage Doubles Apples & Cinnamon
  Lowfat - Cottage Cheese & Topping
Cottage Doubles Blueberry Lowfat -
  Cottage Cheese & Topping
Cottage Doubles Peach Lowfat -
  Cottage Cheese & Topping
Cottage Doubles Pineapple Lowfat -
  Cottage Cheese & Topping
Cottage Doubles Raspberry Lowfat -
  Cottage Cheese & Topping
Cottage Doubles Strawberry Lowfat -
  Cottage Cheese & Topping
Large Curd Lowfat 2% Milkfat Cottage
  Cheese
Large Curd Smooth & Creamy 4%
  Milkfat Min Cottage Cheese
Liveactive Lowfat with Mixed Berries
  Cottage Cheese
Liveactive Lowfat with Pineapple
  Cottage Cheese
Small Curd 2% Milkfat Low Fat Snack

Size Cottage Cheese
Small Curd 4% Milkfat Min Cottage
  Cheese
Small Curd 4% Milkfat Min Snack Size
  Cottage Cheese
Small Curd Fat Free Cottage Cheese
Small Curd Fat Free Snack Size Cottage
  Cheese
Small Curd Lowfat 2% Milkfat Cottage
  Cheese
Small Curd Smooth & Creamy 4%
  Milkfat Min Cottage Cheese

Creamland Dairies
Cottage Cheese (All)

Crowley Foods
Cottage Cheese

Daisy Brand
Daisy Brand (All)

Friendship Dairies
Friendship Products (All BUT Toasted
  Onion Flavored Sour Cream)

Giant
Cottage Cheese - Low Fat ()
Cottage Cheese - No Salt Added ()
Cottage Cheese - Nonfat ()
Cottage Cheese - Pineapple ()
Cottage Cheese - Regular ()

Hood
Cottage Cheese (All)

Kemps ()
Cottage Cheese

Knudsen 〰
Cottage Doubles Apples & Cinnamon
  Lowfat Cottage Cheese & Topping
Cottage Doubles Blueberry Lowfat
  Cottage Cheese & Topping
Cottage Doubles Peach Lowfat Cottage
  Cheese & Topping
Cottage Doubles Pineapple Lowfat
  Cottage Cheese & Topping
Cottage Doubles Raspberry Lowfat
  Cottage Cheese & Topping
Cottage Doubles Strawberry Lowfat
  Cottage Cheese & Topping
Free Nonfat Cottage Cheese
Free Nonfat Cottage Cheese On The Go

Liveactive Cottage Cheese
Liveactive Lowfat with Mixed Berries
  Cottage Cheese
Liveactive Lowfat with Pineapple
  Cottage Cheese
Lowfat & Pineapple Cottage Cheese
Lowfat Small Curd Cottage Cheese
Single Serve Lowfat Cottage Cheese On
  The Go
Small Curd Lowfat 2% Milkfat Cottage
  Cheese
Small Curd Lowfat Cottage Cheese

Kroger ()
Cottage Cheeses

Lactaid
Cottage Cheese

Laura Lynn (Ingle's)
Cottage Cheese (All Sizes)

Light n' Lively 🔊
Fat Free Cottage Cheese
Lowfat Cottage Cheese
Lowfat Snack Size Cottage Cheese

Lucerne (Safeway)
Cottage Cheese (All BUT Fruit Added)

Nancy's
Cultured Dairy and Soy Products (All)

Penn Maid
Cottage Cheese

Publix ()
Fat Free
Large Curd, 4% Milkfat
Low Fat
Low Fat with Pineapple
Small Curd, 4% Milkfat

South Beach Living 🔊
1% Milkfat w/Calcium Cottage Cheese

Stop & Shop
Cottage Cheese - Calcium Added ()
Cottage Cheese - Lowfat ()
Cottage Cheese - Nonfat with Pineapple ()

CREAM

Creamland Dairies
Whipping Cream (All)

Giant
20% Light Whipping Cream
Heavy Whipping Cream
Sweetened Whipped Light Cream

Hood
Creams (All)

Lucerne (Safeway)
Whipping Cream - Heavy
Whipping Cream - Light
Whipping Cream - Regular

Meijer
Ultra Pasteurized Heavy Whipping
  Cream

Publix ()
Heavy Whipping Cream
Whipping Cream

Stop & Shop
Heavy Whipping Cream
Light Cream
Whipping Cream

CREAM CHEESE

Albertsons
Cream Cheese

Crystal Farms
Aerosol Cream Cheese (All Flavors)
Cream Cheese (All Flavors and
  Varieties)

Giant
Cream Cheese - Fat Free ()
Cream Cheese - Garden Vegetable ()
Cream Cheese - Lite ()
Cream Cheese - Regular ()
Cream Cheese - Sour Cream & Chive
  ()
Cream Cheese - Strawberry ()
Cream Cheese - Whipped ()

Hy-Vee
1/3 Less Fat Than Cream Cheese
Blueberry Cream Cheese
Cream Cheese
Fat Free Cream Cheese
Fat Free Soft Cream Cheese
Fat Free Strawberry Cream Cheese

Garden Vegetable Cream Cheese
Onion/Chive Cream Cheese
Soft Cream Cheese
Soft Light Cream Cheese
Strawberry Cream Cheese
Whipped Cream Cheese

Kroger ()
Cream Cheeses

Laura Lynn (Ingle's)
Cream Cheese Bar
Fat Free Cream Cheese Bar
Neufchatel Bar
Onion & Chive Cream Cheese
Soft Cream Cheese (Cup)
Strawberry Cream Cheese
Whipped Cream Cheese

Lifeway
Lifeway (All)

Lucerne (Safeway)
Cream Cheese - Fat Free
Cream Cheese - Garden Vegetable
Cream Cheese - Light
Cream Cheese - Neufchatel
Cream Cheese - Onion/Chive
Cream Cheese - Soft Bars
Cream Cheese - Strawberry
Cream Cheese - Whipped Spread

Nancy's
Cultured Dairy and Soy Products (All)

Nature's Promise (Giant)
Organic Cream Cheese ()

Nature's Promise (Stop & Shop)
Organic Cream Cheese ()

Philadelphia Cream Cheese ⌒
Blueberry Cream Cheese
Chive & Onion Light Cream Cheese
Cream Swirls Peaches 'N Cream Cream Cheese
Fat Free Cream Cheese
Garden Vegetable Cream Cheese
Honey Nut Cream Cheese
Light Cream Cheese
Light Garden Vegetable Cream Cheese
Neufchatel 1/3 Less Fat
Original Cream Cheese
Pineapple Cream Cheese

Regular Cream Cheese
Regular Whipped Cream Cheese
Roasted Garlic Light Cream Cheese
Salmon Cream Cheese
Strawberry Cream Cheese
Strawberry Fat Free Cream Cheese
Whipped Cinnamon 'N Brown Sugar Cream Cheese
Whipped Cream Cheese
Whipped Garlic 'N Herb Cream Cheese
Whipped Mixed Berry Cream Cheese
Whipped Ranch Cream Cheese
Whipped with Chives

Publix ()
Fat Free
Light - Soft (All Flavors)
Neufchatel
Regular
Regular - Soft (All Flavors)

Stop & Shop
Cream Cheese - Chive & Onion (Lite, Regular & Whipped) ()
Fat Free Cream Cheese ()
Garden Vegetable Cream Cheese (Lite, Regular & Whipped) ()
Honey Walnut Cream Cheese (Lite, Regular & Whipped) ()
Neufchatel Cheese ()
Plain Cream Cheese (Lite, Regular & Whipped) ()
Strawberry Cream Cheese (Lite, Regular & Whipped) ()

Trader Joe's ()
Cream Cheese (All)

Ukrop's
Dips/Spreads/Sauces - Cream Cheese and Olive Spread

EGG SUBSTITUTES

Albertsons
Egg Substitute

All Whites
All Whites

Better'n Eggs
Better'N Eggs

Ener-G
Egg Replacer

Giant
100% Egg Whites
Eggs Made Simple

Hy-Vee
Refrigerated Egg Substitute

Laura Lynn (Ingle's)
Egg Starts (All)

Lucerne (Safeway)
Best of The Egg

Meijer
Egg Substitute (Refrigerated)

Nulaid
ReddiEgg Fat Free & Cholesterol Free
Real Egg Product (All)

OrgraN
OrgraN (All)

Stop & Shop
100% Egg Whites
Eggs Made Simple

Trader Joe's ()
Quick Scrambled Egg Whites (Deli)

EGGNOG & OTHER NOGS

Borden Egg Nog
Borden Egg Nog

Hood
Cinnamon Eggnog
Gingerbread Eggnog
Golden Eggnog
Light Eggnog
Pumpkin Eggnog
Vanilla Eggnog

Kroger ()
Eggnog - Liquid
Eggnog - Powdered

Lucerne (Safeway)
Egg Nog

Publix ()
Low Fat Eggnog
Original Eggnog

Stop & Shop
Egg Nog - Light
Egg Nog - Regular

HALF & HALF

Creamland Dairies
Half and Half (All)

Giant
Half & Half - Fat Free
Half & Half - Regular

Hood
Simply Smart Fat Free Half & Half

Laura Lynn (Ingle's)
Half & Half (All Sizes)

Lucerne (Safeway)
Half & Half

Meijer
Ultra Pasteurized Heavy Half & Half

Publix ()
Fat Free Half & Half
Half & Half

Stop & Shop
Half & Half - Fat Free
Half & Half - Regular

HUMMUS

Athenos 🖎
Artichoke & Garlic Hummus
Black Olive Hummus
Cucumber Dill Hummus
Greek Style with Lemon Garlic &
Oregano Hummus
Neo Classic Original Hummus
Neo Classic Original w/Sesame Seeds
& Parsley Hummus
Neo Classic Roasted Garlic w/Garlic &
Parsley Hummus
Neo Classic Roasted Red Pepper w/Red
Peppers & Parsley Hummus
Original Hummus
Original Party Size Hummus
Pesto Hummus
Roasted Eggplant Hummus
Roasted Garlic Hummus
Roasted Garlic Party Size Hummus

Roasted Red Pepper Hummus
Roasted Red Pepper Party Size
   Hummus
Scallion Hummus
Spicy Three Pepper Hummus

Cedar's Mediterranean Foods
Hummus (All)

Emerald Valley Kitchen
Emerald Valley Kitchen (All)

Fantastic World Foods ()
Original Hummus

Guiltless Gourmet
Hummus (All) ᵞ

Manischewitz
Hummus (Ready to Serve)

Trader Joe's ()
Hummus (All; Refrigerated)

Tribe Hummus
Hummus (All Flavors)

MARGARINE & SPREADS

Benecol
Light Spread
Regular Spread

Canoleo
Canoleo (All)

Country Crock
Spread and Spreadable Butter Products
   (All)

Crystal Farms
Margarine and Spreads (All Types)

Giant
48% Margarine Spread

Hy-Vee
100% Corn Oil Margarine
Best Thing Since Butter
Rich & Creamy Soft Margarine
Soft Margarine
Soft Spread
Vegetable Margarine Quarters

I Can't Believe It's Not Butter!
Margarine and Spread Products (All)

Kroger ()
Margarine
Vegetable Spreads

Laura Lynn (Ingle's)
Lite Spread Margarine (Tub)
Margarine Quarters
Margarine Spread
Margarine Spread (Tub)
Taste Like Butter Spread

Manitoba Harvest ᵞ
Manitoba Harvest (All)

Meijer
Margarine Corn Oil Quarters
Margarine Soft Sleeve
Margarine Soft Tub
Spread - 48% Crock
Spread - 70% Quarters
Spread No Ifs Ands Or Butter

Promise
Margarine and Spread Products (All)

Publix ()
Corn Oil Margarine Quarters
Homestyle Spread - 48% Vegetable Oil
Homestyle Squeeze Spread - 60%
   Vegetable Oil
It Tastes Just Like Butter Spread - 70%
   Vegetable Oil
Original Spread Quarters - 70%
   Vegetable Oil

Safeway
Light Homestyle Spread
Margarine
Vegetable Oil Spreads - 70%,
   37% Light & 70% 1/4 Lb Sticks
   (Homestyle)

MILK, CHOCOLATE & FLAVORED

Giant
1% Low Fat Chocolate Milk

Hood
Calorie Countdown Dairy Beverages
   (All Flavors & Fat Levels)
Chocolate Milk - Full Fat (All Sizes)
Chocolate Milk - Low Fat (All Sizes)
Simply Smart Fat Free Chocolate Milk

Louis Trauth Dairy
Louis Trauth Dairy (All BUT Lowfat
   Buttermilk, Cookies N Cream Ice
   Cream, Chocolate Chip Cookie Dough

Ice Cream, Ice Cream Sandwiches, and Sundae Nut Cones)

Lucerne (Safeway)
Chocolate Milk

Meijer
1% Chocolate Milk Single Serve
Chocolate Milk
Strawberry Milk

Nesquik ()
Ready-to-Drink Milk (All Flavors)

Publix ()
Chocolate Milk
Low Fat Chocolate Milk

Safeway
Milk Drinks - Chillin Chocolate
Milk Drinks - Marvelous
Milk Drinks - Mocha Cappuccino
Milk Drinks - Vanilla Shake
Milk Drinks - Very Berry Strawberry

Turkey Hill
All Natural Recipe - Chocolate
Cool Moos - Strawberry

MILK, LACTOSE-FREE

Giant
Lactose Free Milk - Calcium Added
Lactose Free Milk - Skim
Lactose Free Milk - Whole

Lactaid
Milk Lactaid

Laura Lynn (Ingle's)
Lactose Reduced Milk

Lucerne (Safeway)
Lactose Free Fat Free Milk

Meijer
Lactose Free Milk - 2% with Calcium
Lactose Free Milk - Fat Free with Calcium

Stop & Shop
Lactose Free Milk - Calcium Fortified Fat Free
Lactose Free Milk - Whole

SOUR CREAM

Albertsons
Sour Creams

Axelrod
Sour Cream

Breakstone's ᨆ
All Natural Sour Cream
Free Fat Free Sour Cream
Grade A Pasteurized Homogenized Sour Cream
Reduced Fat Sour Cream

Cascade Fresh ᨆ
Cascade Fresh (All)

Creamland Dairies
Sour Cream (All)
Sour Cream Dips (All)

Crowley Foods
Sour Cream

Daisy Brand
Daisy Brand (All)

Friendship Dairies
Friendship Products (All BUT Toasted Onion Flavored Sour Cream)

Giant
Sour Cream - Lite
Sour Cream - Nonfat

Hood
Sour Cream (All)

Hy-Vee
Light Sour Cream
Sour Cream

Kemps ()
Sour Cream

Knudsen ᨆ
Fat Free Sour Cream
Hampshire 100% Natural Sour Cream
Hampshire Sour Cream
Light Sour Cream

Kroger ()
Sour Cream

Laura Lynn (Ingle's)
Sour Cream (All Sizes)

Lucerne (Safeway)
Sour Cream - Low Fat
Sour Cream - Non Fat

Sour Cream - Regular

Nancy's
Cultured Dairy and Soy Products (All)

Penn Maid
Sour Cream

Publix ()
Fat Free
Light
Regular

Stop & Shop
Sour Cream - Light
Sour Cream - Nonfat

Tillamook
Sour Cream (All)

Trader Joe's ()
Sour Cream (All)

SOYMILK & MILK ALTERNATIVES

Blue Diamond Growers () 𝄪 𝄪
Almond Breeze Non-Dairy Almond
Milk 𝄪

Eden Foods
EdenBlend
Edensoy Unsweetened

Health Market (Hy-Vee)
Organic Chocolate Soy Milk
Organic Original Soy Milk
Organic Vanilla Soy Milk

Hy-Vee
Chocolate Soy Milk
Enriched Original Rice Milk
Enriched Vanilla Rice Milk
Original Soy Milk
Refrigerated Chocolate Soymilk
Refrigerated Original Soy Milk
Refrigerated Vanilla Soy Milk
Vanilla Soy Milk

Kroger ()
Rice Drink - Plain
Rice Drink - Vanilla
Soy Drink- Plain
Soy Drink- Vanilla

Laura Lynn (Ingle's)
Soy Milk

Manitoba Harvest 𝄪
Manitoba Harvest (All)

Nature's Promise (Giant)
Ricemilk - Plain
Ricemilk - Vanilla
Soymilk - Chocolate
Soymilk - Plain
Soymilk - Vanilla

Nature's Promise (Stop & Shop)
Chocolate Soymilk
Organic Soymilk - Chocolate
Organic Soymilk - Plain
Organic Soymilk - Vanilla
Ricemilk - Plain
Ricemilk - Vanilla

Pacific Natural Foods
Almond Non-Dairy Beverages -
Original
Almond Non-Dairy Beverages - Vanilla
Hazelnut
Low Fat Rice - Plain
Low Fat Rice - Vanilla
Organic Soy - Unsweetened, Original
Select Soy - Plain
Select Soy - Vanilla
Ultra Soy - Plain
Ultra Soy - Vanilla

Publix GreenWise Market ()
Soy Milk - Chocolate
Soy Milk - Plain
Soy Milk - Vanilla

Rice Dream
Classic Carob
Classic Original
Classic Vanilla
Enriched Chocolate
Enriched Original
Enriched Vanilla
Heartwise Original
Heartwise Vanilla
Horchata

Select Brand (Safeway)
Organic Soy Beverage
Organic Vanilla Soy Beverage (Low
Fat)

Trader Joe's ()
Rice Milk

Soy Beverages (All)
Soymilks (All; Refrigerated)

WHIPPED TOPPINGS

Albertsons
Whipping Toppings
Axelrod
Aerosol Topping
Cool Whip 🗫
Chocolate Whipped Topping
Extra Creamy Whipped Topping
Free Whipped Topping
French Vanilla Whipped Topping
Regular Whipped Topping
Strawberry Whipped Topping
Sugar Free Whipped Topping
Whipped Topping Lite
Crowley Foods
Aerosol Topping
Crystal Farms
Aerosol Whip Cream
Dream Whip 🗫
Regular Whipped Topping Mix
Twin Pk. Whipped Topping Mix
Giant
Frozen Whipped Topping - Fat Free
Frozen Whipped Topping - Lite
Frozen Whipped Topping - Nondairy
Frozen Whipped Topping - Regular
Frozen Whipped Topping - Vanilla
Hood
Instant Whipped Cream
Sugar Free Light Whipped Cream
Hy-Vee
Frozen Extra Creamy Whipped Topping
Frozen Fat Free Whipped Topping
Frozen Lite Whipped Topping
Frozen Whipped Topping
Real Whipped Cream
Real Whipped Lite Cream
Ingles Markets
Frozen Whipped Toppings
Kroger ()
Whipping Cream

Laura Lynn (Ingle's)
Whipping Cream (All Sizes)
Lucerne (Safeway)
Aerosol Whipping Cream - Light &
Non Dairy
Whipped Topping - Lactose Free
Whipped Topping - Light
Whipped Topping - Regular
Meijer
Frozen Whipped Topping
Frozen Whipped Topping - Lite
Frozen Whipped Topping Fat Free
Ultra Pasteurized Non Dairy Aerosol
Ultra Pasteurized Whip Cream Aerosol
Penn Maid
Aerosol Topping
Publix ()
Whipped Heavy Cream (Aerosol Can)
Whipped Light Cream (Aerosol Can)
Whipped Topping - Fat Free (Aerosol
Can)
Stop & Shop
Frozen Whipped Topping - Fat Free
Frozen Whipped Topping - French
Vanilla
Frozen Whipped Topping - Lite
Frozen Whipped Topping - Non Dairy
Frozen Whipped Topping - Regular
Sweetened Whipped Light Cream

YOGURT

Axelrod
Yogurt
Brown Cow 🍼
Yogurts (All BUT Fruit & Whole
Grains)
Cascade Fresh 🍼
Cascade Fresh (All)
Coburn Farms (Save-A-Lot)
Yogurt - Low Fat & Lite
Crowley Foods
Yogurt
Dannon
Plain Activia
Plain DanActive

Plain Lowfat
Plain Natural
Plain Nonfat

Friendship Dairies

Friendship Products (All BUT Toasted Onion Flavored Sour Cream)

Giant

Grab'Ums Yogurt To Go - Cotton Candy/Melon ()

Grab'Ums Yogurt To Go - Strawberry/Blueberry ()

Grab'Ums Yogurt To Go - Tropical Punch/Raspberry

Punch/Raspberry ()

Lowfat Blended - Blueberry ()

Lowfat Blended - Cherry ()

Lowfat Blended - Peach ()

Lowfat Blended - Raspberry ()

Lowfat Blended - Strawberry ()

Lowfat Blended - Strawberry-Banana ()

Lowfat Blended - Vanilla ()

Lowfat Fruit on the Bottom - Blueberry ()

Lowfat Fruit on the Bottom - Boysenberry ()

Lowfat Fruit on the Bottom - Cherry ()

Lowfat Fruit on the Bottom - Lemon ()

Lowfat Fruit on the Bottom - Mixed Berry ()

Lowfat Fruit on the Bottom - Pineapple ()

Lowfat Fruit on the Bottom - Raspberry ()

Lowfat Fruit on the Bottom - Strawberry ()

Lowfat Fruit on the Bottom - Strawberry/Banana ()

Lowfat Plain ()

Lowfat Vanilla ()

Nonfat Light - Banana ()

Nonfat Light - Blueberry ()

Nonfat Light - Caramel ()

Nonfat Light - Cherry ()

Nonfat Light - Cherry Vanilla ()

Nonfat Light - Coffee ()

Nonfat Light - Raspberry ()

Nonfat Light - Strawberry ()

Nonfat Light - Strawberry/Banana ()

Nonfat Light - Vanilla ()

Hy-Vee

Banana Cream Non Fat Yogurt
Black Cherry Low Fat Yogurt
Blueberry Low Fat Yogurt
Blueberry Non Fat Yogurt
Cherry Non Fat Yogurt
Cherry-Vanilla Low Fat Yogurt
Fat Free Plain Yogurt
Key Lime Pie Fat Free Yogurt
Lemon Chiffon Non Fat Yogurt
Lemon Low Fat Yogurt
Mixed Berry Low Fat Yogurt
Non Fat Vanilla Yogurt
Peach Non Fat Yogurt
Peach Yogurt
Plain Low Fat Yogurt
Raspberry Low Fat Yogurt
Raspberry Non Fat Yogurt
Strawberry Banana Low Fat Yogurt
Strawberry Banana Non Fat Yogurt
Strawberry Low Fat Yogurt
Strawberry Non Fat Yogurt
Whipped Low Fat Cherry Yogurt
Whipped Low Fat Key Lime Pie Yogurt
Whipped Low Fat Orange Cream Yogurt
Whipped Low Fat Peaches N Cream Yogurt
Whipped Low Fat Raspberry Yogurt
Whipped Low Fat Strawberry Yogurt
Yogurt To Go Strawberry
Yogurt To Go Strawberry & Blueberry
Yogurt To Go Strawberry/Banana & Cherry

Kemps ()

Yogurt

Laura Lynn (Ingle's)

Low Fat Yogurt
Non Fat Yogurt

Lifeway

Lifeway (All)

Lucerne (Safeway)
Fat Free Yogurt (All Varieties)
Pre-Stirred Low Fat Yogurt (All Varieties)
Yo Cups (All Varieties)
Yo On The Go (All Varieties)

Meijer
Blended Boysenberry
Blended Strawberry
Blended Strawberry-Banana
Blended Tropical Fruit
Fruit/Bottom Blueberry
Fruit/Bottom Peach
Fruit/Bottom Raspberry
Fruit/Bottom Strawberry
Lite Banana Crème
Lite Black Cherry
Lite Blueberry
Lite Cherry-Vanilla
Lite Coconut Cream
Lite Lemon Chiffon
Lite Mint Chocolate
Lite Peach
Lite Raspberry
Lite Strawberry
Lite Strawberry-Banana
Lite Vanilla
Lowfat Blended Blueberry
Lowfat Blended Cherry
Lowfat Blended Mixed Berry
Lowfat Blended Peach
Lowfat Blended Pina Colada
Lowfat Blended Raspberry
Lowfat Vanilla
Tube-Yo-Lar Strw/Blue
Tube-Yo-Lar Troppnch/Rasp
Tube-Yo-Lar Wtr/Strw/Ban

Nancy's
Cultured Dairy and Soy Products (All)

Old Chatham Sheepherding Company
Yogurts (All)

Penn Maid
Yogurt

Publix ()
Apple Pie Light - Fat Free
Banana Crème Pie Light - Fat Free
Banana Fruit On The Bottom

Black Cherry Creamy Blend
Black Cherry Fruit On The Bottom
Black Cherry with Chocolate - Limited Edition
Blackberry Fruit On The Bottom
Blueberry - No Sugar Added
Blueberry Creamy Blend
Blueberry Fruit On The Bottom
Blueberry Light - Fat Free
Cappuccino Light - Fat Free
Caramel Crème Light - Fat Free
Cherry Fruit On The Bottom
Cherry Light - Fat Free
Cherry Vanilla Light - Fat Free
Coconut Crème Pie Light - Fat Free
Cranberry Raspberry - No Sugar Added
Creamy Blends Black Cherry & Mixed Berry - Multi Pack
Creamy Blends Blueberry & Strawberry Banana - Multi Pack
Creamy Blends Peach and Strawberry - Multi Pack
Egg Nog - Limited Edition
Fat Free Light "Active" Peach
Fat Free Light "Active" Strawberry
Fat Free Light "Active" Vanilla
Fat Free Plain Yogurt
Guava Fruit On The Bottom
Honey Almond Light - Fat Free
Key Lime Pie Light - Fat Free
Kids/Blue Raspberry & Cotton Candy - Multi Pack
Kids/Grape Bubblegum & Watermelon - Multi Pack
Kids/Strawberry & Blueberry - Multi Pack
Kids/Strawberry Banana & Cherry - Multi Pack
Lemon Chiffon Light - Fat Free
Mandarin Orange Light - Fat Free
Mango Fruit On The Bottom
Mixed Berry Fruit On The Bottom
Peach - No Sugar Added
Peach Creamy Blend
Peach Fruit On The Bottom
Peach Light - Fat Free
Piña Colada Light - Fat Free
Pineapple Fruit On The Bottom

Pumpkin Pie - Limited Edition
Raspberry Fruit On The Bottom
Raspberry Light - Fat Free
Strawberry - No Sugar Added
Strawberry Creamy Blend
Strawberry Fruit On The Bottom
Strawberry Light - Fat Free
Strawberry with Chocolate - Limited Edition
Strawberry/Banana Fruit On The Bottom
Strawberry/Banana Light - Fat Free
Tropical Blend Fruit On The Bottom
Vanilla - No Sugar Added
Vanilla Creamy Blend
Vanilla Light - Fat Free

Redwood Hill Farm
Redwood Hill Farm & Creamery (All)

Stonyfield Farm ♔
Soy Yogurts (All BUT Frozen Yogurt, Oikos Greek Yogurt, YoBaby Plus Fruit & Cereal and YoKids Squeezers)
Yogurts (All BUT Frozen Yogurt, Oikos Greek Yogurt, YoBaby Plus Fruit & Cereal and YoKids Squeezers)

Stop & Shop
Grab'Ums Yogurt To Go - Cotton Candy/Melon ()
Grab'Ums Yogurt To Go - Strawberry/Blueberry ()
Grab'Ums Yogurt To Go - Tropical Punch/Raspberry ()
Lowfat Blended Blueberry ()
Lowfat Blended Peach ()
Lowfat Blended Raspberry ()
Lowfat Blended Strawberry ()
Lowfat Blended Vanilla ()
Lowfat Fruit On The Bottom - Blueberry ()
Lowfat Fruit On The Bottom - Peach ()
Lowfat Fruit On The Bottom - Raspberry ()
Lowfat Fruit On The Bottom - Strawberry ()
Lowfat Fruit On The Bottom -

Strawberry/Banana ()
Nonfat Light Banana ()
Nonfat Light Blueberry ()
Nonfat Light Cherry ()
Nonfat Light Cherry Vanilla ()
Nonfat Light Coffee ()
Nonfat Light Peach ()
Nonfat Light Raspberry ()
Nonfat Light Strawberry ()
Nonfat Light Strawberry/Banana ()
Nonfat Light Vanilla ()
Nonfat Plain ()

Tillamook
Yogurt (All)

Trader Joe's ()
Non-Dairy Soy Yogurt (All; Deli)
Yogurt (All)

Wallaby Yogurt Company
Yogurt (All)

WholeSoy & Co. ♔
Yogurt (All)

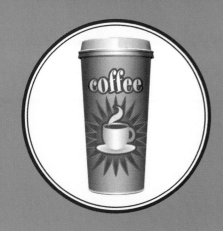

BEVERAGES

Beer

Bard's Tale Beer
Bard's
Dragon's Gold Beer

Green's
Discovery Gluten-Free Amber Ale
Endeavour Gluten-Free Dubbel Ale
Quest Gluten-Free Tripel Ale

Lakefront Brewery
New Grist

Rampao Valley Brewery 🏅
Honey Beer

Redbridge 🏅
Redbridge Beer

Sprecher's
Mbege
Shakparo

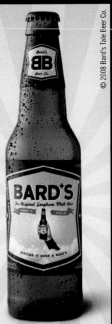
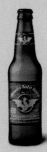

Carbonated

7Up
7Up (All)
A&W
A&W (All)
Adirondack Beverages
Adirondack Beverages (All)
Albertsons
A+ Soda (All Flavors)
Seltzers
Sparkling Water
Barq's
Barq's Root Beer
Caffeine Free Barq's Root Beer
Diet Barq's Red Crème Soda
Diet Barq's Root Beer
Boylan's
Boylan Products (All)
Canada Dry
Canada Dry (All)
China Cola
China Cola
Coca-Cola Company, The
Caffeine Free Coca-Cola Classic
Caffeine Free Diet Coke
Cherry Coke
Cherry Coke Zero
Coca-Cola Blak
Coca-Cola Classic
Coca-Cola Zero
Diet Cherry Coke
Diet Coke
Diet Coke Plus
Diet Coke Sweetened with Splenda
Diet Coke with Lime
Vanilla Coke
Vanilla Coke Zero
Crush
Crush (All)
Diet Rite
Diet Rite (All)
Dr. Pepper
Dr. Pepper (All)
Fanta
Grape
Orange Zero

Faygo
Faygo Products (All)
Fresca
Fresca
Hansen's
Hansen's Beverages (All)
Hires
Hires (All)
Hy-Vee
Cherry Cola
Club Soda
Cola
Cream Soda
Diet Cola
Diet Heee Haw
Diet Orange
Diet Root Beer
Diet Tonic
Dr. Hy-Vee
Gingerale
Grape
Heee Haw
Lemon Lime
Orange
Root Beer
Seltzer Water
Strawberry
Tonic Water
IBC
IBC (All)
Izze
Izze (All)
Knouse Foods
Sparkling Apple Cider
Kroger ()
Big K Soft Drinks
Manzanita Sol
Soft Drinks
Martinelli's
Martinelli's (All)
Meijer
C/F Dt Encore Red
DT Caffeine-Free Encore Red
DT Cherry Encore
DT Encore Blue
DT Encore Red

Encore Blue
Encore Cherry Red
Encore Red
Red Pop

Mirinda
Carbonated Beverages

Mountain Dew
Carbonated Soft Drinks

Mug
Carbonated Beverages (All)

Nutrisoda
Calm
Energize
Flex
Focus
Immune
Radiant
Renew
Slender

Pepsi
Carbonated Beverages (All)

Publix ( )
Black Cherry Soda
Cherry Cola
Citrus Hit Soda
Club Soda
Cola
Cream Soda
Diet Cola
Diet Ginger Ale
Diet Tonic Water
Ginger Ale
Grape Soda
Lemon Lime Seltzer
Lemon Lime Soda
Orange Soda
Raspberry Seltzer
Root Beer
Tonic Water

RC Cola
RC Cola (All)

Reed's
Reed's (All)

Santa Cruz Organic
Santa Cruz Organic (All)

Save-A-Lot
Diet & Regular Sodas ( )

Schweppes
Schweppes (All)

Select Brand (Safeway)
Soda (All Varieties)

Shasta
Shasta

Sierra Mist
Carbonated Beverages (All)

Sonoma Sparkler
Sonoma Sparkler (All)

Sprite
Sprite
Sprite Zero

Squirt
Squirt (All)

Stewart's
Stewart's (All)

Stop & Shop
100% Natural Sparkling Apple Juice
(Shelf Stable)

Sundrop
Sundrop (All)

Sunkist
Sunkist (All)

Tava
Carbonated Beverages

Trader Joe's ( )
Organic Sparkling Beverages -
Grapefruit
Organic Sparkling Beverages - Lemon
Refreshers - Blueberry
Refreshers - Pomegranate
Refreshers - Tangerine
Sparkling Waters (All)

Tropicana Twister Soda
Carbonated Beverages

Tubz (Save-A-Lot)
Diet Root Beer

Vernors
Vernors (All)

Virgil's
Virgil's (All)

Welch's (Dr. Pepper/Snapple Group)
Welch's (All)

Chocolate Drinks

Yoo-hoo
Yoo-hoo (All)

Cider (Alcoholic)

Ace Cider
Ace Cider (All)
Cider Jack
Cider Jack
Fox Barrel
Fox Barrel (All)
J.K. Scrumpy's Organic Gate Gold Organic Hard Cider
J.K. Scrumpy's Organic Gate Gold
Organic Hard Cider
Original Sin Hard Cider
Original Sin Hard Cider
Samuel Smith's Organic Cider
Samuel Smith's Organic Cider
Woodchuck Draft Cider
Woodchuck Draft Cider
Woodpecker Cider
Woodpecker Cider

Coffee Creamers & Flavorings

Albertsons
Coffee Creamers - Dry (All Flavors)
Coffee Creamers - Liquid (All Flavors)
Non-Dairy Creamer
Coffee-Mate ()
Liquid - Flavored & Non-Flavored
Powder - Flavored & Non-Flavored
Cremora ()
Cremora (All)
Giant
Coffee Cream
Nondairy Creamer
Hood
Country Creamer

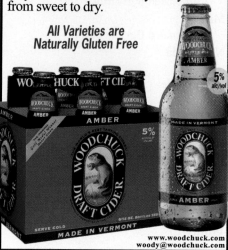

Hy-Vee
Fat Free Coffee Creamer
French Vanilla Coffee Creamer
Hazelnut Coffee Creamer
Original Coffee Creamer
Refrigerated Fat Free French Vanilla
Coffee Creamer
Refrigerated Fat Free Hazelnut Coffee
Creamer
Refrigerated French Vanilla Coffee
Creamer
Refrigerated Hazelnut Coffee Creamer
Laura Lynn (Ingle's)
Non Dairy Creamer (Refrigerated)
Lucerne (Safeway)
Coffee Creamer - French Vanilla
Coffee Creamer - Original
Coffee Creamer - Powdered
French Vanilla Liquid Creamer
Hazelnut Liquid Creamer
Irish Cream Liquid Creamer
Light Non Dairy Creamer
Meijer
Ultra Pasteurized Nondairy Creamer

Nescafé ()
Ice Java Coffee Syrup (All Flavors)

Publix ()
Coffee Creamer
Fat Free Non-Dairy Creamer
Non-Dairy Creamer (Powder)
Non-Dairy French Vanilla Flavored
Creamer (Powder)
Non-Dairy Lite Creamer (Powder)

Stop & Shop
Fat Free Nondairy Creamer

COFFEE DRINKS & MIXES

Alter Eco Fair Trade
Coffee (All)

Bolthouse Farms
Hazelnut Latte
Mocha Cappuccino

Caribou
Caribou Iced Coffee

Eight O'Clock Coffee
Coffee (All)

Folgers
Coffees (All)

General Foods International Coffees ✐
Cafe Francais
Cafe Francais - Dark Mayan Chocolate
Cafe Francais - French Vanilla Café
Cafe Francais - Pumpkin Spice
Cafe Mocha 100 Calorie Packs -
Cappuccino
Cafe Vienna
Chai Latte
Crème Caramel Coffee Drink Mix
Decaffeinated French Vanilla Café
Decaffeinated Sugar Free French
Vanilla Café
Decaffeinated Sugar Free Suisse Mocha
French Vanilla 100 Calorie Packs -
Cappuccino
French Vanilla Café
French Vanilla Cappuccino Coolers
French Vanilla Nut
Hazelnut Belgian Cafe
Hazelnut Cappuccino Coolers
Italian Cappuccino

On The Go Cafe Mocha Sugar Free -
Coffee House Drink Mix
On The Go Hazelnut Cappuccino Sugar
Free - Coffee House Drink Mix
On The Go Vanilla Latte Sugar Free -
Cappuccino Coolers
Orange Cappuccino
Sugar Free - Cafe Vienna
Sugar Free - French Vanilla Cafe
Sugar Free - Suisse Mocha
Suisse Mocha
Swiss White Chocolate
Viennese Chocolate Cafe

Green Mountain Coffee Roasters
Coffees (All)

Hy-Vee
100% Colombian Coffee
Breakfast Blend Coffee
Coffee
Decaffeinated Coffee
Decaffeinated Instant Coffee
French Roast Coffee
Instant Coffee

Illy
Coffee (All)

JavaSoy Coffee
JavaSoy Coffee

JFG Coffee
Decaf Instant Coffee
Instant Coffee
Rich French Roast (Bag)

Kava
Kava Coffee

Kroger ()
Coffee - Instant
Coffee - Unflavored Ground
Coffee - Whole

Laura Lynn (Ingle's)
Coffees (All)

Luzianne
Bonus Blend Dark Roast
Bonus Blend Decaf
Bonus Blend Medium Roast
Coffee Partner (Package Chicory)
Dark Roast
Dark Roast Pure
Decaf

Medium Roast

Maxwell House ⌒

Breakfast Blend Coffee
Cafe Collection Decaffeinated Coffee
Cafe Collection French Roast Coffee
Cafe Collection Hazelnut Coffee
Cafe Collection House Blend Coffee
Colombian Supreme Ground Coffee
Colombian Supreme Ground Coffee - Vacuum Bags
Dark Roast Coffee
Decaffeinated Instant Bags - Coffee Singles
Filter Packs Original Coffee
Filter Packs Original Decaffeinated Coffee
French Roast Coffee - Vacuum Bags
French Roast Decaffeinated Coffee - Vacuum Bags
French Roast Ground Coffee
Hazelnut Flavored Ground Coffee
Instant Original Decaffeinated Coffee
Lite - Vacuum Bags
Lite Ground Coffee
Master Blend Coffee - Vacuum Bags
Master Blend Decaffeinated Coffee
Master Blend Ground Coffee
Original Coffee Singles
Original Decaffeinated Coffee - Vacuum Bags
Original Decaffeinated Ground Coffee
Original Ground Coffee
Original Rich Coffee
Slow Roast Coffee
Slow Roast Ground Coffee
Vanilla Coffee

Meijer

Coffee - Decaf
Coffee - French Roast
Coffee - French Roast Ground
Coffee - Ground Colombian
Coffee - Ground Lite 50%
Coffee - Ground Lite 50% Decaf
Coffee - Regular
Coffee - Colombian Ground

Melitta

Coffee (All)

Millstone

Millstone Coffees (All)

Mountain Blend ()

Instant Coffee

Nescafé ()

Classic Instant Coffee

Newman's Own Organics

Coffees (All)

Publix ()

Coffee (All Varieties)

Safeway

Coffee - Decaffeinated Classic Roast
Espresso Coffee Beans

Sanka ⌒

Naturally Decaffeinated Coffee

Select Brand (Safeway)

Coffee - Creamy Hazelnut
Coffee Beverage - Instant Flavored
Whole Bean Flavored Coffees

Soyfee

Soyfee

Tassimo

Tassimo (All)

Taster's Choice (Nescafé) ()

Instant Coffee - Flavored & Non-flavored

Trader Joe's ()

Coffee (All)
Matcha Latte

Yuban ⌒

100% Arabica Hazelnut Single Serve Coffee Pods
100% Colombian Coffee
100% Colombian Dark Roast Coffee
100% Colombian Decaffeinated Coffee
100% Colombian Decaffeinated Single Serve Coffee
100% Colombian Organic Rich Medium Roast Coffee
100% Colombian Original Coffee
100% Colombian Single Serve Coffee

DIET & NUTRITIONAL

Boost

Glucose Control Nutritional Drink

High Protein Nutritional Energy Drink
Nutritional Energy Drink
Plus Nutritional Energy Drink

Ensure
Liquid Products (All)

Gatorade ()
Nutrition Shakes

Glucerna
Glucerna Shakes (All Flavors)
Glucerna Snack Shakes (All Flavors)

Hy-Vee
Chocolate Nutritional Supplement
Chocolate Nutritional Supplement Plus
Strawberry Nutritional Supplement
Strawberry Nutritional Supplement Plus
Vanilla Nutritional Supplement
Vanilla Nutritional Supplement Plus

Kashi
Go Lean Shake Mix - Chocolate
Go Lean Shake Mix - Vanilla

Meijer
Chocolate DND
Diet Quick Chocolate Extra Thin
Diet Quick Strawberry Extra Thin
Diet Quick Vanilla Extra Thin
Gluco-Burst - Strawberry DND
Gluco-Burst - Vanilla DND
Strawberry DND
Vanilla DND

Metamucil
Metamucil Powders

Safeway
Nutritional Shake/Drinks (All Flavors, including Plus)
Weight Loss Shakes - Chocolate Royale
Weight Loss Shakes - Milk Chocolate
Weight Loss Shakes - Vanilla

Slim-Fast
Slim-Fast Easy To Digest Shakes - Chocolate
Slim-Fast Easy To Digest Shakes - Coffee
Slim-Fast Easy To Digest Shakes - Vanilla

ENERGY

Full Throttle
Full Throttle Mother

Fuze ()
Fuze

Gatorade ()
Energy Drink

Hansen's
Hansen's Beverages (All)

Inko
Inko's (All)

Monster Energy
Monster Beverage Products (All)

Red Bull
Red Bull Energy Drink
Red Bull Sugarfree

SoBe
SoBe (All)

Syzmo
Syzmo Energy Line

Turkey Hill
T-Fusion Energy Tea

Vitaminenergy
Vitaminenergy Products (All)

FLAVORED OR ENHANCED WATER

Adirondack Beverages
Adirondack Beverages (All)

Capri Sun
Roarin' Waters Grape Fruit Flavored Water Beverage
Roarin' Waters Strawberry Kiwi Fruit Flavored Water Beverage
Roarin' Waters Tropical Fruit Fruit Flavored Water Beverage
Roarin' Waters Variety Pk Fruit Flavored Water Beverage
Roarin' Waters Wild Cherry Fruit Flavored Water Beverage

Dasani
Dasani Lemon
Dasani Plus Cleanse + Restore
Dasani Plus Refresh + Revive

Emerge Nutrient Infused Water
Emerge (All Flavors)

Fruitwater
Fruitwater Products (All)

Hy-Vee
Black Cherry Water Cooler
Key Lime Water Cooler
Kids Size Purified Water with Fluoride Added
Kiwi Strawberry Water Cooler
Mixed Berry Water Cooler
Peach Melba Water Cooler
Peach Water Cooler
Raspberry Water Cooler
Strawberry Water Cooler
White Grape Water Cooler

Kellogg's
Special K2O Protein Water

Kroger ( )
Crystal Clear Flavored Waters

Propel ( )
Propel Fit Water

Smartwater
Smartwater Products (All)

Vitaminwater
Vitaminwater Products (All)

HOT COCOA & CHOCOLATE MIXES

Best Friends Cocoa
Hot Cocoa - Cinnamon Twist
Hot Cocoa - Marshmallow Cloud
Hot Cocoa - Raspberry Truffle
Hot Cocoa - Traditional

Coburn Farms (Save-A-Lot)
Hot Cocoa Mix

DariFree
Chocolate

Equal Exchange ( )
Cocoa Products ( )

Ghirardelli ( )
Powdered Hot Cocoa

Giant
Hot Cocoa - Mini Marshmallows
Hot Cocoa - Regular

Hy-Vee
Instant Chocolate Flavored Drink Mix
Instant Hot Cocoa Mix
No Sugar Added Instant Hot Cocoa Mix

Kroger ( )
Instant Cocoa

Laura Lynn (Ingle's)
Cocoa

Meijer
Chocolate Flavor Drink Mix
Cocoa Hot Instant Marshmallow
Hot Cocoa Mix
Hot Cocoa Mix - No Sugar Added
Hot Cocoa Mix - Sugar Free
Hot Cocoa Mix - w/Marshmallows
Organic Hot Cocoa Regular

Midwest Country Fare (Hy-Vee)
Hot Cocoa Mix
Instant Chocolate Flavored Drink Mix

Nestlé ( )
Hot Cocoa Mix (All BUT Double Chocolate Meltdown [47 & 60 oz], Rich Chocolate Flavor [60 oz], Fat Free & Fat Free with Marshmallows)

Safeway
Instant Chocolate Drink Mix

Select Brand (Safeway)
Cocoa Mix - European

Stop & Shop
Hot Cocoa - Fat Free No Sugar Added
Hot Cocoa - Light
Hot Cocoa - Mini Marshmallows
Hot Cocoa - Regular

Tassimo
Tassimo (All)

Trader Joe's ( )
Conacado Organic Cocoa
Sipping Chocolate

INSTANT BREAKFAST

Carnation Instant Breakfast ( )
Carnation Instant Breakfast Powder (All BUT Chocolate Malt)

Safeway
Instant Breakfast

JUICE DRINK MIXES

Alpine
Cider Drink Mixes

Country Time (Kraft) ❧
Lemonade Drink Mix
Lemonade Flavor Drink Mix
Lemonade Iced Tea Classic Drink Mix
Lemonade Iced Tea Raspberry Drink
  Mix
Lemonade Lite Drink Mix
On The Go Lemonade Drink Mix
  Packets
Pink Lemonade Drink Mix
Pink Lemonade Flavor Drink Mix
Pink Lemonade Lite Drink Mix
Raspberry Lemonade Drink Mix
Strawberry Lemonade Drink Mix

Crystal Light ❧
Energy Wild Strawberry On the Go
Fruit Punch Drink Mix
Fruit Punch Sugar Free On the Go
Fusion Fruit Punch Fruit Drinks
Hydration Lightly Lemon On the Go
Immunity Cherry Pomegranate On the
  Go
Immunity Natural Cherry Pomegranate
  Drink Mix
Lemonade Sugar Free
Lemonade Sugar Free On the Go
Lemonade Value Pack Sugar Free
Liveactive For Digestive Health Mixed
  Berry Drink Mix
Liveactive For Digestive Health
  Raspberry Peach Drink Mix
Natural Lemonade Drink Mix
Pineapple-Orange Sugar Free Fruit
  Drinks
Pink Lemonade Sugar Free
Raspberry Ice Sugar Free Fruit Drinks
Raspberry Ice Sugar Free On the Go
Raspberry Lemonade Sugar Free
Raspberry Lemonade Sugar Free On
  The Go
Raspberry Peach Sugar Free Calcium
Ruby Red Grapefruit Sunrise
Strawberry-Kiwi Sugar Free Fruit
  Drinks

Strawberry-Orange-Banana Sugar Free
  Fruit Drinks
Sunrise Classic Orange On the Go
Sunrise Classic Orange Sugar Free
Tangerine Strawberry Sugar Free
  Calcium
Tangerine Strawberry Sunrise
White Grape Drink Mix
White Grape Drink Mix On The Go

Giant
Cherry Drink Mix
Grape Drink Mix
Lemonade Drink Mix
Orange Drink Mix
Pink Lemonade Drink Mix
Strawberry Drink Mix
Sugar Free Drink Mix - Fruit Punch
Sugar Free Drink Mix - Iced Tea
Sugar Free Drink Mix - Lemon Lime
Sugar Free Drink Mix - Lemonade
Tropical Punch Drink Mix

Hy-Vee
Splash Cherry Drink Mix
Splash Grape Drink Mix
Splash Lemonade Drink Mix
Splash Orange Drink Mix
Splash Tropical Fruit Punch Drink Mix

Kool-Aid ❧
Berry Blue Unsweetened Twists Soft
  Drink Mix
Black Cherry Unsweetened Powdered
  Soft Drink Mix
Blastin' Berry Cherry Unsweetened
  Twists Soft Drink Mix
Cherry Sugar Free Powdered Soft Drink
  Mix
Cherry Sugar-Sweetened Powdered Soft
  Drink Mix
Grape Sugar Free Powdered Soft Drink
  Mix
Grape Sugar-Sweetened Powdered Soft
  Drink Mix
Grape Unsweetened Powdered Soft
  Drink Mix
Ice Blue Raspberry Lemonade Sugar
  Sweetened Twists Soft Drink Mix
Ice Blue Raspberry Lemonade

Unsweetened Twists Soft Drink Mix

Invisible Changin' Cherry Sugar
Sweetened Powdered Soft Drink Mix

Invisible Changin' Cherry Unsweetened
Powdered Soft Drink Mix

Invisible Grape Illusion Sugar
Sweetened Powdered Soft Drink Mix

Invisible Grape Illusion Unsweetened
Powdered Soft Drink Mix

Invisible Unsweetened Wild
Watermelon Kiwi Mad Scientwists
Soft Drink Mix

Lemonade Sugar-Sweetened Powdered
Soft Drink Mix

Lemonade Unsweetened Powdered Soft
Drink Mix

Lemon-Lime Unsweetened Powdered
Soft Drink Mix

On The Go Cherry Powdered Soft
Drink Mix

On The Go Tropical Punch Powdered
Soft Drink Mix

On The Go Tropical Punch Sugar Free
Powdered Soft Drink Mix

Orange Sugar-Sweetened Powdered
Soft Drink Mix

Orange Unsweetened Powdered Soft
Drink Mix

Pink Lemonade Unsweetened Powdered
Soft Drink Mix

Raspberry Reaction Invisible
Unsweetened Mad Scientwists Soft
Drink Mix

Singles Cherry Powdered Soft Drink
Mix

Singles Grape Powdered Soft Drink
Mix

Singles Orange Powdered Soft Drink
Mix

Singles Tropical Punch Powdered Soft
Drink Mix

Slammin' Strawberry Kiwi
Unsweetened Twists Soft Drink Mix

Soarin' Strawberry Lemonade
Unsweetened Powdered Soft Drink
Mix

Strawberry Sugar-Sweetened Powdered
Soft Drink Mix

Strawberry Unsweetened Powdered Soft
Drink Mix

Tropical Punch Powdered Soft Drink
Mix

Tropical Punch Sugar Free Powdered
Soft Drink Mix

Tropical Punch Sugar-Sweetened
Powdered Soft Drink Mix

Tropical Punch Unsweetened Powdered
Soft Drink Mix

Twists Blastin' Berry Cherry Sugar Free
Envelope Powdered Soft Drink Mix

Watermelon Cherry Unsweetened
Twists Soft Drink Mix

Kroger ( )

Drink Aid Canisters

Instant Spiced Cider

Laura Lynn (Ingle's)

Orange Breakfast Drink

Meijer

Crystal Quencher - Black Cherry

Crystal Quencher - Key Lime

Crystal Quencher - Kiwi Strawberry

Crystal Quencher - Peach

Crystal Quencher - Raspberry

Crystal Quencher - Tangerine Lime

Crystal Quencher - White Grape

Drink Mix - Breakfast Orange

Drink Mix - Cherry

Drink Mix - Grape

Drink Mix - Lemon Sugar Free

Drink Mix - Lemonade

Drink Mix - Lemonade Stix

Drink Mix - Orange

Drink Mix - Orange Free & Light

Drink Mix - Pink Lemonade

Drink Mix - Pink Lemonade Sugar Free

Drink Mix - Punch

Drink Mix - Raspberry Stix

Drink Mix - Raspberry Sugar Free

Drink Mix - Strawberry

Drink Mix - Strawberry Orange Banana

Strawberry Flavor Drink Mix

Metamucil

Metamucil Powders

Safeway

Spiced Cranberry Apple Cider Mix

Strawberry Star Fruit Drink Mix
Sugar Free Raspberry and Lemonade
Drink Mix

South Beach Living ☙
Natural Strawberry Banana (On The Go
Drink Mix)
Natural Tropical Breeze (On The Go
Drink Mix)

Stop & Shop
Cherry Drink Mix
Grape Drink Mix
Lemonade Drink Mix
Orange Drink Mix
Pink Lemonade Drink Mix
Strawberry Drink Mix
Sugar Free Drink Mix - Fruit Punch
Sugar Free Drink Mix - Iced Tea
Sugar Free Drink Mix - Lemon Lime
Sugar Free Drink Mix - Lemonade
Tropical Punch Drink Mix

Tang ☙
Grape Drink Mix
Orange Drink Mix
Orange Kiwi Drink Mix
Orange Pineapple Drink Mix
Orange Strawberry Drink Mix
Orange Sugar Free Drink Mix
Tangerine Strawberry Drink Mix
Tropical Passionfruit Drink Mix
Watermelon Wallop Juice Drink
Wild Berry Drink Mix

JUICES & FRUIT DRINKS

After the Fall
After The Fall Beverages
Albertsons
Juices (All BUT Orange)
Apple & Eve
100% Juice Products (All)
Bionaturae
Fruit Nectars
Bolthouse Farms
Carrot Juice
Clementine Juice
Cranberry Lemonade
Mango Lemonade

Orange Juice
Passion Fruit Apple Carrot
Prickly Pear Cactus Lemonade
Vedge

Bom Dia
Acai-Blueberry
Acai-Cacao
Acai-Mangosteen
Acai-Pomegranate

Bossa Nova ☷
Açai Juices (All)

Campbell's
Tomato Juice (All)

Capri Sun ☙
Apple Splash 100% Fruit Juice
Berry Breeze 100% Fruit Juice
Coastal Cooler Juice Drink
Fruit Dive 100% Fruit Juice
Fruit Punch Juice Drink
Grape Juice Drink
Grape Tide 100% Fruit Juice
Lemonade Juice Drink
Mountain Cooler Juice Drink
Orange Juice Drink
Pacific Cooler Juice Drink
Red Berry Juice Drink
Splash Cooler Juice Drink
Strawberry Juice Drink
Strawberry Kiwi Juice Drink
Surfer Cooler Juice Drink
Tropical Punch Juice Drink
Variety Pk 100% Fruit Juice
Wild Cherry Juice Drink

Ceres
Juices (All)

Clamato
Clamato (All BUT Clamato Red Eye)

Country Time (Dr. Pepper/Snapple Group)
Country Time (All)

Country Time (Kraft) ☙
Large Ready To Drink Pouches
Lemonade

Crystal Light ☙
Berry Pomegranate Immunity Sugar
Free Bottles
Energy Wild Strawberry Sugar Free

Bottles
Focus Citrus Splash Multi-Serve Bottle
Hydration Pink Lemonade Sugar Free
Bottles
Immunity Berry Pomegranate Sugar
Free Bottles
Lemonade Multi-Serve Bottle
Lemonade Sugar Free Bottles
Pink Lemonade Hydration Sugar Free
Bottles
Raspberry Ice Multi-Serve Bottle
Raspberry Ice Sugar Free Bottles
Raspberry Ice/Classic Orange/
Lemonade Bottles
Sunrise Classic Orange Bottles
Sunrise Classic Orange Multi-Serve
Bottles
Sunrise Classic Orange Sugar Free
Sunrise Classic Orange Sugar Free
Bottles
Wild Strawberry Energy Sugar Free
Bottles

Del Monte ()
100% Fruit Juices
Tomatoes & Tomato Products (All BUT
Del Monte Spaghetti Sauce Flavored
with Meat)

Dole
100% Juices

Eden Foods
Apple Concentrate
Apple Juice
Cherry Concentrate
Cherry Juice (Montmorency Tart
Cherries)

Florida's Natural
Premium Orange Juice
Ruby Red Grapefruit Juice

Gardner Groves (Save-A-Lot)
Grapefruit Juice (100% Juice)

Giant
100% Natural Sparkling Apple Juice
(Shelf-Stable)
Apple Juice Cocktail From Concentrate
(Shelf-Stable)
Berry Berry Cooler (Shelf-Stable)
Big Apple Cooler (Shelf-Stable)

Cosmic Orange Cooler (Shelf-Stable)
Fruit Punch Juice Drink (Shelf-Stable)
Fruity Punch Cooler (Shelf-Stable)
Goofy Grape Cooler (Shelf-Stable)
Grapefruit Juice (Chilled)
Kids Happy Drinks (Shelf-Stable)
Orange Cranberry Juice (Chilled)
Orange Juice (Added Calcium)
(Chilled)
Orange Juice (from Concentrate)
(Chilled)
Orange Juice (Not Concentrate)
(Chilled)
Orange Juice (with Pulp) (Chilled)
Orange Strawberry Juice (Chilled)
Premium Ruby Red Grapefruit Juice -
Not From Concentrate (Chilled)
Prune Juice with Pulp (Shelf-Stable)
Strawberry Kiwi Juice (Shelf-Stable)
Tomato Juice (Shelf-Stable)
Tropical Juice Drink (Shelf-Stable)
Wild Cherry Juice Drink (Shelf-Stable)

Goya ()
Bitter Orange
Coconut Water
Nectars
Sugar Cane Juice

Hansen's
Hansen's Beverages (All)

Hawaiian Punch
Hawaiian Punch (All)

Hood
Juices (All)

Hy-Vee
100% Apple Juice From Concentrate
100% Cranberry Juice Blend
100% Cranberry/Apple Juice Blend
100% Cranberry/Raspberry Juice Blend
100% Unsweetened Prune Juice From
Concentrate
100% White Grape Juice From
Concentrate
All Natural Tomato Juice
All Natural Vegetable Juice
Concord Grape Juice
Cranberry Apple Juice Cocktail From
Concentrate

Cranberry Grape Juice Cocktail From Concentrate
Cranberry Juice Cocktail From Concentrate
Cranberry Raspberry Juice Cocktail
Cranberry Strawberry Juice Cocktail
Fruit Punch
Fruit Punch Coolers
Grapefruit Juice From Concentrate
Just Juice - Apple
Just Juice - Berry
Just Juice - Cherry
Just Juice - Grape
Just Juice - Punch
Just Juice - Strawberry
Lemon Juice
No Concentrate Country Style Orange Juice
No Concentrate Orange Juice
No Concentrate Orange Juice with Calcium
Not From Concentrate Ruby Red Grapefruit Juice
Ruby Red Grapefruit Juice Cocktail From Concentrate
Splash Cherry
Splash Grape
Splash Lemonade
Splash Orange
Splash Raspberry
Splash Strawberry
Splash Tropical Punch
Tomato Juice From Concentrate
Tropical Punch Coolers
Vegetable Juice From Concentrate

Ingles Markets
Apple
Cocktail Juice
Cranberry
Cranberry Blend Juices
Grape
Grapefruit Juices
Lemon Juice
Light Cranberry Blends
Light Fruit Punch
Organic Juices
Peach Juice
Prune Juices

Vegetable Juice
White Cranberry Blend Juices
White Cranberry Juices
White Grape

Knouse Foods
Apple Cider
Apple Juice
Apple Juice Drink
Fruit Punch
Grape Drink
Natural Apple Juice
Orange Pineapple Drink
Papaya Punch Drink
Premium Apple Juice

Kool-Aid ✑
Blue Raspberry Jammers Juice Drink
Cherry Bursts Soft Drink
Cherry Jammers Juice Drink
Grape Bursts Soft Drink
Grape Jammers Juice Drink
Green Apple Jammers Juice Drink
Kiwi Strawberry Jammers Juice Drink
Lime Bursts Soft Drink
Orange Jammers Juice Drink
Tropical Punch Bursts Soft Drink
Tropical Punch Jammers Juice Drink

Kroger ()
Fruit Juices
Shelf Stable Juices
Vegetable Juice

Langers
Juices (All)

Louis Trauth Dairy
Louis Trauth Dairy (All BUT Lowfat Buttermilk, Cookies N Cream Ice Cream, Chocolate Chip Cookie Dough Ice Cream, Ice Cream Sandwiches, and Sundae Nut Cones)

Manischewitz
Grape Juice

Martinelli's
Martinelli's (All)

Meijer
Acai & Blueberry Juice Blend (Shelf Stable)
Acai & Grape Juice Blend (Shelf Stable)

Apple Juice (Shelf Stable)
Apple Juice From Concentrate (Shelf Stable)
Apple Juice Natural (Shelf Stable)
Apple Juice Not From Concentrate (Shelf Stable)
Cherry Juice (Shelf Stable)
Cran Grape Juice Light (Shelf Stable)
Cran/Rasp Juice w/3 Fruit Juices (Shelf Stable)
Cranberry Apple Juice Cocktail (Shelf Stable)
Cranberry Flavored w/2 Fruit Juices (Shelf Stable)
Cranberry Grape Flavored w/2 Juices (Shelf Stable)
Cranberry Grape Juice Cocktail (Shelf Stable)
Cranberry Grape Juice Drink (Shelf Stable)
Cranberry Juice Cocktail (Shelf Stable)
Cranberry Juice Cocktail Light (Shelf Stable)
Cranberry Raspberry 100% (Shelf Stable)
Cranberry Raspberry Juice Cocktail (Shelf Stable)
Cranberry Strawberry Cocktail (Shelf Stable)
Drink - Berry Blend Splash (Shelf Stable)
Drink Cranberry Raspberry (Shelf Stable)
Drink Cranberry Strawberry (Shelf Stable)
Drink Thirst Quencher - Fruit Punch (Shelf Stable)
Drink Thirst Quencher - Lemon Lime (Shelf Stable)
Drink Thirst Quencher - Orange (Shelf Stable)
Fruit Punch (Shelf Stable)
Fruit Punch Genuine (Shelf Stable)
Fruit Punch Light (Shelf Stable)
Grape Cranberry Juice Cocktail Light (Shelf Stable)
Grape Juice From Concentrate (Shelf Stable)

Grapefruit Juice (Shelf Stable)
Juice - Berry 100% (Shelf Stable)
Juice - Cherry 100% (Shelf Stable)
Juice - Cranapple Cocktail (Shelf Stable)
Juice - Cranberry White Cocktail (Shelf Stable)
Juice - Cranberry White Peach (Shelf Stable)
Juice - Grape (Shelf Stable)
Juice - Grape 100% Genuine (Shelf Stable)
Juice - Grape White (Shelf Stable)
Juice - Punch 100% Genuine (Shelf Stable)
Lemon Juice (Shelf Stable)
Lemon Juice Squeeze Bottle (Shelf Stable)
Light Grape Juice Cocktail w/Splenda (Shelf Stable)
Lime Juice (Shelf Stable)
Orange Juice (Shelf Stable)
Orange Premium Carafe (Refrigerated)
Orange Premium Hi Pulp Carafe (Refrigerated)
Orange Premium w/Cal Carafe (Refrigerated)
Orange Premium w/Calcium (Refrigerated)
Orange Reconstituted (Refrigerated)
Orange Reconstituted + Pulp (Refrigerated)
Orange Reconstituted w/Calcium (Refrigerated)
Orange w/Calcium (Refrigerated)
Organic Apple Juice (Shelf Stable)
Organic Concord Grape Juice (Shelf Stable)
Organic Cranberry Juice (Shelf Stable)
Organic Lemonade (Shelf Stable)
Pink Grapefruit Juice (Shelf Stable)
Pomegranate & Blueberry Blend (Shelf Stable)
Pomegranate & Cranberry Blend (Shelf Stable)
Prune Juice (Shelf Stable)
Raspberry Cran Juice Cocktail Light (Shelf Stable)

Ruby Red Grapefruit Cocktail Light (Shelf Stable)

Ruby Red Grapefruit Cocktail Light 22% (Shelf Stable)

Ruby Red Grapefruit Juice Cocktail (Shelf Stable)

Strawberry/Kiwi Splash (Shelf Stable)

White Cran/Straw Juice Cocktail (Shelf Stable)

White Cranberry Flavored Juice Blend (Shelf Stable)

White Cranberry Juice Cocktail (Shelf Stable)

White Cranberry Peach Juice Cocktail (Shelf Stable)

White Grape Juice From Concentrate (Shelf Stable)

White Grape Peach Juice Blend (Shelf Stable)

White Grape Raspberry Juice Blend (Shelf Stable)

White Grapefruit Juice (Shelf Stable)

White Grapefruit Juice Cocktail (Shelf Stable)

Midwest Country Fare (Hy-Vee)

100% Unsweetened Apple Cider

100% Unsweetened Apple Juice

Cranberry Apple Juice Cocktail

Cranberry Juice Cocktail

Cranberry Raspberry Juice

Grape Juice From Concentrate

Ruby Red Grapefruit Juice Cocktail

Minute Maid

Active Orange Juice

Light Lemonade

Multi-Vitamin Orange Juice

Mott's

Mott's (All)

Naked Juice

Naked Juice Products (All BUT Green Machine)

Nantucket Nectars

Nantucket Nectars (All)

Nature's Promise (Giant)

Organic Cranberry Juice From Concentrate

Pomegranate Juice - Blueberry Blend

Pomegranate Juice - Cranberry Blend

Pomegranate Juice - Regular

Nature's Promise (Stop & Shop)

Organic Cranberry Juice From Concentrate (Shelf Stable)

Nestlé Juicy Juice ()

Juicy Juice (All Flavors)

Juicy Juice Harvest Surprise (All Flavors)

Newman's Own

Gorilla Grape

Grape Juice

Lemonade

Lightly Sweetened Lemonade

Limeade

Orange Mango Tango

Organic Lemonade

Pink Lemonade

Razz-Ma-Tazz Raspberry Juice Cocktail

Ocean Spray

Beverages (All)

Odwalla

Juices (All BUT Super Protein Vanilla Al Mondo & Superfood)

Old Orchard

Old Orchard Juices

Orangina

Orangina (All)

POM Wonderful

POM Wonderful

Publix ()

Apple Juice

Cranberry Apple Juice Cocktail

Cranberry Juice Cocktail

Deli Old Fashion Lemonade

Grape Juice

Grape-Cranberry Juice Cocktail

Orange Juice From Concentrate

Orange Juice with Calcium From Concentrate

Pineapple Juice

Premium Orange Juice - Calcium Plus (Not from Concentrate)

Premium Orange Juice - Grove Pure (Not from Concentrate)

Premium Orange Juice - Old Fashioned

(Not from Concentrate)
Premium Orange Juice - Original (Not from Concentrate)
Premium Ruby Red Grapefruit (Not from Concentrate)
Raspberry Cranberry Juice Cocktail
Reduced Calorie Cranberry Juice Cocktail
Ruby Red Grapefruit Juice
Ruby Red Grapefruit Juice from Concentrate
Tomato Juice
White Grape Juice

Publix GreenWise Market ()
Organic Tomato Juice

R.W. Knudsen Beverages
R.W. Knudsen Beverages (All BUT Very Veggie Line)

Raley's ()
100% Acai Sour Cherry Juice Blend
100% Apple Juice
100% Cranberry & Concord Grape
100% Cranberry Raspberry
100% Grape Juice
100% Pomegranate Cranberry Juice Blend
100% Vegetable Juice
100% White Grape Juice
Blueberry Juice Cocktail
Cranberry Apple Juice Cocktail
Cranberry Juice Cocktail
Grape Cranberry Juice Cocktail (CA+CRV)
Grapefruit Juice
Light Cranberry Juice Cocktail
Light Grape Juice Cocktail
Light White Grape Juice Cocktail
Low Sodium Vegetable Juice
Prune Juice
Raspberry Cranberry JC Cocktail
Reconstituted Lemon Juice
Ruby Red Grapefruit Juice Drink
Tomato Juice

ReaLemon
ReaLemon (All)

Safeway
Apple Cider

Apple Juice
Apple/Cranberry Juice
Berry Splash
Cranberry Cocktail Juice
Cranberry/Raspberry Juice
Grape/Cranberry Cocktail
Grapefruit Juice
Grapefruit/Tangerine Cocktail Juice
Lemon Juice
Lemonade
Light Cranberry Cocktail Juice
Limeade
Orange Juice
Pink Grapefruit Juice
Prune Juice
Ruby Red Grapefruit Cocktail
Strawberry/Kiwi Splash
Tropical Splash
Vegetable Juice
White Grape Juice
White Grapefruit Juice

Santa Cruz Organic
Santa Cruz Organic (All)

Shelby's (Save-A-Lot)
Shelby's Grove Apple Juice (100% Juice)

Simply Lemonade
Simply Lemonade

Simply Limeade
Simply Limeade

Simply Orange Juice Company
Country Stand Medium Pulp with Calcium

Snapple
Snapple (All)

SoBe
SoBe (All)

Squeez-Eez
Lemon Juice
Lime Juice

Stop & Shop
100% Apple Juice From Concentrate - Regular & Vitamin C Added (Shelf Stable)
100% Berry Juice (Shelf Stable)
100% Cherry Juice (Shelf Stable)
100% Cranberry Juice Blend (Shelf

Stable)
100% Grape Cranberry Juice (Shelf Stable)
100% Grape Juice Blend (Shelf Stable)
100% Raspberry Cranberry Juice Blend (Shelf Stable)
100% Unsweetened Grapefruit Juice (Shelf Stable)
100% White Grape Juice (Shelf Stable)
100% White Grapefruit Juice (Shelf Stable)
Apple Juice Cocktail From Concentrate (Shelf Stable)
Artificially Flavored Fruit Drink From Concentrate (Shelf Stable)
Berry Berry Cooler (Shelf Stable)
Big Apple Cooler (Shelf Stable)
Cosmic Orange Cooler (Shelf Stable)
Cran/Apple Juice Cocktail (Shelf Stable)
Cranberry Grape Juice Cocktail (Shelf Stable)
Cranberry Lime Juice Cocktail From Concentrate (Shelf Stable)
Cranberry Raspberry Juice Cocktail (Shelf Stable)
Fruit Punch/Juice Drink (Shelf Stable)
Fruity Punch Cooler (Shelf Stable)
Goofy Grape Cooler (Shelf Stable)
Grape Drink (Shelf Stable)
Grapefruit Juice (Chilled)
Lemon Juice Reconstituted (Chilled)
Lemon Lime Drink (Shelf Stable)
Light Cranberry Juice Cocktail From Concentrate (Shelf Stable)
Lite CranRaspberry Juice Cocktail (Shelf Stable)
Lite Grape Juice Cocktail (Shelf Stable)
Natural Apple Juice - Unsweetened & Added Calcium (Shelf Stable)
Orange Cranberry Juice (Chilled)
Orange Drink (Shelf Stable)
Orange Strawberry Juice (Chilled)
Pink Lemonade (Shelf Stable)
Prune Juice with Pulp (Shelf Stable)
Ruby Red Grapefruit Tangerine Juice (Shelf Stable)
Strawberry Kiwi Juice (Shelf Stable)

Tomato Juice (Shelf Stable)
Tropical Carrot/Strawberry/Kiwi Blend (Shelf Stable)
Tropical Juice Drink (Shelf Stable)
Unsweetened Apple Juice with Added Vitamin C (Shelf Stable)
Vegetable Juice From Concentrate (Shelf Stable)
White Cranberry Juice Cocktail (Shelf Stable)
White Cranberry Peach Juice Drink (Shelf Stable)
White Cranberry Strawberry Juice Drink (Shelf Stable)
Wild Cherry Juice Drink (Shelf Stable)
Wildberry Drink (Shelf Stable)

SunnyD
SunnyD (All)

Sunrise Valley (Stop & Shop)
Orange Juice - Calcium Added (Chilled)
Orange Juice - Regular (Chilled)

Trader Joe's ()
French Market Lemonade (All Flavors)
Organic Mango Lemonade

Tree Ripe
Apple Juice
Orange Juice
Orange Juice Plus Calcium & Vitamins
Orange Juice with Pulp
Organic Orange Juice
Pineapple Orange Juice

Tree Top
Juices

Turkey Hill
Lemonade
Limonade
Orangeade
Pink Lemonade
Strawberry Kiwi Lemonade

V8
Diet Splash Juice Blends (All)
Splash Juice Blends (All)
Vegetable Juices (All)
V-Fusion Blends (All)

Welch's
Welch's (All)

Wyman's
Wyman's (All)

MIXERS

Faygo
Faygo Products (All)
Margaritaville
Margaritaville (All)
Mr. & Mrs. T
Mr. & Mrs. T (All BUT Pina Colada Drink Mix)
Rose's
Rose's (All)
Simply Enjoy (Giant)
Cosmopolitan Mixer
Lemon Drop Martini Mixer
Margarita Cocktail Mixer
Mojito Cocktail Mixer
Watermelon Martini Mixer
Simply Enjoy (Stop & Shop)
Cosmopolitan Mixer
Lemon Drop Martini Mixer
Margarita Cocktail Mixer
Mojito Cocktail Mixer
Watermelon Martini Mixer
Trader Joe's ()
Margarita Mix

PROTEIN POWDER

Bob's Red Mill 🍴
Soy Protein Powder
Manitoba Harvest 🍴
Manitoba Harvest (All)
MetRx
Protein Plus Powder - Chocolate
Protein Plus Powder - Vanilla

SMOOTHIES & SHAKES

Bolthouse Farms
Berry Boost
Blue Goodness
C-Boost
Strawberry Banana

Vanilla Chai
Cascade Fresh 🍴
Cascade Fresh (All)
Lucerne (Safeway)
Smoothies - Light (All Flavors)
Luna
Sport Smoothies
Nesquik ()
MilkShake
Publix ()
Fat Free Light Mixed Berry Yogurt Smoothie
Fat Free Light Strawberry Yogurt Smoothie
Stonyfield Farm 🍴
Smoothies (All BUT Frozen Yogurt, Oikos Greek Yogurt, YoBaby Plus Fruit & Cereal and YoKids Squeezers)
Tillamook
Yogurt Smoothies (All)
V8
Splash Smoothies - Strawberry Banana

SPORTS

Albertsons
Sport Drinks (Albertson's Brand Only)
Capri Sun 〰
Berry Ice All Natural Sports Drink
Lightspeed Lemon Lime with Electrolytes Sports Drink
Thunder Punch All Natural Sports Drink
Variety Pk Sports Drink
Gatorade ()
Endurance Formula
G2
Thirst Quencher
Ingles Markets
Sports Drinks
Luna
Sport Electrolyte Drinks
POWERade
Grape
Mountain Blast

Select Brand (Safeway)
- Amazon Freeze Winners Thirst Quencher
- Fruit Punch Winners Thirst Quencher
- Glacier Wave Winners Thirst Quencher
- Lemon Ice Winners Thirst Quencher
- Lemon Lime Winners Thirst Quencher
- Lemon Winners Thirst Quencher
- Orange Winners Thirst Quencher
- Tangerine Freeze Winners Thirst Quencher
- Tropical Winners Thirst Quencher

Zico
- Zico (All)

Tea & Tea Mixes

Adagio Teas
- Teas (All)

Alter Eco Fair Trade
- Teas (All)

Bigelow Tea
- Bigelow Tea (All BUT the following Herb Teas [Blueberry Harvest, Chamomile Mango, Cinnamon Spice, formerly Sinfully Cinnamon, Fruit & Berries, Specially Strawberry], Herbal Garden Teas [Apple & Spice, Hibiscus & Rose Hips, Strawberry], and Take-A-Break Loose Tea, and Fruit & Berries Ice Tea)

Boston Tea
- Boston Tea (All)

Crystal Light
- Antioxidant Honey Lemon Green Tea On the Go
- Antioxidant Raspberry Green Tea On the Go
- Antioxidant Raspberry Green Tea Sugar Free Iced Tea
- Decaffeinated Lemon Iced Tea
- Decaffeinated Sugar Free Iced Tea
- Iced Tea - Sugar Free
- Iced Tea - Sugar Free On the Go
- Lemon Iced Tea Sugar Free
- Peach Sugar Free Iced Tea
- Peach Tea Sugar Free On the Go
- Raspberry Sugar Free Iced Tea

Eden Foods
- Lotus Root Tea Powder
- Mu 16 Herb Tea
- Organic Chamomile Herb Tea
- Organic Genmaicha Tea
- Organic Hojicha Chai Roasted Green Tea
- Organic Hojicha Tea
- Organic Kukicha Tea - Loose (Reclosable Pouch)
- Organic Kukicha Twig Tea
- Organic Matcha Tea Refill
- Organic Sencha Ginger Green Tea
- Organic Sencha Green Tea
- Organic Sencha Green Tea - Loose (Reclosable Pouch)
- Organic Sencha Mint Green Tea
- Organic Sencha Rose Green Tea

Giant
- Iced Tea Mix

Health Market (Hy-Vee)
- Green Tea Extract

Hy-Vee
- Decaffeinated Green Tea
- Decaffeinated Tea Bags
- Family Size Tea Bags
- Green Tea
- Green Tea Bags
- Orange & Spice Specialty Tea
- Tea Bags

JFG Tea
- Tea Bags

Kroger
- Tea - Bagged
- Tea - Instant

Laura Lynn (Ingle's)
- Cold Brew Tea
- Decaf Tea
- Family Decaf Tea
- Family Tea
- Green Tea
- Tagless Tea
- Tea Bags

Luzianne
- Decaf Tea Bags
- Diet Peach (Ready-To-Drink Tea)

Family Decaf Tea Bags
Family Tea Bags
Flavored Tea Bags - Lemon
Flavored Tea Bags - Peach
Flavored Tea Bags - Raspberry
Lemon Sweet (Ready-To-Drink Tea)
Liquid Flavoring - Peach Mango
Liquid Flavoring - Raspberry
Raspberry Sweet (Ready-To-Drink Tea)
Sweet (Ready-To-Drink Tea)
Tea Bags

Meijer
Iced Tea Mix
Instant Tea
Tea Bags
Tea Bags - Decaffeinated
Tea Bags - Green
Tea Bags - Green Decaffeinated

Midwest Country Fare (Hy-Vee)
Tea Bags

Mighty Leaf Tea ()
Mighty Leaf Teas

Nestea (Nestlé) ()
Nestea (All Flavors)

Newman's Own Organics
Teas (All)

Numi Organic Tea
Numi Organic Tea (All)

Oi Ocha
Oi Ocha (All)

Oregon Chai
Oregon Chai (All BUT Vanilla Dry Mix)

Orient Emporium Tea Co.
Orient Emporium Teas (All)

Original Ceylon Tea Company, The
Teas (All)

Publix ()
Decaffeinated Tea Bags
Tagless Tea Bags
Tea Bags (All Varieties)

Red Rose
Red Rose Teas

Republic of Tea, The
Full Leaf Teas (All)
Teabags (All)

Revolution Tea
Revolution Tea (All)

Rishi Tea
Teas (All)

Safeway
Iced Tea Mix (All Flavors)

Salada
100% Green Decaf Tea
100% Green Tea
Asian Plum White Tea
Decaffeinated Black Tea
Green Chai Tea
Regular Black Tea
White Decaf Tea
White Tea

Select Brand (Safeway)
Chai Tea
Chamomile Herbal Tea
Evening Delight Herbal Tea
Green Tea
Lemon Herbal Tea
Orange Spice Black Tea
Peppermint Herbal Tea
Specialty Tea

Somerset (Save-A-Lot)
Iced Tea Mix
Instant Tea

Stash Tea
Teas (All)

Stop & Shop
Iced Tea Mix

Tassimo
Tassimo (All)

Teance
Teas (All)

Trader Joe's ()
Chai - No Sugar Added
Green Tea Unsweetened
Tea (All)

Twinings
Teas (All)

Yogi Tea
Yogi Tea (All BUT Calming Tea, Fasting Tea, Kava Stress Relief Tea & Stomach Ease Tea)

Tea Drinks

AriZona
Tea Products (All)

Crystal Light 🔄
Lemon Tea Sugar Free Bottles
Metabolism Plus Green Tea Peach
Mango Multi-Serve Bottle

Dr. Andrew Weil for Tea
Dr. Weil for Tea - Brewed Tea

Enviga
Berry Sparkling Green Tea
Sparkling Green Tea

Fuze ()
Fuze

Gold Peak
Lemon Iced Tea

Hansen's
Hansen's Beverages (All)

Hy-Vee
Thirst Splashers Raspberry Tea

Inko
Inko's (All)

Nature's Promise (Stop & Shop)
Organic Fair Trade Green Tea - Decaf
(Shelf Stable & Ready-To-Drink)
Organic Fair Trade Green Tea - Lemon
(Shelf Stable & Ready-To-Drink)
Organic Fair Trade Green Tea - Regular
(Shelf Stable & Ready-To-Drink)

Nestea (Coca-Cola Company, The)
Citrus Green Tea
Diet Citrus Green Tea
Diet Lemon
Diet White Tea Berry Honey
Lemon Sweet (Hot Fill)
Sweetened Lemon Tea
White Tea Berry Honey

Newman's Own
Lemon Aided Ice Tea

POM Wonderful 🎖
POM Wonderful

Publix ()
Deli Iced Tea - Sweetened
Deli Iced Tea - Unsweetened

Sencha Shot
Sencha Shot

Snapple
Snapple (All)

SoBe
SoBe (All)

Teas' Tea ()
Teas' Tea (All)

Turkey Hill
Diet Decaffeinated Iced Tea
Diet Iced Tea
Iced Tea
Lemonade Tea
Nature's Accent - Blueberry Oolong Tea
Nature's Accent - Diet Green Tea
Nature's Accent - Diet Green Tea
Mango
Nature's Accent - Diet Peach White Tea
Nature's Accent - Green Tea
Nature's Accent - Green Tea Mango
Nature's Accents - Tangerine White Tea
Nature's Accents - Zero Calorie Chai
Spiced Tea
Nature's Accents - Zero Calorie
Pomegranate Açaí White Tea
Orange Tea
Peach Tea
Raspberry Tea
Southern Brew Extra Sweet Tea

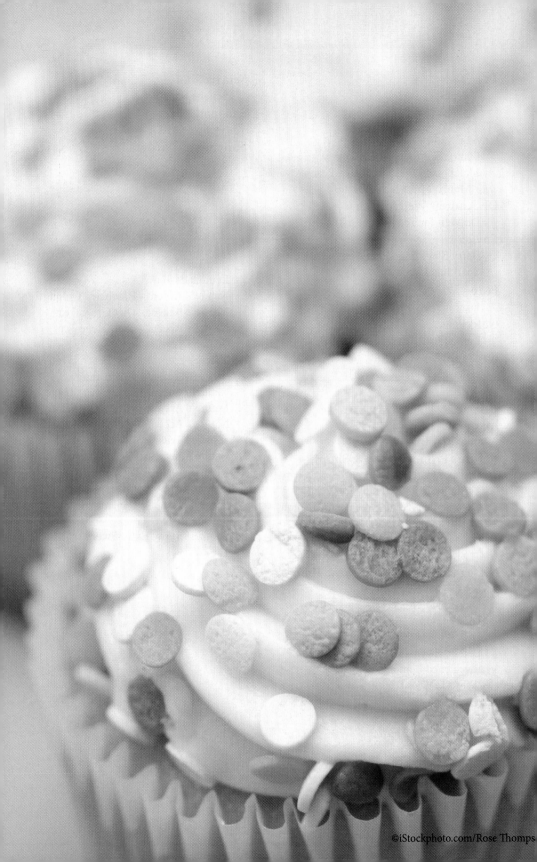

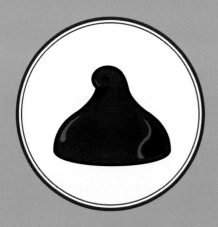

BAKING AISLE

BAKING CHIPS & BARS

Baker's 〰
  Bittersweet Squares Baking Chocolate
  German's Sweet Chocolate Bar
  Premium White Squares Baking
    Chocolate
  Real Dark Semi-Sweet Dipping
    Chocolate
  Real Milk Dipping Chocolate
  Semi-Sweet Baking Chocolate
  Semi-Sweet Chocolate Chunks
  Unsweetened Squares Baking Chocolate

Ener-G
  Chocolate Chips (seasonal)

Enjoy Life Foods 😊 😊
  Semi-Sweet Chocolate Chips

Ghirardelli ()
  Baking Chips

Giant
  Semi-Sweet Chocolate Chips

Guittard
  Guittard (All)

Hershey's
  Semi-Sweet Baking Chocolate
  Semi-Sweet Chocolate Chips
  Unsweetened Baking Chocolate

Hy-Vee
  Butterscotch Chips
  Milk Chocolate Chips
  Peanut Butter Chips
  Semi Sweet Chocolate Chips

Kroger ()
  Butterscotch Morsels
  Chocolate Chunks

  Milk Chocolate Chips
  Peanut Butter Chips
  Semi Sweet Chips
  White and Chocolate Bark Coating

Manischewitz
  Chocolate Morsels

Meijer
  Butterscotch Baking Chips
  Chocolate Chips Semi-Sweet
  Milk Chocolate Chips
  Peanut Butter Chips
  White Baking Chips

Midwest Country Fare (Hy-Vee)
  Chocolate Flavored Chips

Nestlé Toll House ()
  Semi-Sweet Chocolate Chunks
  Semi-Sweet Chocolate Mini Morsels
  Semi-Sweet Morsels

Publix ()
  Butterscotch Morsels
  Milk Chocolate Morsels
  Semi-Sweet Chocolate Morsels

Rapunzel
  Dark Baking Chocolate (Semisweet)
  Dark Chocolate Chips (Baking
    Chocolate)
  Extra Dark Baking Chocolate
    (Bittersweet)
  Extra Dark Chocolate Chips 70%
    (Semisweet) (Baking Chocolate)

Safeway
  Butterscotch Chips
  Chocolate Chips - Milk Chocolate
  Chocolate Chips - Real Chocolate
  Chocolate Chips - Semi Sweet

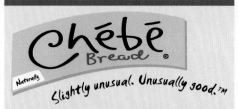
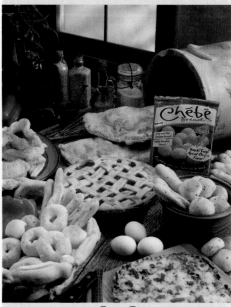
Scharffen Berger
Couverture Bars
Home Baking Bars
Propacks

Select Brand (Safeway)
Chocolate Chips

Stop & Shop
Semi-Sweet Chocolate Chips

Trader Joe's ()
Chocolate Chips - Milk
Chocolate Chips - Semi-Sweet
Chocolate Chips - White Chocolate
Milk Chocolate Peanut Butter Chips
Pound Plus Chocolate Bars
Unsweetened Belgian Baking Chocolate

Tropical Source
Baking Chips

BAKING MIXES

1-2-3 Gluten-Free
1-2-3 Gluten-Free Baking Mixes

Arrowhead Mills
Gluten Free Brownie Mix
Gluten Free Chocolate Chip Cookie Mix
Gluten Free Pancake & Waffle Mix
Gluten Free Pizza Crust Mix
Gluten Free Vanilla Cake Mix
Wild Rice Pancake & Waffle Mix

Bob's Red Mill

GF Brownie Mix
GF Chocolate Cake Mix
GF Chocolate Chip Cookie Mix
GF Cinnamon Raisin Bread Mix
GF Cornbread Mix
GF Hearty Whole Grain Bread Mix
GF Homemade Bread Mix
GF Pancake Mix
GF Pizza Crust Mix
Wheat-Free Biscuit Mix

Breads from Anna
Bread Mix (All)
Piecrust Mix

Chebe
All-Purpose Bread Mix

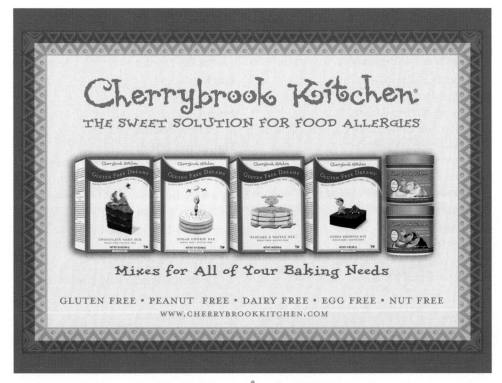

Cinnamon Roll-Up Mix
Foccacia Mix
Garlic-Onion Breadstick Mix
Original Bread Mix
Pizza Crust Mix

Cherrybrook Kitchen
Gluten Free Dreams - Chocolate Chip
  Cookie Mix
Gluten Free Dreams - Fudge Brownie
  Mix
Gluten Free Dreams - Pancake Mix
Gluten Free Dreams - Sugar Cookie
  Mix
Gluten-Free Dreams - Chocolate Cake
  Mix

Chi-Chi's
Fiesta Sweet Corn Cake Mix

Dowd & Rogers
Gluten-Free Dark Vanilla Cake Mix
Gluten-Free Dutch Chocolate Cake Mix
Gluten-Free Golden Lemon Cake Mix

El Torito
Sweet Corn Cake Mix

Food-Tek
Food-Tek (All)

Gluten-Free Pantry, The
Brown Rice Pancake And Waffle Mix
Chocolate Chip Cookie & Cake Mix
Chocolate Truffle Brownie Mix
Coffee Cake Mix
Crisp & Crumble Topping Mix
Decadent Chocolate Cake Mix
Favorite Sandwich Bread Mix
French Bread & Pizza Mix
Muffin & Scone Mix
Old Fashioned Cake & Cookie
Perfect Pie Crust Mix
Spice Cake & Gingerbread Mix
Yankee Cornbread And Muffin Mix

Hodgson Mill
Apple Cinnamon Muffin Mix
Multi Purpose Baking Mix

Hol-Grain
Gluten-Free Chocolate Brownie Mix
Gluten-Free Pancake & Waffle Mix

Junket
Junket (All BUT Hansen Island
Microwavable Fudge Mix)

OrgraN
OrgraN (All)

Pamela's Products
Baking & Pancake Mix
Chocolate Brownie Mix
Chocolate Cake Mix
Chocolate Chunk Cookie Mix
Classic Vanilla Cake Mix
Pamela's Gluten Free Bread Mix

Safeway
Glazed Cake Mix

Trader Joe's ()
Gluten Free Brownie Mix
Gluten Free Pancake & Waffle Mix

BAKING POWDER

Bob's Red Mill ♉
Baking Powder

Clabber Girl
Baking Powder

Davis Baking Powder
Baking Powder

Durkee
Baking Powder

Ener-G
Baking Powder

Hain Pure Foods
Gluten Free Feather Weight Baking
Powder

Hearth Club
Baking Powders

Hilltop Mills (Save-A-Lot)
Baking Powder

Hy-Vee
Double Acting Baking Powder

Kroger ()
Baking Powder

Laura Lynn (Ingle's)
Baking Powder

Rumford
Baking Powder

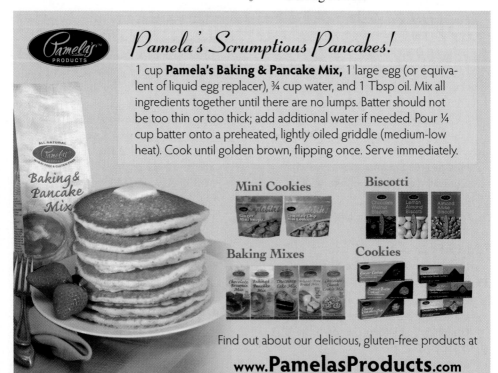

Pamela's Scrumptious Pancakes!

1 cup **Pamela's Baking & Pancake Mix,** 1 large egg (or equivalent of liquid egg replacer), ¾ cup water, and 1 Tbsp oil. Mix all ingredients together until there are no lumps. Batter should not be too thin or too thick; add additional water if needed. Pour ¼ cup batter onto a preheated, lightly oiled griddle (medium-low heat). Cook until golden brown, flipping once. Serve immediately.

Mini Cookies

Biscotti

Baking Mixes

Cookies

Find out about our delicious, gluten-free products at

www.PamelasProducts.com

Safeway
Baking Powder

BAKING SODA

Albertsons
Baking Soda

Arm & Hammer
Baking Soda (Yellow Box)

Bob's Red Mill 🍴
Baking Soda

Durkee
Baking Soda

Hilltop Mills (Save-A-Lot)
Baking Soda

Hy-Vee
Baking Soda

Kroger ()
Baking Soda

Laura Lynn (Ingle's)
Baking Soda

Meijer
Baking Soda

Stop & Shop
Baking Soda

BREAD CRUMBS & OTHER COATINGS

Ener-G
Bread Crumbs

Grandmas ()
Bag N Bake Chicken

Hol-Grain
Brown Rice Bread Crumbs
Gluten-Free Chicken Coating Mix

Luzianne
Seafood Coating Mix

Mary's Gone Crackers 🍴 🍴
Original "Gone Crackers" Crumbs

Nu-World Amaranth
Amaranth 'Bread Crumbs' - Original
Amaranth 'Breadings' - Fiesta
Amaranth 'Breadings' - Southern BBQ

Shake 'N Bake 〰
Barbecue Glaze with Shaker Bag

Sun-Bird ()
Tempura Batter

Williams Foods ()
Bag-N-Bake Chicken

COCOA POWDER

Equal Exchange ()
Cocoa Products ()

Ghirardelli ()
Baking Cocoa Powder

Guittard
Guittard (All)

Hershey's
Cocoa

Hy-Vee
Baking Cocoa

Kroger ()
Baking Cocoa

Stop & Shop
Baking Cocoa

Trader Joe's ()
Organic Cocoa Powder

COCONUT

Baker's 〰
Angel Flake Sweetened Coconut

Hy-Vee
Coconut
Flake Coconut

Kroger ()
Coconut - Regular
Coconut - Sweetened

Laura Lynn (Ingle's)
Coconut

Let's Do…Organic 🍴 ()
Organic Coconut Flakes
Organic Reduced Fat Shredded Coconut
Organic Shredded Coconut

Publix ()
Coconut Flakes

Safeway
Sweetened Coconut

Corn Syrup

Brer Rabbit
Syrup - Full
Syrup - Light
Karo
Syrups (All)
Maple Ridge (Save-A-Lot)
White Corn Syrup
Meijer
Syrup Lite Corn

Cornmeal

Arrowhead Mills
Blue Corn Meal
Yellow Corn Meal
Goya ()
Corn Meal ()
Pinol (Ground Toasted Corn)
Hodgson Mill
Organic Yellow Corn Meal (Plain)
White Corn Meal (Plain)
Yellow Corn Meal (Plain)
Publix ()
Plain Yellow Corn Meal
Safeway
Yellow Corn Meal ()

Extracts and Flavorings

Albertsons
Pure Vanilla Extract
Durkee
Liquid Extracts (All)
Liquid Flavorings (All)
Hy-Vee
Imitation Vanilla
Kroger ()
Extracts
Marcin (Save-A-Lot)
Imitation Vanilla
Pure Vanilla
Marcum Spices (Save-A-Lot) ()
Vanilla

Meijer
Imitation Vanilla
Vanilla Extract
Midwest Country Fare (Hy-Vee)
Imitation Vanilla Flavor
Nielsen-Massey
Nielsen-Massey (All)
Publix ()
Almond Extract
Lemon Extract
Vanilla Extract
Rodelle
Rodelle (All)
Spice Islands Specialty
Vanilla Bean
Trader Joe's ()
Vanilla Extract (All)
Wright's Liquid Smoke
Liquid Smoke - Hickory
Liquid Smoke - Mesquite

Flax Meal

Arrowhead Mills
Flax Seed Meal
Bob's Red Mill
Flaxseed Meal - Brown
Organic Flaxseed Meal - Brown
Organic Golden Flaxseed Meal
Hodgson Mill
Milled Flax Seed
Organic Golden Milled Flax Seed
Travel Flax Milled Flax Seed
Travel Flax Organic Golden Milled Flax Seed

Flours & Flour Mixes

Arrowhead Mills
Buckwheat Flour
Gluten Free All Purpose Baking Mix
Long Grain Brown Rice Flour
Millet Flour
Soy Flour
White Rice Flour

Bob's Red Mill
  Almond Meal/Flour
  Black Bean Flour
  Brown Rice Flour
  Fava Bean Flour
  Garbanzo Bean Flour
  Garbanzo/Fava Bean Flour
  GF All Purpose Baking Flour
  Green Pea Flour
  Hazelnut Meal/Flour
  Millet Flour
  Millet Grits/Meal
  Organic Amaranth Flour
  Organic Brown Rice Flour
  Organic Coconut Flour
  Organic Quinoa Flour
  Organic White Rice Flour
  Potato Flour
  Sorghum Flour
  Sweet White Rice Flour
  Tapioca Flour
  Teff Flour
  White Bean Flour
  White Rice Flour

Dowd & Rogers
  Italian Chestnut Flour

Ener-G
  Corn Mix
  Brown Rice Flour
  Gluten Free Gourmet Blend
  Potato Flour
  Potato Mix
  Potato Starch Flour
  Rice Mix
  Sweet Rice Flour
  Tapioca Flour
  White Rice Flour

Fearn Natural Foods
  Brown Rice Baking Mix
  Rice Baking Mix
  Rice Flour

Gluten-Free Pantry, The
  Beth's All Purpose Flour Mix

Goya ()
  Mandioca ()
  Masarepa ()

  Rice Flour ()
  Yuca Flour ()

Hodgson Mill
  Brown Rice Flour
  Buckwheat Flour
  Organic Soy Flour
  Soy Flour

Lundberg Family Farms
  Rice Flours & Grinds

Manitoba Harvest
  Manitoba Harvest (All)

Nu-World Amaranth
  Amaranth Flour
  Amaranth Toasted Bran Flour

OrgraN
  OrgraN (All)

Tom Sawyer
  All Purpose Gluten Free Flour

FOOD COLORING

Durkee
  Food Coloring (All)

Hy-Vee
  Assorted Food Coloring

Kroger ()
  Food Colors

Safeway
  Food Coloring - Assorted

FROSTING

Cherrybrook Kitchen ()
  Chocolate Frosting
  Chocolate Frosting Mix
  Vanilla Frosting
  Vanilla Frosting Mix

Ginger Evans (Save-A-Lot)
  RTS Frostings (All Flavors BUT
    Coconut Pecan)

Pamela's Products
  Confetti Frosting Mix
  Dark Chocolate Frosting Mix
  Vanilla Frosting Mix

HONEY

Albertsons
Honey
Bramley's (Save-A-Lot)
Bramley's Golden Honey
Hy-Vee
Honey
Squeeze Bear Honey
Meijer
Honey
Honey Squeeze Bear
Honey Squeeze Bottles
Publix ()
Clover Honey
Orange Blossom Honey
Wildflower Honey
Publix GreenWise Market ()
Organic Honey
Raley's ()
Grade A Pure Honey
Grade A Pure Honey (Squeeze Bear)
Safeway
Creamed Honey
Pure Honey
Select Brand (Safeway)
Honey
Trader Joe's ()
Honey (All)
Wholesome Sweeteners 🥛
Organic Amber or Raw Honey

MARSHMALLOWS

Albertsons
Marshmallows
Hy-Vee
Colored Miniature Marshmallows
Marshmallows
Miniature Marshmallows
Jet-Puffed 〰️
Chocomallows Marshmallows
Funmallows 4 Fun Flavors Miniature
  Marshmallows
Marshmallows
Marshmallows Crème

Mini Variety Pack Marshmallows
Miniature Choco Mallows
  Marshmallows
Miniature Marshmallows
Miniature Strawberry Mallows
  Marshmallows
Strawberrymallows Marshmallows
Toasted Coconut Marshmallows
Kroger ()
Colored Marshmallows
Large Marshmallows
Marshmallow Cream
Miniature Marshmallows
Laura Lynn (Ingle's)
Regular Marshmallows
Lunar (Save-A-Lot)
Mini Marshmallows
Manischewitz
Marshmallows
Marshmallow Fluff
Marshmallow Fluff
Meijer
Marshmallows - Mini
Marshmallows - Mini Flavored
Marshmallows - Regular
Publix ()
Marshmallows
Safeway
Marshmallows - Large
Marshmallows - Mini

MILK, CONDENSED

Albertsons
Sweetened Condensed Milk
Borden Eagle Brand
Sweetened Condensed Milk (All)
Hy-Vee
Sweetened Condensed Milk
Laura Lynn (Ingle's)
Sweetened Condensed Milk
Meijer
Milk - Sweetened Condensed
Nestlé Carnation ()
Sweetened Condensed Milk

Safeway
Sweetened Condensed Milk

MILK, EVAPORATED

Coburn Farms (Save-A-Lot)
Evaporated Milk
Hy-Vee
Evaporated Milk
Fat Free Evaporated Milk
Laura Lynn (Ingle's)
Evaporated Milk
Meijer
Milk - Evaporated Lite Skimmed
Milk - Evaporated Small
Milk - Evaporated Tall
Nestlé Carnation ()
Evaporated Milk
Fat Free Evaporated Milk
Low Fat Evaporated Milk
PET Evaporated Milk
PET Evaporated Milk

MILK, INSTANT OR POWDERED

Albertsons
Milk (includes Instant/Powdered)
DariFree
Original
Giant
Instant Nonfat Dry Milk
Hy-Vee
Instant Non Fat Dry Milk
Kroger ()
Milks - Powdered
Laura Lynn (Ingle's)
Instant Dry Milk
Meijer
Milk - Instant (Bulk)
Milk - Instant (Pouches)
Meyenberg
Meyenberg Goat Milk Products (All)
Publix ()
Instant Nonfat Dry Milk
Safeway
Instant Milk

Stop & Shop
Instant Nonfat Dry Milk

MOLASSES

Brer Rabbit
Molasses - Blackstrap
Molasses - Full
Molasses - Mild
Crosby's Molasses
Molasses (All)
Grandma's Molasses
Original
Robust
Holly Sugar
Sugar Products (All)
Wholesome Sweeteners 𝟾
Organic Blackstrap Molasses

OIL & OIL SPRAYS

Albertsons
Cooking/Pan Sprays
Oils
Annie's Naturals ()
Basil Flavored Olive Oil
Dipping Oil Herb Flavored Olive Oil
Organic Meyer Lemon Flavored Extra
Virgin Olive Oil
Organic Sicilian Orange Flavored Extra
Virgin Olive Oil
Roasted Garlic Flavored Extra Virgin
Olive Oil
Roasted Pepper Flavored Olive Oil
Bionaturae
Olive Oil
Blue Plate
Oil
Carapelli ()
Olive Oil
Crisco
Crisco (All BUT Cooking Spray with
Flour)
Dynasty
Sesame Oil
Stir Fry Oil

Eden Foods
Extra Virgin Olive Oil - Spanish
Hot Pepper Sesame Oil
Organic Safflower Oil
Organic Sesame Oil
Organic Soybean Oil
Toasted Sesame Oil

Filippo Berio
Olive Oils

Giant
Blended Oil
Canola Oil
Extra Light Olive Oil
Grill Spray
Peanut Oil
Pure Olive Oil
Soybean Oil

Goya ()
Olive Oil

Grand Selections (Hy-Vee)
100% Pure & Natural Olive Oil
Extra Virgin Olive Oil
Olive Oil Lemon

House Of Tsang ()
Hot Chili Sesame Oil
Mongolian Fire Oil
Sesame Oil
Wok Oil

Hy-Vee
100% Pure Canola Oil
100% Pure Corn Oil
100% Pure Vegetable Oil
Natural Blend Oil

Ingles Markets
Blended Oil
Canola Oil
Corn Oil
Peanut Oil
Vegetable Oil

Kroger ()
Canola Oil
Corn Oil
Olive Oil
Sunflower Oil
Vegetable Oil

Lapas
Olive Oils

Manischewitz
Cooking Sprays (All Varieties)
Vegetable Oil

Manitoba Harvest 8
Manitoba Harvest (All)

Mazola
Oils (All)
Sprays (All)

Meijer
Cooking Spray - Butter
Cooking Spray - Olive Oil Extra Virgin
Cooking Spray - Vegetable Oil
Oil - Blended Canola/Vegetable
Oil - Canola
Oil - Corn
Oil - Olive
Oil - Olive 100% Pure-Italian Classic
Oil - Olive Extra Virgin
Oil - Olive Extra Virgin-Italian Classic
Oil - Olive Infused Garlic & Basil
    Italian
Oil - Olive Infused Roasted Garlic-
    Italian
Oil - Olive Infused Spicy Red Pepper
    Italian
Oil - Olive Milder Tasting
Oil - Peanut
Oil - Sunflower
Oil - Vegetable
Olive-Italian Select Prem. Extra Virgin

MiCasa (Stop & Shop)
Corn Oil
Vegetable Oil

Midwest Country Fare (Hy-Vee)
100% Pure Vegetable Oil
Vegetable Oil

Montebello
Olive Oils

Newman's Own Organics
Olive Oil

Nunez de Prado
Olive Oils

Nutiva
Nutiva (All)

Publix ()
- Butter Flavored Cooking Spray
- Canola Oil
- Corn Oil
- Garlic Flavored Cooking Spray
- Lemon Flavored Cooking Spray
- Olive Oil
- Olive Oil Cooking Spray
- Original Canola Cooking Spray
- Peanut Oil
- Vegetable Oil

Rapunzel
- Canola Oil
- Hazelnut Oil
- Safflower Oil
- Sesame Oil
- Spanish Olive Oil
- Sunflower Oil

Robert Rothschild Farm
- Gourmet Dipping Oil
- Rosemary and Garlic Oil

Safeway
- Cooking Spray - Butter Flavored
- Oils

Simply Enjoy (Giant)
- Flavored Extra Virgin Olive Oil - Basil
- Flavored Extra Virgin Olive Oil - Garlic
- Flavored Extra Virgin Olive Oil - Lemon
- Flavored Extra Virgin Olive Oil - Orange
- Flavored Extra Virgin Olive Oil - Pepper
- Regional Extra Virgin Olive Oil - Apulian
- Regional Extra Virgin Olive Oil - Sicilian
- Regional Extra Virgin Olive Oil - Tuscan
- Regional Extra Virgin Olive Oil - Umbrian

Stop & Shop
- Blended Oil
- Butter Flavored Cooking Spray
- Canola Cooking Spray
- Canola Oil
- Corn Oil

- Extra Light Olive Oil
- Garlic Flavored Cooking Spray
- Grill Spray
- Olive Oil Cooking Spray
- Pure Olive Oil
- Soybean Oil
- Vegetable Cooking Spray
- Vegetable Oil

Trader Joe's ()
- Canola Oil Spray (All)
- Oils (All)

Villa Flor
- Olive Oils

RICE SYRUP

Lundberg Family Farms
- Rice Syrup - Eco-Farmed Sweet Dreams
- Rice Syrup - Organic Sweet Dreams

SHORTENING & OTHER FATS

Albertsons
- Shortening

Crisco
- Crisco (All BUT Cooking Spray with Flour)

Empire Kosher
- Rendered Chicken Fat

Hy-Vee
- Vegetable Oil Shortening
- Vegetable Shortening - Butter Flavor

Ingles Markets
- Shortening
- Vegetable Shortening

Meijer
- Shortening

Midwest Country Fare (Hy-Vee)
- Pre-Creamed Shortening

Publix ()
- Vegetable Shortening

Stop & Shop
- Meat Fat/Vegetable Shortening
- Vegetable Shortening

SPICE MIXES & PACKETS

Ac'cent
Ac'cent Flavor Enhancer

Albertsons
Chopped Onion Seasoning

Andy's Seasoning
Seasoned Salt

Bone Suckin' Sauce 🍴
Bone Suckin' Rib Rub

Cali Fine Foods
Dill Delight Gourmet Seasoning
Garlic Gusto Gourmet Seasoning
Herb Medley Gourmet Seasoning
Spicy Fiesta Gourmet Seasoning
Sweet & Spicy BBQ Rub

Chi-Chi's ()
Fiesta Restaurante Seasoning Mix

Cholula Hot Sauce
Cholula (All)

Chugwater Chili
Chugwater Chili (All)

Durkee
Apple Pie Spice
Chicken & Rib Rub
Chicken Seasoning
Chili Powder
Crazy Dave's Lemon Pepper
Crazy Dave's Pepper & Spice
Crazy Dave's Salt & Spice
Curry Powder
Garlic Pepper
Garlic Salt
Italian Seasoning
Jamaican Jerk Seasoning
Lemon & Herb
Lemon Garlic Seasoning
Lemon Pepper
Lime Pepper
Mr. Pepper
Onion Salt
Oriental 5-Spice
Pickling Spice
Pizza Seasoning
Poultry Seasoning
Pumpkin Pie Spice
Rosemary Garlic Seasoning

Salt Free Garden Seasoning
Salt Free Garlic & Herb
Salt Free Lemon Pepper
Salt Free Original All-Purpose
  Seasoning
Salt Free Veg. Seasoning
Seasoned Pepper
Six Pepper Blend
Smokey Mesquite Seasoning
Spaghetti/Pasta Seasoning
Spicy Spaghetti Seasoning
Steak Seasoning

Durkee California Style Blends
Garlic Salt
Onion Salt

Dynasty
Chinese Five Spices

Eden Foods
Organic Garlic Gomasio (Sesame Salt)
Organic Gomasio (Sesame Salt)
Organic Seaweed Gomasio (Sesame
  Salt)

Emeril's
Chicken Rub
Essence - Asian
Essence - Baby Bam
Essence - Bayou Blast
Essence - Italian
Essence - Original
Essence - Southwest
Fish Rub
Rib Rub
Steak Rub

Gayelord Hauser
Spice Garden Spices and Herbs

Goya ()
Adobo Goya
Chili Powder
Garlic Salt
Jamaican Curry Powder
Salad and Vegetable Seasoning
Sazón Goya
Seasonings
Sofrito

Grandmas ()
Chili
Spaghetti

Hy-Vee
- Chicken Grill Seasoning
- Chili Powder
- Garlic Salt
- Italian Seasoning
- Lemon Pepper
- Seasoned Salt
- Steak Grilling Seasoning
- Taco Mix

Jimmy Dean Chili ()
- Jimmy Dean Chili

KONRIKO
- Chipotle Seasoning
- Creole Seasoning
- Greek Seasoning
- Gulf Coast Seasoning Blend
- Jalapeno Seasoning
- Mojo Seasoning

Laura Lynn (Ingle's)
- Steak Seasoning

Luzianne
- Cajun Seasoning

Lydia's Organics
- Lydia's Organics (All)

Manischewitz
- Brisket & Steak Seasoning
- Fish Seasoning
- Poultry Seasoning

Marcum Spices (Save-A-Lot) ()
- Canadian Steak Seasoning
- Chili Powder
- Fried Chicken Seasoning
- Seasoned Meat Tenderizer
- Soul Seasoning

Mayacamas
- Black Olive Pesto Skillet Toss
- Dried Tomato Skillet Toss
- Garden Style Skillet Toss
- Green Olive Pesto Skillet Toss
- Seafood Skillet Toss
- Spicy Skillet Toss

Meijer
- Chili Powder
- Garlic Salt
- Mild Taco
- Onion Salt
- Seasoned Salt
- Spaghetti Mix
- Taco Seasoning

Midwest Country Fare (Hy-Vee)
- Chili Powder
- Italian Seasoning
- Season Salt

Morton Salt
- Hot Salt
- Nature's Seasons Seasoning Blend
- Seasoned Salt Substitute
- Tender Quick Mix

Nueva Cocina
- Picadillo Seasoning
- Taco Fresco Seasoning w/Chipotle
- Taco Fresco Seasonings

Old Bay
- Old Bay Seasoning

Oriental Classics ()
- Sweet & Sour Pork

Oven Fry
- Fish Fry For Fish Seasoned Coating

Publix ()
- Chili Powder
- Garlic Powder with Parsley
- Garlic Salt
- Italian Seasonings
- Lemon & Pepper
- Seasoned Salt
- Taco Seasoning Mix

Safeway
- Fajita Seasoning Mix

Spice Hunter
- Spice Blends (All)

Spice Islands Specialty
- Beau Monde
- Chili Powder
- Fines Herbs
- Garlic Pepper Seasoning
- Grilling Gourmet & World Flavors (All)
- Italian Herb Seasoning
- Summer Savory

Spike
- Spike 5Herb Magic!
- Spike Garlic Magic!
- Spike Hot 'N Spicy Magic!

ALWAYS READ LABELS

Spike Onion Magic!
Spike Original Magic!
Spike Salt Free Magic!
Spike Vegit Magic!

Stir N's (Save-A-Lot)
Chili & Taco Seasoning Mixes

Sun-Bird ()
Beef & Broccoli
Chinese Chicken Salad
Chop Suey
Chow Mein
Fried Rice
General Tso's Chicken
Honey Sesame Chicken
Honey Teriyaki
Hot & Spicy Fried Rice
Hot & Spicy Kung Pao
Hot & Spicy Szechwan
Lemon Chicken Stir Fry
Mongolian Beef
New Hot & Sour Soup
Oriental Vegetable Stir Fry
Pad Thai
Spare Rib
Spicy Orange Beef
Stir Fry
Sweet & Sour
Thai Chicken
Thai Fried Rice
Thai Red Curry
Thai Spicy Beef
Thai Stir Fry

Swanson (Williams Food) ()
Swanson Chicken Salad

Taste of Thai, A
Chicken & Rice Seasoning

Tempo
Chili Mix
Sloppy Joe Mix

Tradiciones ()
Carne Adovada
Chimichurri
Green Mole
Guajillo Enchilada
Red Mole

TryMe
Tiger Seasoning

Wagners ()
Hollandaise

Wick Fowler's
Taco Seasoning

Williams Foods ()
Chili Makins
Chili with Onions
Chipotle Chili
Chipotle Taco
Country Store Chili Soup
Country Store Tortilla Soup
Fancy Chili
Original Chili
Sloppy Joe
Spaghetti
Taco
Tex-Mex Chili
Tex-Mex Taco - Hot
White Chicken Chili

SPICES

Albertsons
Iodized Salt

B&G Foods
Capers

Durkee
Allspice
Alum
Anise Seed
Basil
Bay Leaves
Caraway Seed
Cardamom
Cayenne Pepper
Celery Flakes
Celery Seed
Chives
Cilantro
Cinnamon
Cloves
Coriander
Cream of Tartar
Crushed Red Pepper
Cumin
Dill Seed/Weed
Fennel

Garlic - Minced
Garlic Powder
Ginger
Hickory Smoke Salt
Mace
Marjoram
Meat Tenderizer
Mint Leaves
MSG
Mustard
Nutmeg
Onion - Minced
Onion Powder
Orange Peel
Oregano
Paprika
Parsley
Pepper - Black/White (All)
Pepper - Green Bell
Poppy Seed
Rosemary
Sage
Sesame Seed
Tarragon
Thyme
Turmeric

Durkee California Style Blends
Garlic Powder
Onion Powder

Eden Foods
Sea Salt - French Coast
Sea Salt - Portuguese Coast

Giant
Iodized Salt
Plain Salt

Goya ()
All Spice
Anis Seed
Bay Leaf
Chamomile Manzanilla
Crushed Peppers
Cumin Seed
Garlic Powder
Ground Black Pepper
Ground Cinnamon
Ground Cumin
Ground Oregano

Ground Pepper
Onion Powder
Oregano Leaf
Paprika
Spices
Star Anis
Stick Cinnamon
Whole Black Pepper
Whole Cloves

Hy-Vee
Basil Leaf
Bay Leaves
Black Pepper
Chopped Onion
Dill Weed
Garlic Powder
Ground Cinnamon
Ground Cloves
Ground Mustard
Iodized Salt
Meat Tenderizer
Oregano Leaf
Paprika
Parsley Flakes
Plain Salt
Red Crushed Pepper
Rosemary
Salt & Pepper Shaker Set
Thyme

Kroger ()
Salt

Laura Lynn (Ingle's)
Black Pepper

Litehouse
Freeze-Dried Basil
Freeze-Dried Chives
Freeze-Dried Dill
Freeze-Dried Garlic
Freeze-Dried Oregano
Freeze-Dried Parsley
Freeze-Dried Red Onion
Freeze-Dried Salad Herb Blend

Manischewitz
Salt

Marcum Spices (Save-A-Lot) ()
Black Pepper
Coarse Ground Black Pepper

Crushed Oregano
Crushed Red Pepper
Garlic Powder
Garlic Salt
Ground Cinnamon
Italian Seasoning
Lemon Pepper
Minced Onion
Onion Powder
Onion Salt
Paprika
Parsley Flakes
Rubbed Sage

Meijer
Black Pepper
Cinnamon
Garlic Powder
Minced Onion
Oregano Leaves
Paprika
Parsley Flakes
Salt Iodized
Salt Plain

Midwest Country Fare (Hy-Vee)
Chopped Onion
Cinnamon
Garlic Powder
Garlic Salt
Ground Black Pepper
Onion Powder
Parsley Flakes
Pure Ground Black Pepper

Morton Salt
Coarse Kosher Salt
Iodized Salt
Lite Salt Mixture
Pickling & Canning Salt
Popcorn Salt
Salt & Pepper Shakers
Salt Substitute
Sea Salt
Table Salt (Non-Iodized)

No Salt
No Salt Salt Substitute

Para MiCasa (Giant)
Adobo - Pepper
Adobo - Regular

Polaner
Ready To Use Wet Spices - Basil
Ready To Use Wet Spices - Garlic
Ready To Use Wet Spices - Jalapenos

Publix ()
Adobo Seasoning with Pepper
Adobo Seasoning Without Pepper
Black Pepper
Cinnamon
Garlic Powder
Ground Ginger
Ground Red Pepper
Minced Onion
Onion Powder
Paprika
Parsley Flakes
Salt
Whole Bay Leaves
Whole Black Pepper
Whole Oregano

Spice Hunter
Spices (All)

Spice Islands Specialty
Crystallized Ginger
Old Hickory Smoked Salt
Saffron
Salt-Free (All)

Stop & Shop
Iodized Salt
Plain Salt

Trader Joe's ()
Private Label Spices (All)

SPRINKLES

Kroger ()
Rainbow Sprinkles
Sugar Sprinkles

Laura Lynn (Ingle's)
Chocolate Sprinkles Toppings
Rainbow Sprinkles Toppings

Let's Do... ()
Carnival Sprinkelz
Chocolatey Sprinkelz
Confetti Sprinkelz

Safeway
- Sprinkles - Easter
- Sprinkles - Halloween
- Sprinkles - Holiday
- Sprinkles - Sand Sugar Party
- Sprinkles - Valentines

STARCHES

Argo
- Corn Starch

Benson's
- Corn Starch

Bob's Red Mill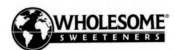
- Arrowroot Starch
- Cornstarch
- Potato Starch

Canada
- Corn Starch

Durkee
- Arrowroot

Eden Foods
- Organic Kuzu Root Starch

Hy-Vee
- Cornstarch

Kingsford
- Corn Starch

Kroger ()
- Corn Starch

Laura Lynn (Ingle's)
- Corn Starch

Let's Do…Organic ⅋ ()
- Organic Tapioca Starch

Manischewitz
- Potato Starch

Meijer
- Corn Starch

Safeway
- Corn Starch

Streit's
- Potato Starch

SUGAR & SUGAR SUBSTITUTES

Albertsons
- Aspartame

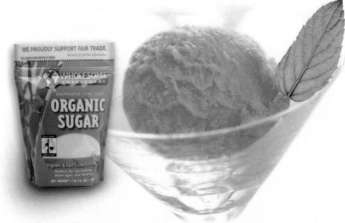

ALWAYS READ LABELS

Saccharin

Alter Eco Fair Trade
Sugar (All)

Billington's 𝄞
Dark Muscovado Sugar
Demerara Sugar
Light Muscovado Sugar
Milled Golden Cane Sugar (All Types)

Dixie Crystals
Sugar Products (All)

Equal
Equal

Equal Exchange ()
Sugar

Florida Crystals 𝄞
Sugar Products (All)

Giant
Granulated Sugar
Sucralose

Holly Sugar
Sugar Products (All)

Hy-Vee
Aspartame Sweetener
Confectioners Powdered Sugar
Dark Brown Sugar
Light Brown Sugar
Pure Cane Sugar
Saccharin Sugar Substitute

Imperial Sugar
Sugar Products (All)

Ingles Markets
Brown Sugar
Confectioner's Sugar
Sugar

Kroger ()
Dark Brown Sugar
Granulated Sugar
Light Brown Sugar
Powdered Sugar
Sugar Substitutes

Meijer
Sugar
Sugar - Confectioners
Sugar - Dark Brown
Sugar - Light Brown

Nielsen-Massey
Nielsen-Massey (All)

NutraSweet
NutraSweet (All)

Publix ()
Dark Brown Sugar
Granulated Sugar
Light Brown Sugar
Powdered - 10X & 4X Sugar

Safeway
Aspartame Sweetener
Sugar - Brown, Granulated & Powdered

Savannah Gold
Savannah Gold (All)

Splenda
Splenda
Splenda Brown Sugar Blend
Splenda Flavor Blends For Coffee -
Caramel
Splenda Flavor Blends For Coffee -
Cinnamon Spice
Splenda Flavor Blends For Coffee -
French Vanilla
Splenda Flavor Blends For Coffee -
Hazelnut
Splenda Flavor Blends For Coffee -
Mocha
Splenda No Calorie Sweetener (Packets,
Café Sticks and Granulated)
Splenda Sugar Blend

Stop & Shop
Granulated Sugar
Sucralose
Sweet Measure

Sweet 'N Low
Sweet 'N Low

Trader Joe's ()
Sugar (All)

Wholesome Sweeteners 𝄞
Organic Blue Agave Syrups
Organic Sucanat (All Types)
Organic Sugars (Evaporated or
Dehydrated Cane Juice) (All Types)
Sucanat (All Types)
Organic Zero/Organic Erythritol/Sugar
Substitute

Whole Grains

Alter Eco Fair Trade
Quinoa (All)

Arrowhead Mills
Amaranth
Buckwheat Groats
Flax Seed
Golden Flax Seed
Hulled Millet
Quinoa

Bob's Red Mill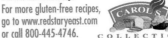
Flaxseed (Brown)
Hulled Millet
Organic Amaranth Grain
Organic Buckwheat Berries
Organic Buckwheat Groats
Organic Buckwheat Kernels - Kasha
Organic Flaxseed - Brown
Organic Golden Flaxseed
Organic Quinoa Grain
Teff Grain

Eden Foods
Quinoa

Trader Joe's
Organic Quinoa

Yeast

Bakipan
Active Dry Yeast (ADY)
Bread Machine Yeast
Instant Yeast

Bob's Red Mill
Yeast - Active Dry
Yeast - Nutritional T6635 Lg Flake

Fleischmann's Yeast
Fleischmann's Yeast (All)

Gayelord Hauser
Brewers Yeast

Hodgson Mill
Active Dry Yeast
Fast Rise Yeast

Kroger
Yeast Packets

Red Star Yeast
Active Dry Yeast (ADY)
Bread Machine Yeast
Quick Rise Yeast
Vegetarian Support Nutritional Yeast
Flakes

SAF
Active Dry Yeast (ADY)
Bread Machine Yeast
Gourmet Perfect Rise

Miscellaneous

Bob's Red Mill
Guar Gum
Organic Textured Soy Protein
Rice Bran
Soy Lecithin
Textured Vegetable Protein (TVP)
Xanthan Gum

Certo
Liquid Fruit Pectin

Ener-G
- Calcium Carbonate
- Crumbles
- Rice Bran
- Xanthan Gum

Fearn Natural Foods
- Lecithin Granules
- Liquid Lecithin
- Natural Soya Powder
- Soya Granules
- Soya Protein Isolate

Fibersure
- Fibersure

Let's Do...Organic ♀ ()
- Organic Tapioca Granules
- Organic Tapioca Pearls

MCP ↝
- Fruit Pectin - Premium For Homemade Jams & Jellies

None Such
- Mince Meat

Nu-World Amaranth
- Puffed Amaranth

OrgraN
- OrgraN (All)

Sure.Jell ↝
- Fruit Pectin - Premium For Homemade Jams & Jellies
- Fruit Pectin - Premium For Lower Sugar Recipes
- No Cook Jam Pectin

Williams Foods ()
- Jel Ease - Pectin

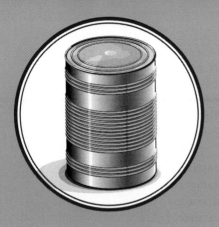

CANNED AND PRE-PACKAGED FOODS

Asian Specialty Items

Eden Foods
Agar Agar Bars
Agar Agar Flakes
Arame
Bonito Flakes
Daikon Radish - Dried & Shredded
Eden Shake (Furikake) Seasoning
Hiziki
Instant Wakame Flakes
Kombu
Lotus Root
Maitake Dried Mushrooms
Mekabu Wakame
Nori
Organic Dulse Flakes
Organic Shiro Miso
Pickled Daikon Radish
Shiitake Dried Sliced Mushrooms
Shiitake Dried Whole
Shiso Leaf Powder (Pickled Beefsteak
   Leaf)
Sushi Nori
Toasted Nori Krinkles
Ume Plum Balls
Ume Plum Concentrate (Bainiku Ekisu)
Umeboshi Paste
Umeboshi Plums
Wakame
Wasabi Powder
Yansen Dandelion Root Concentrate

Beans, Baked

Albertsons
Baked Beans
Amy's Kitchen
Organic Vegetarian Baked Beans
B&M Baked Beans
B&M Baked Beans (All)
Bush's Best
Bush's Best (All BUT Chili Beans,
   Chili Magic Chili Starter &
   Homestyle Chili Lines)
Eden Foods
Baked Beans with Sorghum & Mustard
Giant
Brown Sugar & Bacon Baked Beans
Pork & Beans
Vegetarian Baked Beans
Halstead Acres (Save-A-Lot)
Pork & Beans
Health Market (Hy-Vee)
Organic Baked Beans
Organic Maple & Onion Baked Beans
Heinz ()
Vegetarian Beans
Hormel ()
Kid's Kitchen - Beans & Wieners
Hy-Vee
Home Style Baked Beans
Onion Baked Beans
Original Baked Beans
Pork & Beans

Ingles Markets
Beans & Franks
Pork & Beans

Meijer
Baked Beans Organic
Pork & Beans

Midwest Country Fare (Hy-Vee)
Pork & Beans

Publix ()
Baked Beans
Pork & Beans

Safeway
Pork & Beans

Stop & Shop
Brown Sugar & Bacon Baked Beans
Homestyle Baked Beans
Vegetarian Baked Beans

BEANS, OTHER

Albertsons
Canned Beans
Dry Packed Beans

Arrowhead Mills
Adzuki Beans
Garbanzo Beans
Green Lentils
Red Lentils
Split Peas, Green

Bush's Best
Bush's Best (All BUT Chili Beans, Chili Magic Chili Starter & Homestyle Chili Lines)

Eden Foods
Aduki Beans
Black Beans
Black Eyed Peas
Butter Beans (Baby Lima)
Cannellini (White Kidney) Beans
Caribbean Black Beans
Garbanzo Beans (Chick Peas)
Great Northern Beans
Kidney Beans
Navy Beans
Pinto Beans
Rice & Cajun Small Red Beans
Rice & Caribbean Black Beans
Rice & Garbanzo Beans
Rice & Kidney Beans
Rice & Lentils
Rice & Pinto Beans
Small Red Beans

Fantastic World Foods ()
Instant Black Beans

Furmano's
Furmano's (All)

Giant
Black Beans
Chick Peas
Kidney Beans - Dark & Light Red
Kidney Beans - No Added Salt
Kidney Beans - Regular
Lima Beans
Organic Black Beans
Organic Garbanzo Beans
Organic Light Kidney Beans
Pink Beans
Pinto Beans
Red Beans

Goya ()
Blue-Labeled Canned Beans

Halstead Acres (Save-A-Lot)
Great Northern Beans
Pinto Beans

HamBeens ()
Baby Lima

HamPeas ()
California Blackeye Peas
Green Split Pea
Large Lima

Health Market (Hy-Vee)
Organic Black Beans
Organic Dark Red Kidney Beans
Organic Garbanzo Beans
Organic Pinto Beans

Hy-Vee
Baby Lima Beans
Black Beans
Black-Eyed Peas
Butter Beans
Chili Style Beans
Dark Red Kidney Beans

Garbanzo Beans Chick Peas
Great Northern Beans
Large Lima Beans
Lentils
Light Red Kidney Beans
Navy Beans
Pinto Beans
Red Beans
Red Kidney Beans

Ingles Markets
Canned Blackeye Peas
Canned Kidney Beans
Canned Lima Beans
Chili Beans
Dried Beans (All)

Joan of Arc
Black Beans
Butter Beans
Garbanzo Beans
Great Northern Beans
Light & Dark Red Kidney Beans
Pinto Beans
Red Beans

Kroger ()
Unseasoned Beans - Canned
Unseasoned Beans - Dry

Meijer
Beans - Mexican Style
Black Beans
Black Beans Organic
Blackeye Peas
Butter Beans
Garbanzo Beans
Garbanzo Beans - Organic
Great Northern Beans
Kidney Beans - Dark Red
Kidney Beans - Dark Red Organic
Kidney Beans - Light Red
Pinto Beans
Pinto Beans - Organic
Red Beans

Midwest Country Fare (Hy-Vee)
Chili Style Beans

Publix ()
Kidney Beans - Dark and Light

Publix GreenWise Market ()
Black Beans - Organic Vegetables

Dark Red Kidney Beans - Organic
Vegetables
Garbanzo Beans - Organic Vegetables
Pinto Beans - Organic Vegetables

Safeway
Black Beans
Black-Eyed Beans
Light Red Kidney Dried Beans
Mexican Style Chili Beans
Pinto Beans

Stop & Shop
Black Beans
Black Eyed Peas
Chick Peas
Kidney Beans - Light & Dark Red
Lima Beans
Pink Beans
Pinto Beans
Red Beans
Romano Beans

Taco Bell ↫
Home Originals - Bean Con Queso

Trader Joe's ()
Beans (All)

Williams Foods ()
Hot Chili Beans
Medium Chili Beans
Mild Chili Beans

BEANS, REFRIED

Albertsons
Refried Beans

Amy's Kitchen
Organic Refried Beans with Green
Chiles
Organic Refried Black Beans
Organic Traditional Refried Beans
Organic Traditional Refried Beans -
Light in Sodium

Eden Foods
Refried Black Beans
Refried Black Soy & Black Beans
Refried Kidney Beans
Refried Pinto Bean
Refried Spicy Black Beans
Refried Spicy Pinto Beans

Fantastic World Foods ()
Instant Refried Beans
Health Market (Hy-Vee)
Organic Refried Beans
Hy-Vee
Black Refried Beans
Fat Free Refried Beans
Traditional Refried Beans
Vegetarian Refried Beans
Ingles Markets
Fat Free Refried Beans
Refried Beans
Meijer
Fat Free Refried Beans
Refried Beans
Refried Beans - Fat Free
Refried Beans - Organic Black Bean
Refried Beans - Organic Blk Bean/
Jalapeno
Refried Beans - Organic Roasted Chili/
Lime
Refried Beans - Organic Traditional
Refried Beans - Vegetarian
Safeway
Refried Beans
Taco Bell 🐾
Fat Free Refried Beans
Vegetarian Blend Refried Beans

BOUILLON

Edward & Sons 🍴 ()
Garden Veggie Bouillon Cubes
Low Sodium Veggie Bouillon Cubes
Not-Beef Bouillon Cubes
Not-Chick'N Bouillon Cubes
Giant
Beef Flavored Bouillon Cubes - Instant
Beef Flavored Bouillon Cubes - Regular
Chicken Flavored Bouillon Cubes -
Instant
Chicken Flavored Bouillon Cubes -
Regular
Goya ()
Consomme-Chicken Bouillon
Cubito - Beef Bouillon

Cubito - Chicken Bouillon
Ham Flavored Concentrate
Herb-Ox Bouillon ()
Beef
Chicken
Garlic Chicken
Vegetable
Hy-Vee
Beef Bouillon Cubes
Chicken Bouillon Cubes
Instant Beef Bouillon
Instant Chicken Bouillon
Rapunzel
Vegetable Bouillon (No Salt Added/
Low Sodium) ()
Vegetable Bouillon w/Herbs ()
Vegetable Bouillon w/Sea Salt ()
Stop & Shop
Beef Flavored Bouillon Cubes - Instant
Beef Flavored Bouillon Cubes - Regular
Chicken Flavored Bouillon Cubes -
Instant
Chicken Flavored Bouillon Cubes -
Regular

BROTH & STOCK

College Inn ()
Garden Vegetable Broth
Organic Beef Broth
Giant
Beef Broth
Chicken Broth
Imagine
Beef Broth
Free Range Chicken Broth
No-Chicken Broth
Vegetable Broth
Kitchen Basics
Beef Stock (All)
Chicken Stock (All)
Clam Stock (All)
Ham Stock (All)
Pork Stock (All)
Seafood Stock (All)
Turkey Stock (All)

Vegetable Stock (All)

Manischewitz
Chicken Broth

Meijer
Broth - Chicken
Broth Chicken (First Line)

Nature's Promise (Giant)
All Natural Beef Broth
Organic Chicken Broth
Organic Vegetable Broth

Nature's Promise (Stop & Shop)
All Natural Beef Broth
Organic Chicken Broth
Organic Vegetable Broth

Pacific Natural Foods
Beef Broth
Natural Free Range Chicken
Organic Free Range Chicken
Organic Low Sodium Chicken
Organic Mushroom
Organic Vegetable Broth

Raley's ()
Chicken Broth

Safeway
Chicken Broth

Shelton's
Chicken Broth Fat Free
Chicken Broth Regular
Fat Free Organic Chicken Broth
LS/FF Organic Turkey Broth
Regular Organic Chicken Broth
Regular Organic Turkey Broth

Stop & Shop
Beef Broth
Chicken Broth

Swanson (Campbell's)
Chicken with Roasted Garlic Broth
Lower Sodium Beef Broth (All)
Natural Goodness Chicken Broth (All)
Organic Broths - Beef
Organic Broths - Chicken
Organic Broths - Vegetable
Regular Beef Broth (All)
Regular Chicken Broth (All)
Vegetable Broth

Trader Joe's ()
Organic Chicken Broth - Low Sodium
Organic Chicken Broth - Regular
Organic Hearty Vegetable Broth
Roasted Beef in Beef Broth

Valley Fresh ()
Broth

Wolfgang Puck's
All Natural Roasted Chicken Stock
Organic Beef Broth
Organic Chicken Broth
Organic Vegetable Broth

CHILI & CHILI MIXES

Amy's Kitchen
Organic Black Bean Chili
Organic Medium Chili
Organic Medium Chili - Light in
Sodium
Organic Medium Chili with Vegetables
Organic Spicy Chili
Organic Spicy Chili - Light in Sodium

Bean Cuisine
Bean Soups Bag - Chili

Bush's Best
Bush's Best (All BUT Chili Beans,
Chili Magic Chili Starter &
Homestyle Chili Lines)

Carroll Shelby Chili
Original Texas Chili Kit

Chugwater Chili
Chugwater Chili (All)

Del Monte ()
Homestyle Chili with Beans

Halstead Acres (Save-A-Lot)
Chili Hot Beans

Healthy Advantage (Safeway)
Vegetarian Chili

Hormel ()
Chili with Beans - Chunky
Chili with Beans - Hot
Chili with Beans - Regular

Hy-Vee
Chili with Beans
Hot Chili with Beans

Meijer
Chili with Beans (Regular)
Chili with No Beans (Regular)
Pacific Natural Foods
All Natural Beef Steak Chili with Beans
Shelton's
Chicken Chili Mild
Chicken Chili Spicy
Turkey Chili Mild
Turkey Chili Spicy
Taco Bell 𝒢
Home Originals - Chili Con Queso with
Meat
Texas Pete
Chili No Bean
Hot Dog Chili
Trader Joe's ()
3 Bean and Beef Chili
Chicken Chili with Beans
Organic Vegetarian Chili
Vegetarian 3 Bean Chili
Wick Fowler's
2-Alarm Chili Kit
False Alarm Chili Kit
One Step Wick Fowler Chili

COCONUT MILK

Goya ()
Coconut Milk
Cream of Coconut
Let's Do…Organic 🥛 ()
Organic Creamed Coconut
Native Forest 🥛 ()
Organic Coconut Milk
Organic Light Coconut Milk
Taste of Thai, A
Coconut Milk
Lite Coconut Milk
Thai Kitchen
Coconut Milk Lite - Thailand
Coconut Milk Lite Organic - Thailand
Premium Coconut Milk - Thailand
Premium Coconut Milk Organic -
Thailand

Trader Joe's ()
Light Coconut Milk

CRANBERRY SAUCE

Hy-Vee
Jellied Cranberry Sauce
Whole Berry Cranberry Sauce
Manischewitz
Cranberry Sauce
Ocean Spray
Sauces (All)
Publix ()
Whole Cranberry Sauce
Safeway
Cranberry Sauce - Jellied
Cranberry Sauce - Whole
Stop & Shop
Cranberry Sauce - Jellied
Cranberry Sauce - Whole Berry
Wild Thymes
Wild Thymes (All BUT Toasted Sesame
Wasabi Vinaigrette, Indonesian Peanut
Sesame Dipping Sauce, Hawaiian
Teriyaki Marinade and Korean Ginger
Scallion Marinade.)

FRUIT

Albertsons
Canned Apricots
Canned Peaches
Canned Pears
Canned Pineapple
Del Monte ()
Canned/Jarred Fruits (All)
Giant
Apricots - Heavy Syrup
Apricots - Island in Light Syrup
Bartlett Pear Halves - Heavy Syrup
Bartlett Pear Halves - Juice
Bartlett Pear Halves - Light Syrup
Bartlett Pear Halves - Pear Juice
Bartlett Pear Halves - Splenda
Blueberries in Syrup
Fruit Cocktail - Heavy Syrup

Fruit Cocktail - Pear Juice
Fruit Cocktail - Splenda
Fruit Mix in Heavy Syrup
Peaches - Heavy Syrup
Peaches - Pear Juice
Peaches - Yellow Cling
Red Tart Pitted Cherries in Water
Sweet Cherries in Heavy Syrup - Dark
Sweet Cherries in Heavy Syrup - Light
Very Cherry Fruit Mix in Light Syrup
Whole Plums in Heavy Syrup

Goya ()
Guava Paste

Hy-Vee
Bartlett Pear Halves
Bartlett Pears
Chunk Pineapple
Crushed Pineapple
Diced Peaches
Fruit Cocktail
Lite Chunk Mixed Fruit
Lite Fruit Cocktail
Lite Peach Halves
Lite Peach Slices
Lite Pears
Lite Unpeeled Apricot Halves
    Sweetened with Splenda
Mandarin Oranges
Mandarin Oranges in Light Syrup
Mandarin Oranges in Orange Gel
Mixed Fruit
Natural Lite Diced Bartlett Pears
Natural Lite Diced Peaches
Peach Halves
Peach Slices
Peaches in Strawberry Gel
Pineapple in Lime Gel
Pumpkin
Purple Plums
Sliced Bartlett Pears
Sliced Pineapple
Unpeeled Apricot Halves
Yellow Cling Lite Sliced Peaches

Ingles Markets
Canned Pineapple

Knouse Foods
Dutch Baked Apples

Fried Apples
Red Tart Pitted Cherries
Sliced Apples
Spiced Apple Rings
Spiced Crab Apples

Kroger ()
Fruit - Canned

Meijer
Apricot Halves Unpeeled in Pear Juice
Fruit Cocktail in Heavy Syrup
Fruit Cocktail in Pear Juice Lite
Fruit Cocktail Juice
Fruit Cocktail Juice Easy Open
Fruit Mix Juice
Fruit Salad Tropical
Grapefruit Sections in Syrup
Grapefruit Sections Juice
Mandarin Oranges Light Syrup
Peaches - Cling Halves in Heavy Syrup
Peaches - Cling Halves in Juice (Lite)
Peaches - Cling Halves Pear Juice Lite
Peaches - Cling Sliced in Heavy Syrup
Peaches - Cling Sliced in Juice
Peaches - Cling Slices Pear Juice Lite
Peaches - Yellow Sliced in Heavy Syrup
Pear Halves - Juice Easy Open
Pear Halves - Lite
Pear Halves in Heavy Syrup
Pear Slices in Heavy Syrup
Pears - Halves in Heavy Syrup
Pears - Halves in Juice (Lite)
Pears - Sliced Heavy Syrup
Pears - Slices in Heavy Syrup
Pears - Slices in Juice (Lite)
Pineapple - Crushed Heavy Syrup
Pineapple - Crushed in Juice
Pineapple - Sliced Heavy Syrup
Pineapple - Sliced in Juice
Pineapple Chunks - Heavy Syrup
Pineapple Chunks in Juice
Pineapple Juice
Pumpkin

Midwest Country Fare (Hy-Vee)
Bartlett Pear Halves in Light Syrup
Crushed Pineapple
Fruit Cocktail
Lite Peach Halves

Lite Peach Slices
Peach Slices
Pineapple Chunks
Pineapple Slices
Pineapple Tidbits

Native Forest ⚠ ()

Organic Mango Chunks
Organic Papaya Chunks
Organic Pineapple Chunks
Organic Pineapple Crushed
Organic Pineapple Mini Rings
Organic Pineapple Slices
Organic Tropical Fruit Salad

Oregon Fruit Products

Canned Fruit Products (All)

Publix ()

Apricot Halves - Unpeeled in Heavy
    Syrup
Bartlett Pears in Heavy Syrup (Halves
    and Slices)
Chunky Mixed Fruit in Heavy Syrup
Fruit Cocktail in Heavy Syrup
Lite Bartlett Pear Halves in Pear Juice
Lite Chunky Mixed Fruit in Pear Juice
Lite Fruit Cocktail in Pear Juice
Lite Yellow Cling Peaches in Pear Juice
    (Halves and Slices)
Mandarin Oranges in Light Syrup
Pineapple (All Styles)
Yellow Cling Peaches in Heavy Syrup
    (Halves and Slices)

Raley's ()

Chunks Pineapple
Crushed Pineapple
Sliced Pineapple

S&W ()

Canned/Jarred Fruits (All)

Safeway

Canned Pumpkin
Mixed Fruit & Peel
Red Tart Pitted Cherries
Sliced Peaches

Stop & Shop

Apricots - Heavy Syrup and Splenda
Bartlett Pear Halves - Heavy Syrup,
    Light Syrup, Pear Juice & Splenda
Fruit Cocktail - Heavy Syrup, Pear Juice

& Splenda
Fruit Mix in Heavy Syrup
Island Apricots in Light Syrup
Peaches - Yellow Cling, Pear Juice &
    Heavy Syrup (Whole & Slices)
Very Cherry Fruit Mix in Light Syrup
Whole Plums in Heavy Syrup

Trader Joe's ()

Chunky Spiced Apples
Mandarin Oranges in Light Syrup

Wyman's

Wyman's (All)

MEAT

Albertsons

Corned Beef Hash

Giant

Premium Chunk Chicken Breast in
    Water

Hargis House (Save-A-Lot)

Vienna Sausages

Hormel ()

Black Label - Canned Hams
Breast of Chicken Chunk Meats
Chicken Chunk Meats
Corned Beef
Corned Beef Hash
Dried Beef
Ham Chunk Meats
Ham Patties
Turkey Chunk Meats

Kroger ()

Chicken - Canned
Chicken - Pouch

Meijer

Chicken Chunk White
Corned Beef Hash

Safeway

Corned Beef Hash

SPAM ()

Classic
Less Sodium
Lite
Oven Roasted Turkey
Smoke Flavored

Stop & Shop
- Premium Chunk Chicken Breast in Water

Swanson (Campbell's)
- Mixin' Chicken
- Premium Chunk Chicken Breast in Water (All Sizes)
- Premium White & Dark Chunk Chicken (All Sizes)

Underwood
- Deviled Ham Spread

Valley Fresh ()
- Chicken
- Turkey

PIE FILLINGS

Giant
- Blueberry Fruit Filling
- Cherry Pie Filling
- Lite Cherry Pie Filling
- Spiced Apple Pie Filling

Gold Leaf (Save-A-Lot)
- Apple Pie Filling
- Blueberry Pie Filling
- Cherry Pie Filling
- Peach Pie Filling

Hy-Vee
- 100% Natural Pumpkin
- More Fruit Apple Pie Filling Or Topping
- More Fruit Cherry Pie Filling Or Topping

Knouse Foods
- Apple Pie Filling
- Apricot Pie Filling
- Banana Crème Pie Filling
- Blackberry Pie Filling
- Blueberry Pie Filling
- Cherries Jubilee Pie Filling
- Cherry Pie Filling
- Chocolate Crème Pie Filling
- Coconut Crème Pie Filling
- Dark Sweet Cherry Pie Filling
- Key Lime Pie Filling
- Lemon Crème Pie Filling
- Lemon Pie Filling

- Lite Apple Pie Filling
- Lite Cherry Pie Filling
- Peach Pie Filling
- Pineapple Pie Filling
- Raisin Pie Filling
- Strawberry Glaze Pie Filling
- Strawberry Pie Filling
- Vanilla Crème Pie Filling

Kroger ()
- Canned Pie Filling

Libby's ()
- Libby's 100% Pure Pumpkin
- Libby's Easy Pumpkin Pie Mix

Meijer
- Pie Filling - Apple
- Pie Filling - Blueberry
- Pie Filling - Cherry
- Pie Filling - Cherry Lite
- Pie Filling - Peach

Midwest Country Fare (Hy-Vee)
- Apple Pie Filling
- Cherry Pie Filling

SEAFOOD, OTHER

Chicken of the Sea
- Chicken of The Sea (All BUT Ahi Tuna Steak in Grilled Herb Marinade, Ahi Tuna Steak in Teriyaki Sauce, Crabtastic! Imitation Crab, Salmon Steak in Mandarin Orange Glaze, Mandarin Orange Salmon Cups, Teriyaki Tuna Cups & Tuna Salad Kits.)

Crown Prince
- Crown Prince Products (All)

Giant
- Filet of Mackerel
- Portuguese Sardines

Goya ()
- Octopus
- Sardines

Hy-Vee
- Alaska Pink Salmon
- Alaska Red Salmon

Kasilof
- Smoked Salmon Items (All)

Kroger ()
Salmon - Canned
Sardines - Canned

Meijer
Salmon - Pink
Salmon - Sockeye Red

Trader Joe's ()
Pink Salmon - Skinless, Boneless
Skinless & Boneless Sardines in Olive
Oil
Whole Smoked Oysters in Olive Oil

Underwood
Sardines in Mustard Sauce
Sardines in Soybean Oil

SEAFOOD, TUNA

Albertsons
Canned Tuna

Bumble Bee
Canned Seafood Products

Chicken of the Sea
Chicken of The Sea (All BUT Ahi Tuna
Steak in Grilled Herb Marinade, Ahi
Tuna Steak in Teriyaki Sauce, Crab-
tastic! Imitation Crab, Salmon Steak
in Mandarin Orange Glaze, Mandarin
Orange Salmon Cups, Teriyaki Tuna
Cups & Tuna Salad Kits.)

Crown Prince
Crown Prince Products (All)

Grand Selections (Hy-Vee)
Solid White Albacore Tuna

Hy-Vee
Light Chunk Tuna in Oil
Light Chunk Tuna in Water

Ingles Markets
Chunk Tuna
Solid White Albacore Tuna

Kroger ()
Tuna - Canned
Tuna - Pouch

Midwest Country Fare (Hy-Vee)
Light Tuna Chunks Packed in Water

Safeway
Chunk Light Tuna

Select Brand (Safeway)
Tongol Tuna

StarKist Tuna ()
Starkist Tuna (All BUT Tuna Creations
Herb & Garlic, Tuna Fillet Teriyaki &
Lunch Kit Crackers)

Trader Joe's ()
Tuna (All)

SOUPS & SOUP MIXES

Amy's Kitchen
Curried Lentil Soup
Organic Black Bean Vegetable Soup
Organic Chunky Tomato Bisque Soup
Organic Chunky Tomato Bisque Soup -
Light in Sodium
Organic Chunky Vegetable Soup
Organic Cream of Tomato Soup
Organic Cream of Tomato Soup - Light
in Sodium
Organic Fire Roasted Southwestern
Vegetable Soup
Organic Lentil Soup
Organic Lentil Soup - Light in Sodium
Organic Lentil Vegetable Soup
Organic Lentil Vegetable Soup - Light
in Sodium
Organic Split Pea Soup
Organic Split Pea Soup - Light in
Sodium
Organic Summer Corn & Vegetable
Soup
Organic Tuscan Bean & Rice Soup
Thai Coconut Soup

Bean Cuisine
Bean Soups Bag - Island Black Bean
Bean Soups Bag - Lots of Lentil
Bean Soups Bag - Louisiana Cajun
Bean Soups Bag - Santa Fe Corn
Chowder
Bean Soups Bag - Southwest Tortilla
Bean Soups Bag - Thick As Fog Split
Pea
Bean Soups Bag - Thirteen Bean
Bouillabaisse
Bean Soups Bag - White Bean

Provencal

Bear Creek
Cheddar Broccoli
Cheddar Potato
Chili
Creamy Potato
Creamy Wild Rice
Navy Bean

Campbell's
Chicken Broccoli Cheese (Chunky Soup)
Savory Lentil (Select Soup)

Dr. McDougall's Right Foods
Black Bean & Lime Big Cup
Light Sodium Split Pea
Pad Thai Big Cup
Tamale Pie Big Cup
Tortilla Soup Big Cup

Eden Foods
Organic Genmai (Brown Rice) Miso

Ener-G
Cream of Mushroom Soup

Fantastic World Foods ()
Baja Black Bean Chipotle Soup Cup
Blarney Stone Creamy Potato Simmer Soup
Buckaroo Bean Chili Soup Cup
Creamy Potato Leek Soup Cup
Great Lakes Cheddar Broccoli Soup Cup
Southwest Tortilla Bean Soup Cup
Split Pea Soup Cup
Summer Vegetable Rice Soup Cup

Gold's
Borscht
Hungarian Cabbage Borscht
Lo-Cal Borscht
Russian Borscht
Schav
Unsalted Borscht

HamBeens ()
15 Bean Soup - Original (Ensure packaged after 7/2006)
Beef 15 Bean Soup (Ensure packaged after 7/2006)
Cajun 15 Bean Soup (Ensure packaged after 7/2006)

Chicken 15 Bean Soup (Ensure packaged after 7/2006)
Chili 15 Bean Soup (Ensure packaged after 7/2006)
Confetti Lentil Soupreme
El Cantarito De Frijoles
Garlic & Herb Lentils
Great Northern
Great Northern Bean Soup
Navy Bean Soup
Spanish-American Black Bean Soup
Spanish-American Pinto Bean Soup

Hormel ()
Microwave Bean & Ham Soup

Hurst's Brand Soups ()
Black Bean Soup with Ham
Green Split Pea with Ham

Imagine
Crab Bisque
Creamy Broccoli Soup
Creamy Butternut Squash Soup
Creamy Chicken Soup
Creamy Portobello Mushroom Soup
Creamy Potato Leek Soup
Creamy Sweet Corn Soup
Creamy Tomato & Basil Soup
Creamy Tomato Soup
Lobster Bisque
Sweet Potato Soup

Laura Lynn (Ingle's)
Beefy Onion Soup Mix
Onion Soup Mix

Manischewitz
Borscht (All)
Chicken Rice Cup of Soup
Chicken Soup
Condensed Clear Chicken Soup
Hearty Bean Cello Soup Mix
Homestyle Mediterranean Black Bean Soup Mix
Schav
Soup Mix
Split Pea Homestyle Soup Mix
Split Pea Soup Mix with Seasoning Cello Soup Mix
Tomato Vegetable Homestyle Soup Mix
Vegetable Soup & Dip Mix

Mayacamas
Dark Mushroom Soup
French Onion Soup
Lentil Soup
Potato Leek Soup
Tomato Soup

Meijer
Chicken (Aseptic)
Soup Condensed Chicken with Rice
Soup Homestyle Chicken with Rice

Midwest Country Fare (Hy-Vee)
Onion Soup

Miso-Cup
Japanese Restaurant Style
Original Golden Vegetable
Reduced Sodium
Savory Seaweed
Traditional with Tofu

Nueva Cocina
Cuban Black Bean Soup
Cuban Black Bean Soup with Chipotles
Red Bean Soup

OrgraN
OrgraN (All)

Pacific Natural Foods
Creamy Roasted Carrot
Hearty Chicken Tortilla
Organic Creamy Butternut Squash
Organic Creamy Tomato
Organic French Onion
Roasted Red Pepper and Tomato

Publix
Broccoli and Cheddar Soup (Deli)
Chicken Tortilla Soup (Deli)
Organic Moroccan and Chick Pea Soup (Deli)
Organic Tomato and Rice Soup (Deli)
Potato Cheddar and Bacon Soup (Deli)
Spring Vegetable Soup (Deli)

Raley's
Homestyle Chicken and Wild Rice Soup
Homestyle Lentil Soup

Safeway
Chicken with Rice Soup
Condensed Homestyle Chicken with Wild Rice Soup
Onion Soup Mix

Select Brand (Safeway)
Autumn Harvest Butternut Squash Signature Soup
Baked Potato Signature Soup
Black Bean & Rice Soup Mix
Black Bean Soup Cups
Fiesta Chicken Tortilla Signature Soup
Potato Leek Soup Cups
Rosemary Chicken & White Bean Signature Soup
Split Pea Soup Cups
Tex Mex Soup Cups
Tortilla Con Queso Soup Mix

Shelton's
Black Bean & Chicken Soup
Chicken Corn Chowder
Chicken Rice Soup
Chicken Tortilla Soup

Simply Asia
Rice Noodle Soup Bowls - Garlic Sesame
Rice Noodle Soup Bowls - Sesame Chicken
Rice Noodle Soup Bowls - Spring Vegetable

Stop & Shop
Condensed Chicken with Rice Soup
Ready To Serve Chunky Vegetable Soup

Taste of Thai, A
Coconut Ginger Soup Base

Thai Kitchen
Coconut Ginger Soup (Can)
Hot & Sour Soup (Can)
Instant Rice Noodle Soup - Bangkok Curry
Instant Rice Noodle Soup - Garlic & Vegetable
Instant Rice Noodle Soup - Lemongrass & Chili
Instant Rice Noodle Soup - Spring Onion
Instant Rice Noodle Soup - Thai Ginger
Rice Noodle Soup Bowls - Lemongrass & Chili
Rice Noodle Soup Bowls - Mushroom

Rice Noodle Soup Bowls - Roasted Garlic
Rice Noodle Soup Bowls - Spring Onion
Rice Noodle Soup Bowls - Thai Ginger

Trader Joe's ()
Butternut Squash Soup (Deli)
Butternut Squash Soup - Regular
Butternut Squash Soup with Apple
Carrot Ginger Soup
Creamy Corn and Roasted Red Pepper Soup
Creamy Corn Chowder (Potbelly)
Creamy Vegetable Medley Bisque
Green Split Pea Soup (East Coast/ Midwest) (Deli)
India Sambhar Lentil Stew
Instant Rice Noodle Soup - Mushroom
Instant Rice Noodle Soup - Roasted Garlic
Instant Rice Noodle Soup - Spring Onion
Lemon Curry Chicken Soup (East Coast/Midwest) (Deli)
Lentil Soup with Vegetables (All)
Miso Soup
Organic Black Bean Soup
Organic Creamy Corn and Roasted Red Pepper Soup
Organic Creamy Tomato Soup
Organic Sweet Potato Bisque
Organic Tomato and Roasted Red Pepper Soup
Rich Onion Soup (Potbelly)
Spanish Lentils with Vegetables
Sweet Potato Bisque

Wolfgang Puck's
Chicken Tortilla
Hearty Lentil & Vegetables
Organic Black Bean
Organic Chicken with White & Wild Rice
Organic Creamy Butternut Squash
Organic French Onion
Organic Split Pea
Organic Thick Hearty Lentil & Vegetables

Organic Tortilla
Roast Chicken with Wild Rice
Roasted Chicken with Rice & Rosemary

STEWS

Dinty Moore ()
Beef Stew
Chicken Stew
Microwave Meals - Beef Stew

Trader Joe's ()
Premium Chicken Stew
Spanish Chicken Stew

TOMATO PASTE

Albertsons
Tomato Paste - Italian Style
Tomato Paste - Regular

Contadina ()
Tomatoes & Tomato Products (All BUT Contadina Tomato Paste with Italian Herbs)

Del Monte ()
Tomatoes & Tomato Products (All BUT Del Monte Spaghetti Sauce Flavored with Meat)

Giant
Tomato Paste

Hy-Vee
Tomato Paste

Meijer
Tomato Paste - Domestic
Tomato Paste - Organic

Nature's Promise (Stop & Shop)
Organic Tomato Paste

Publix ()
Tomato Paste

Raley's ()
Tomato Paste

S&W ()
Tomatoes & Tomato Products (All)

Safeway
Canned Tomato Products (All)

Stop & Shop
Tomato Paste

TOMATOES

Albertsons
Canned Tomatoes
Diced Tomatoes & Green Chilies
Tomato Sauce

Bionaturae
Canned Tomatoes
Tomatoes in Glass

Contadina ()
Tomatoes & Tomato Products (All BUT
Contadina Tomato Paste with Italian
Herbs)

Del Monte ()
Tomatoes & Tomato Products (All BUT
Del Monte Spaghetti Sauce Flavored
with Meat)

Eden Foods
Crushed Tomatoes
Crushed Tomatoes with Basil
Crushed Tomatoes with Onion & Garlic
Diced Tomatoes
Diced Tomatoes with Basil
Diced Tomatoes with Green Chilies
Diced Tomatoes with Roasted Onion &
Garlic
Whole Tomatoes - Peeled
Whole Tomatoes with Basil - Peeled

Furmano's
Furmano's (All)

Hy-Vee
Crushed Tomatoes
Diced Tomatoes
Diced Tomatoes - Chili Ready
Diced Tomatoes with Chilies
Diced Tomatoes with Garlic & Onion
Italian Style Diced Tomatoes
Italian Style Stewed Tomatoes
Italian Style Tomato Sauce
Mild Diced Tomatoes & Green Chilies
Original Diced Tomatoes & Green
Chilies
Petite Cut Diced Tomatoes
Petite Cut Diced Tomatoes with Garlic
& Olive Oil
Petite Cut Diced Tomatoes with Sweet
Onion

Petite Diced Tomatoes
Stewed Tomatoes
Tomato Sauce
Whole Peeled Tomatoes

Laura Lynn (Ingle's)
Tomato Products

L'Esprit de Campagne 🎖
Dried Tomatoes

Mediterranean Organics
Mediterranean Organics (All)

Meijer
Diced Tomatoes
Diced Tomatoes - Chili Ready
Diced Tomatoes - Organic
Diced Tomatoes in Italian
Diced Tomatoes in Juice
Stewed Tomatoes
Stewed Tomatoes - Italian
Stewed Tomatoes - Mexican
Tomato Puree
Tomato Sauce
Tomato Sauce - Organic
Tomatoes - Crushed in Puree
Tomatoes - Diced Green Chilies Orig
Tomatoes - Diced w/Green Chilies
Tomatoes - Petite Diced
Tomatoes - Whole Peeled
Tomatoes - Whole Peeled No Salt
Tomatoes - Whole Peeled Organic
Tomatoes w/Basil - Organic

Midwest Country Fare (Hy-Vee)
Tomato Sauce

Nature's Promise (Giant)
Organic Crushed Tomatoes with Basil
Organic Diced Tomatoes
Organic Tomato Paste
Organic Whole Peeled Tomatoes

Nature's Promise (Stop & Shop)
Organic Crushed Tomatoes with Basil
Organic Diced Tomatoes
Organic Tomato Sauce
Organic Whole Peeled Tomatoes

Publix ()
Tomato Sauce
Tomatoes - Crushed
Tomatoes - Diced with Green Chilies
Tomatoes - Diced with Roasted Garlic

& Onion
Tomatoes - Peeled Whole
Tomatoes - Sliced, Stewed

Raley's ()
Crushed Tomatoes in Tomato Juice
Diced Tomatoes - No Salt Added
Diced Tomatoes in Juice
Diced Tomatoes w/Green Chili Peppers
Italian Style Stewed Tomatoes
Mexican Style Tomatoes
Stewed Tomatoes
Tomato Sauce
Tomato Sauce - No Salt
Whole Peeled Tomatoes in Juice

S&W ()
Tomatoes & Tomato Products (All)

Saclà
Antipasto Clasico - Sun Dried Tomatoes

Safeway
Canned Tomato Products (All)

Stop & Shop
Crushed Tomatoes - Italian Seasoning
Crushed Tomatoes - No Added Salt
Crushed Tomatoes - Regular
Diced Tomato - Italian Seasonings
Diced Tomato - No Salt Added
Diced Tomato - Regular
Stewed Tomatoes - Italian Seasonings
Stewed Tomatoes - Mexican Style
Stewed Tomatoes - No Salt Added
Stewed Tomatoes - Regular
Tomato Puree
Tomato Sauce - Regular & No Added Salt
Whole Peeled Tomatoes - Regular & No Added Salt

Trader Joe's ()
Sun Dried Tomatoes (All)
Whole Peeled Pear Tomatoes with Basil (All)

VEGETABLES

Albertsons
Canned Broccoli
Canned Carrots
Canned Cauliflower

Canned Green Beans
Canned Peas
Canned Potatoes
Canned Spinach
Canned Squash
Canned Turnip Greens
Canned Vegetables
Domestic Mushrooms

Allens
Canned Items (All)

Alter Eco Fair Trade
Hearts of Palm (All)

Del Monte ()
Canned Vegetables (All)

Furmano's
Furmano's (All)

Giant
Beets - No Salt Added
Beets - Regular
Black Eyed Peas
Carrots
Corn - Cream Style
Corn - Mexican
Corn - No Added Salt
Corn - Whole Kernel
Cut Sweet Potatoes - Light Syrup
Cut Sweet Potatoes - Regular
Golden Cut Wax Beans
Green Beans - French
Spinach - No Salt Added
Spinach - Regular
Succotash
Sweet Peas
Whole Potatoes - No Salt Added
Whole Potatoes - Regular

Goya ()
Artichoke Hearts
Blue-Labeled Canned Peas
Canned Hominy

Grand Selections (Hy-Vee)
Crisp & Sweet Whole Kernel Corn
Fancy Cut Green Beans
Fancy Whole Green Beans
Young, Early June Premium Peas

Health Market (Hy-Vee)
Organic Cut Green Beans
Organic French Cut Green Beans

Organic Sweet Peas
Organic Whole Kernel Corn

Hy-Vee

Blue Lake Cut Green Beans
Blue Lake French Style Green Beans
Blue Lake Whole Green Beans
California Carrots
Cream Style Corn
Cut Green Beans
Diced Green Chilies
Fancy Diced Beets
Fancy Sliced Beets
Golden Hominy
Green Split Peas
Mushrooms - Stems & Pieces
Sliced Carrots
Sliced Hot Jalapenos
Sliced Mushrooms
Sliced Water Chestnuts
Sweet Peas
White Hominy
Whole Green Chilies
Whole Kernel Corn
Whole Kernel White Sweet Corn

Ingles Markets

Canned Spinach
Canned Turnip Greens
Canned Turnip Greens with Diced
   Turnips
Chopped Mustard Greens
Cream Style Corn
Cut Asparagus
Cut Beets
Cut Sweet Potatoes
French Style Green Beans
Gold 'N White Corn
Mixed Vegetables
No Salt - Cut Green Beans
No Salt - Mixed Vegetables
No Salt - Whole Kernel Corn
Pole Beans
Sliced Beets
Sliced Carrots
Sliced Potatoes
Sweet Peas
Tiny June Peas
Vacuum Packed Corn

Whole Baby Carrots
Whole Kernel Corn
Whole Potatoes

Kroger ()

Plain Canned Vegetables
Plain Instant Potatoes

Laura Lynn (Ingle's)

Cut Green Beans
Mushrooms (All)

Meijer

Asparagus Cuts & Tips
Beets - Harvard Sweet Sour
Beets - Sliced
Beets - Sliced, No Salt
Beets - Sliced, Pickled
Beets - Whole Medium
Beets - Whole Pickled
Carrots - Sliced
Carrots - Sliced, No Salt
Chilies - Diced Mild Mexican Style
Corn - Cream Style
Corn - Golden Sweet Organic
Corn - Whole Kernel Crisp & Sweet
Corn - Whole Kernel Golden
Corn - Whole Kernel Golden No Salt
Corn - Whole Kernel White
Green Beans - Cut
Green Beans - Cut Blue Lake
Green Beans - Cut No Salt
Green Beans - Cut Organic
Green Beans - Cut Veri Green
Green Beans - French Style
Green Beans - French Style Blue Lake
Green Beans - French Style No Salt
Green Beans - French Style Organic
Green Beans - French Style Veri Green
Green Beans - Whole
Hominy - White
Kale Greens (Chopped)
Lima Beans
Mixed Vegetables
Mushrooms - Sliced
Mushrooms - Stems & Pieces
Mushrooms - Stems & Pieces No Salt
Mushrooms - Whole
Mustard Greens (Chopped)
Peas & Sliced Carrots

Pimentos - Pieces
Pimentos - Sliced
Small Peas
Spinach
Spinach - Cut Leaf
Spinach - No Salt
Sweet Peas
Sweet Peas - No Salt
Sweet Peas - Organic
Sweet Potatoes Cut - Light Syrup
Turnip Greens, Chopped
Wax Beans Cut
White Potatoes - Sliced
White Potatoes - Whole

Midwest Country Fare (Hy-Vee)
Cream Style Corn
Cut Green Beans
French Style Green Beans
Mushrooms & Stems
No Salt Added Mushrooms & Stems
Sweet Peas
Whole Kernel Corn

Native Forest ⚇ ()
Artichoke Hearts - Marinated
Artichoke Hearts - Quartered
Artichoke Hearts - Whole
Green Asparagus Cuts & Tips
Green Asparagus Spears
Organic Hearts of Palm
White Asparagus Spears

Nature's Promise (Giant)
Organic Corn
Organic Cut Green Beans
Organic Sweet Peas

Nature's Promise (Stop & Shop)
Organic Corn
Organic Cut Green Beans
Organic Sweet Peas

Publix ()
Beets
Carrots
Corn - Cream Style Golden
Corn - Whole Kernel
Green Beans
Green Beans - Veggi-Green
Green Lima Beans
Mixed Vegetables

Potatoes - White
Sweet Peas
Sweet Peas - Small

Publix GreenWise Market ()
Green Beans - Organic Vegetables
Sweet Peas - Organic Vegetables
Whole Kernel Corn - Organic
Vegetables

Raley's ()
Mixed Vegetables
Peas and Diced Carrots
Quartered Artichoke Hearts
Sliced Potatoes
Sweet Peas
Whole Artichoke Hearts
Whole Potatoes

S&W ()
Canned Vegetables (All BUT S&W
Canned Dry Bean products)

Saclà
Antipasto Clasico - Artichokes

Safeway
Button Sliced Mushrooms
Cream Style Corn
Green Beans
Lima Beans
No Salt Whole Kernel Corn
White Hominy

Select Brand (Safeway)
Organic Peas

Stop & Shop
Beets - Sliced
Beets - Whole
Carrots
Cut Sweet Potatoes in Light Syrup
Golden Cut Wax Beans
Green Beans - French Style & No
Added Salt
Mexican Style Corn
Mixed Vegetables - Regular & No
Added Salt
Peas - No Salt Added
Peas and Carrots
Spinach - Regular & No Added Salt
Sweet Peas
Whole Kernel Corn
Whole Potatoes - Regular & No Added

Salt

Trader Joe's ()
Artichoke Hearts in Water
Dolmas in Olive Oil
Hearts of Palm (All)
Marinated Bean Salad
Marinated Mushrooms with Garlic
Steamed Beets (Deli)

Trappey
Okra

MISCELLANEOUS

Del Monte ()
Tomatoes & Tomato Products (All BUT
Del Monte Spaghetti Sauce Flavored
with Meat)

OrgraN
OrgraN (All)

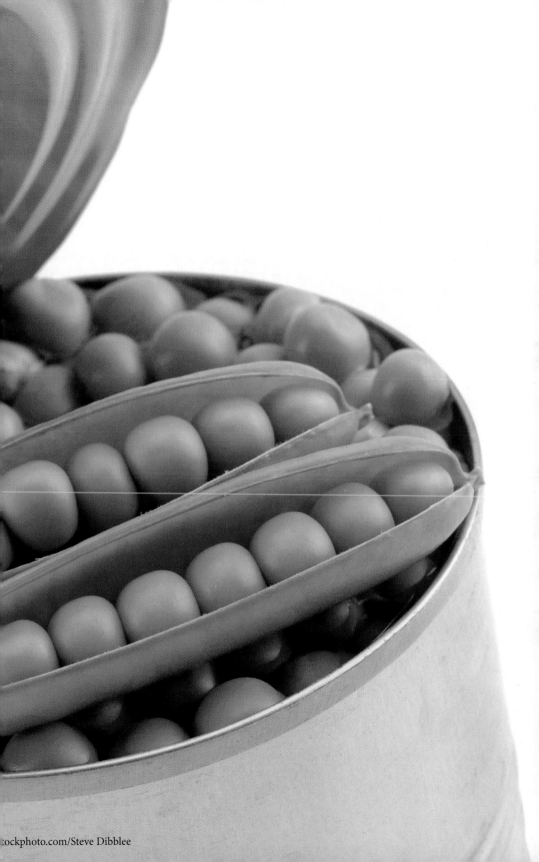

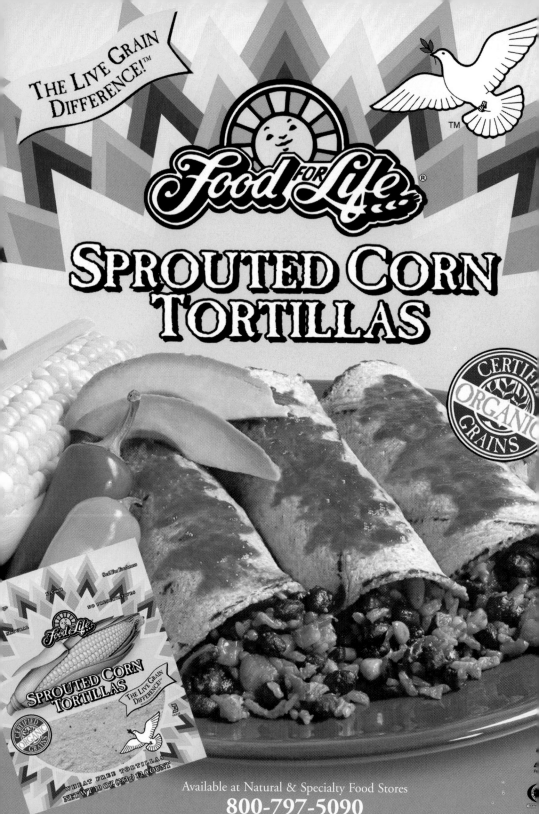

THE LIVE GRAIN DIFFERENCE!™

TM

Food for Life ®

SPROUTED CORN TORTILLAS

CERTIFIED ORGANIC GRAINS

Available at Natural & Specialty Food Stores

800-797-5090
www.foodforlife.com

Food For Life Baking Company, Inc. • 2991 E. Doherty St. • Corona, CA 92879

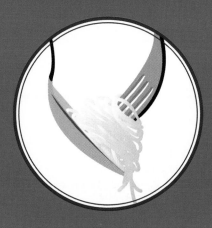

PACKAGED SIDES, MEALS & MEAL HELPERS

Meals & Meal Starters

Annie's Homegrown ()
Gluten-Free & Wheat-Free Rice Pasta
& Cheddar ☷

Del Monte ()
Harvest Selections Santa Fe Style Rice
& Beans

Dinty Moore ()
Microwave Meals - Rice with Chicken
Microwave Meals - Scalloped Potatoes
& Ham

Gluten-Free & Fabulous
Macaroni & Cheese

Hargis House (Save-A-Lot)
Tamales ()

Hormel ()
Beef Tamales
Compleats Microwave Meals - BBQ
Beef & Beans
Compleats Microwave Meals - Chicken
& Rice
Compleats Microwave Meals - Sweet &
Sour Rice

Ian's Natural Foods ☷ ☷ ()
Wheat Free Gluten Free Recipe Pasta
Dinner Kit
Wheat Free Gluten Free Recipe Pizza
Dinner Kit

Luzianne
Creole Dinner Kit
Jambalaya Dinner Kit

Mediterranean Organics
Mediterranean Organics (All)

Nu-World Amaranth
Amaranth Side Serve - Garlic Herb
Amaranth Side Serve - Savory Herb
Amaranth Side Serve - Spanish Tomato

Publix ()
Carrot Salad (Deli)
Chicken Salad (Deli)
Chicken Tarragon Salad (Deli)
Chunky Chicken Salad (Deli)
Cranberry Orange Relish Salad (Deli)
Egg Salad (Deli)
Garlic Redskin Smashed Potatoes (Deli)

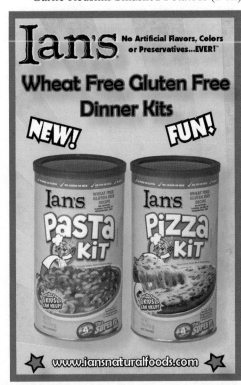

German Potato Salad (Deli)
Greek Potato Salad (Deli)
Ham Salad (Deli)
Homestyle Potato Salad (Deli)
Low Fat Potato Salad (Deli)
Marshmallow Delight Salad (Deli)
New York Style Potato Salad (Deli)
Santa Fe Turkey Salad (Deli)
Southern Style Potato Salad (Deli)

Road's End Organics ⚅ ()
GF Alfredo Chreese Mix
GF Cheddar Chreese Mix
Organic GF Alfredo Mac & Chreese
Organic GF Cheddar Penne & Chreese

Safeway
Classic Potato Salad (Deli Counter) ()
Deviled Egg Potato Salad (Deli
  Counter) ()
Mustard Potato Salad (Deli Counter) ()
Old Fashioned Potato Salad (Deli
  Counter) ()

Select Brand (Safeway)
Signature Broccoli Cheddar Au Gratin

Taste of India, A
Masala Rice & Lentils Quick Meal
Spiced Rice with Raisins Quick Meal

Taste of Thai, A
Red Curry Noodles Quick Meal
Spicy Peanut Bake

Tasty Bite
Agra Peas & Greens
Bengal Lentils
Jaipur Vegetables
Jodhpur Lentils
Kashmir Spinach
Kerala Vegetables
Madras Lentils
Massaman Vegetables
Paneer Makhani
Peas Paneer
Punjab Eggplant
Satay Vegetables
Spinach Dal
Spinach Soy

Thai Kitchen
Noodle Carts - Pad Thai

Noodle Carts - Roasted Garlic
Noodle Carts - Thai Peanut
Noodle Carts - Toasted Sesame
Stir-Fry Rice Noodle Meal Kit -
  Lemongrass & Chili
Stir-Fry Rice Noodle Meal Kit -
  Original Pad Thai
Stir-Fry Rice Noodle Meal Kit - Thai
  Peanut
Take-Out Boxes - Ginger & Sweet Chili
Take-Out Boxes - Original Pad Thai
Take-Out Boxes - Thai Basil & Chili

Trader Joe's ()
Baby Spinach Salad (Deli)
Blissful Bleu Cheese Potato Salad
  (Deli)
Chef Salad (Deli)
Chicken Caesar Salad - NO Croutons
  (Deli)
Chicken Curry Salad (Deli)
Chicken Salad
Chicken Salad with Currants and
  Almonds
Classic Greek Salad (Deli)
Cobb Salad (Deli)
Dolmas (Deli)
Egg White Salad (Deli)
Eggless Egg Salad (Deli)
Eggplant Caponata Appetizer
Garden Fresh Gazpacho (Refrigerated)
Garden Salad (Deli)
Gorgonzola Walnut Salad (Deli)
Greek Salad (Deli)
Grilled Chicken Salad with Orange
  Vinaigrette (Deli)
Indian Fare Meals (All)
Poppy Seed Slaw (Deli)
Pork Tamale with Salsa Colorado (Deli)
Steamed Lentils (Deli)

Ukrop's
Kitchen Entrees - Grilled Bistro
  Chicken Salad
Salads - Blackened Bistro Chicken
  Salad
Salads - Chunky Tuna Salad
Salads - Cranberry Orange Salad
Salads - Egg Salad

Salads - Gazpacho Salad
Salads - Ham Salad Deluxe
Salads - Light Redskin Potato Salad
Salads - Light Tuna Salad
Salads - Loaded Baked Potato Salad
Salads - Mandarin Orange Salad
Salads - Marinated Cucumber Salad
Salads - Marinated Red Beet Salad
Salads - Old Fashioned Potato Salad
Salads - Raspberry Crème Salad
Salads - Red White and Green Salad
Salads - Redskin Potato Salad
Salads - Sour Cream Potato Salad
Salads - Spring Mix Salad with Grilled Chicken
Salads - Spring Mix Salad with Grilled Salmon
Salads - Springtime Strawberry Salad
Salads - Strawberry Crème Salad
Salads - Summer Corn and Basil Salad
Salads - Tarragon Chicken Salad
Salads - Three Bean Salad
Salads - Tropical Lime Salad
Salads - Tuscan Vegetable and Bean Salad
Salads - Virginia Caviar Salad
Salads - Watergate Salad
Salads - White Chicken Salad

PASTA

Ancient Harvest
Ancient Harvest (All BUT Organic Wheat/Quinoa Spaghetti)
Andean Dream
Quinoa Pasta
Annie Chun's
Maifun Rice Noodles
Pad Thai Rice Noodles
Bionaturae
Gluten Free Pasta 🍴
Conte's Pasta ()
Gluten-Free Pasta
DeBoles
Corn Elbows
Corn Spaghetti
Rice Angel Hair

Rice Fettuccine
Rice Lasagna
Rice Penne
Rice Spaghetti
Rice Spirals
Dynasty
Maifun Rice Stick Noodles
Saifun Bean Thread Noodles
Eden Foods
Bifun (Rice) Pasta
Harusame (Mung Bean) Pasta
Kuzu Pasta
Ener-G
White Rice Lasagna
White Rice Macaroni
White Rice Small Shells
White Rice Spaghetti
White Rice Vermicelli
Gluten-Free & Fabulous
Bon Appetit! Quinoa with Marinara
Glutino 🍴
Brown Rice Fusilli
Brown Rice Macaroni
Brown Rice Penne
Brown Rice Spaghetti
Lundberg Family Farms
Penne
Rotini
Spaghetti
Manischewitz
Passover Noodles
OrgraN
OrgraN (All)
Seitenbacher
Gluten Free Golden Ribbon
Gluten Free Rigatoni
Taste of Thai, A
Thin Rice Noodles
Wide Rice Noodles
Thai Kitchen
Stir-Fry Rice Noodles
Thin Rice Noodles
Tinkyada Rice Pasta 🍴
Tinkyada Rice Pasta (All)
Trader Joe's ()
Organic Brown Rice Pasta (All)

ALWAYS READ LABELS

Rice Noodle
Rice Sticks Rice Pasta

PIZZA CRUST

Glutino 𝕏
Premium Pizza Crusts
Rustic Crust 𝕏
Napoli Herb Gluten-Free Pizza Crust

POLENTA

San Gennaro Foods
Basil Garlic Polenta
Sun Dried Tomato and Garlic Polenta
Traditional Polenta
Trader Joe's ()
Organic Polenta

POTATO, INSTANT & MIXES

Hy-Vee
Four Cheese Mashed Potatoes
Instant Mashed Potatoes
Roasted Garlic Mashed Potatoes
Sour Cream & Chive Mashed Potatoes
Idahoan ()
Au Gratin
Baby Reds
Baby Reds Garlic & Parmesan
Butter & Herb
Creamy Home Style
Four Cheese
Hash Browns
Naturally Au Gratin
Naturally Flakes
Naturally Garlic
Naturally Scalloped
Original Flakes
Real
Roasted Garlic
Scalloped
Southwest
Yukon Gold
Laura Lynn (Ingle's)
Herb & Garlic Mashed Potatoes
Mashed Potatoes

Roasted Garlic Mashed Potatoes
Sour Cream & Chives Mashed Potatoes
Manischewitz
Chicken Flavor Instant Mashed Potatoes
Homestyle Potato Latke Mix
Mini Potato Knish Mix
Potato Kugel Mix
Potato Pancake Mix
Sweet Potato Pancake Mix
Meijer
Potatoes - Hash Browns
Potatoes - Instant Mashed
O'Days (Save-A-Lot)
Mashed Potatoes
Safeway
Herb/Butter Instant Mashed Potatoes
Instant Potatoes
Roasted Garlic Instant Mashed Potatoes
Select Brand (Safeway)
Potato Cups - Buttermilk Ranch ()
Potato Cups - Roasted Garlic ()
Potato Cups - Sour Cream Chive ()
Potato Cups - Three Cheese Broccoli ()
Tasty Bite
Bombay Potatoes
Trader Joe's ()
Garlic Mashed Potatoes

RICE & RICE MIXES

Albertsons
Instant Brown Rice
Instant White Rice
Alter Eco Fair Trade
Rice (All)
Annie Chun's
Rice Express Sprouted Brown Rice
Rice Express Sticky White Rice
Arrowhead Mills
Brown Rice, Basmati
Brown Rice, Long Grain
Baji's Products
Jambalaya Rice Meal
Lemongrass & Basil Rice Meal
Lentil Rice Biryani Rice Meal
Nasi Goreng Rice Meal

Paella Rice Meal

Botan Calrose
Botan Calrose Rice

Dynasty
Jasmine Rice

Fantastic World Foods ()
Arborio Rice
Basmati Rice
Jasmine Rice

Giant
Rice - Brown
Rice - Instant White

GoGo Rice
Brown Rice
Harvest
Hawaiian
Jasmine Rice
Rice Medley
Sushi Rice
Thai Peanut
White Rice

Goya ()
Canilla Long Grain Rice
Medium Grain Rice

Hy-Vee
Boil-In-Bag Rice
Enriched Extra Long Grain Rice
Enriched Long Grain Instant Rice
Extra Long Grain Rice
Instant Brown Rice
Natural Long Grain Brown Rice
Spanish Rice

KONRIKO
Long Grain White Rice
Medium Grain White Rice
Original Brown Rice
Quick-Cook Brown Rice
Wild Pecan Rice

Laura Lynn (Ingle's)
Boil N' Bag Rice
Flavored Rice (All)
Instant Rice
Long Grain White Rice

Lotus Foods
Heirloom and Organic Rices (All)

Lundberg Family Farms
Rice (All Varieties)
RiceXpress - Chicken Herb
RiceXpress - Classic Beef
RiceXpress - Santa Fe Grill
Risotto - Butternut Squash
Risotto - Cheddar Broccoli
Risotto - Creamy Parmesan
Risotto - Garlic Primavera
Risotto - Italian Herb
Risotto - Organic Alfredo
Risotto - Organic Florentine
Risotto - Organic Porcini Mushroom
Risotto - Organic Tuscan

Manischewitz
Lentil Pilaf Mix
Spanish Pilaf Mix

Meijer
Rice - Brown
Rice - Long Grain
Rice - Medium Grain

Midwest Country Fare (Hy-Vee)
Pre-Cooked Instant Rice

Nishiki
Nishiki Rice

Nueva Cocina
Chicken Rice Mix
Mexican Rice Mix
Seafood Rice Mix

Publix ()
Long Grain Brown Rice
Long Grain Enriched Rice
Medium Grain White Rice
Precooked Instant Boil in Bag
Precooked Instant Brown Rice
Precooked Instant White Rice
Yellow Rice Mix

RiceSelect ()
Chef's Originals Smokey Cowboy
   Beans & Rice
Organic Garden Vegetable Rice Mix
Organic Roasted Chicken Herb Rice
   Mix
Organic Three Cheese Rice Mix
Organic Toasted Almond Pilaf
Organic Wild Mushroom & Herb Rice
   Mix

Sonoran Mexican Rice

Safeway
Instant Rice
Rice - Long Grain
Rice - White
Risotto - Cheese ()

Select Brand (Safeway)
Basmati Rice

Stop & Shop
Instant Brown Rice
Organic Long Grain Rice - Brown
Organic Long Grain Rice - White

Taste of Thai, A
Coconut Ginger Rice
Jasmine Rice

Tasty Bite
Beans Masala & Basmati Rice
Mexican Fiesta Pilaf
Peas Paneer & Basmati Rice
Pesto Pilaf
Spinach Dal & Basmati Rice
Sprouts Curry & Basmati Rice
Tandoori Pilaf
Vegetable Supreme & Basmati Rice

Thai Kitchen
Jasmine Rice Mixes - Green Chili & Garlic
Jasmine Rice Mixes - Jasmine Rice
Jasmine Rice Mixes - Lemongrass & Ginger
Jasmine Rice Mixes - Roasted Garlic & Chili
Jasmine Rice Mixes - Spicy Thai Chili
Jasmine Rice Mixes - Sweet Chili & Onion
Jasmine Rice Mixes - Thai Yellow Curry

Trader Joe's ()
Organic Brown Rice - Fully Cooked
Rice Pilaf
Riso Gallo Porcini Risotto
Spanish Style Rice
Sprouted Brown Rice - Fully Cooked
Thai Style Lime Pilaf

Ukrop's
Kitchen Entrees - Caribbean Rice and Beans

Side Dishes - Rice Pilaf

Uncle Ben's
Boil-In-Bag Rice
Fast & Natural Whole Grain Instant Brown Rice
Instant Rice
Original Converted Brand Rice
Ready Rice - Original Long Grain Rice
Ready Whole Grain Rice - Whole Grain Brown
Whole Grain Brown Rice

TACO SHELLS

Giant
Taco Shells

Hy-Vee
Taco Shells

Meijer
Taco Shells

Mission Foods 🍴
Taco Shells

Safeway
Jumbo Taco Shells
White Corn Taco Shells

Taco Bell 〰
Taco Shells
Home Originals - Nacho Taco Shells
Home Originals - Ranch Taco Shells

TORTILLAS & WRAPS

Food for Life 🍴 🍴
Organic Sprouted 100% Whole Kernel Flourless Corn Tortillas
Whole Grain Brown Rice Tortillas
Whole Grain Flourless Tortillas
Whole Kernel Flourless Corn Tortillas

Goya ()
3 Dozen Corn Tortillas

Hy-Vee
White Corn Tortilla

La Tortilla Factory
Smart & Delicious Gluten Free Dark Teff Wraps (All)
Smart & Delicious Gluten Free Ivory

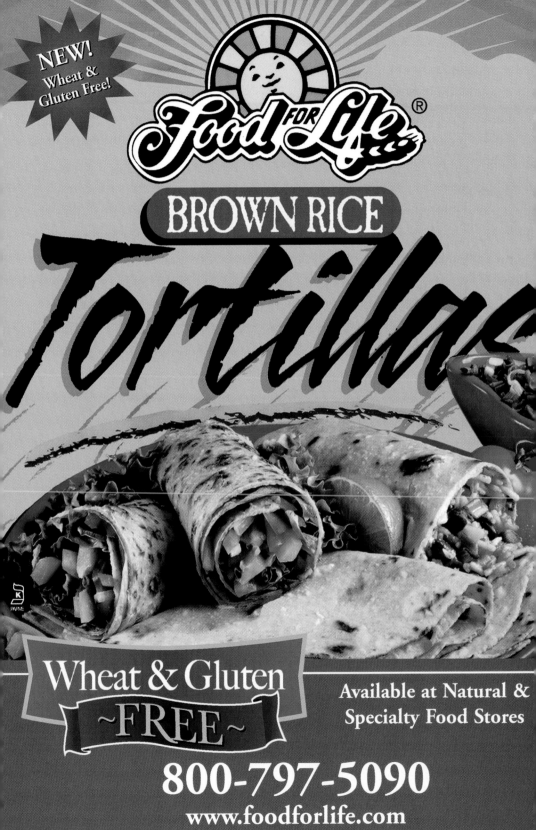

Teff Wraps
Sonoma All Natural Gluten Free Dark
Teff Wraps
Sonoma All Natural Gluten Free Ivory
Teff Wraps

Laura Lynn (Ingle's)
White Corn Tortilla

Manny's ()
Corn Tortillas

Mission Foods
Corn Gorditas
Corn Tortillas
Sopes
Tostadas

Trader Joe's ()
Corn Tortillas - Hand Made
Corn Tortillas - Original

MISCELLANEOUS

Ukrop's
Side Dishes - Bacon and Cheddar
Potato
Side Dishes - Balsamic Glazed Green
Beans
Side Dishes - Broccoli Florets
Side Dishes - Broccoli Slaw
Side Dishes - Cole Slaw
Side Dishes - Collard Greens
Side Dishes - Country Cole Slaw
Side Dishes - Garlic New Potatoes
Side Dishes - Green Beans and Carrots
Side Dishes - Green Beans with Butter
and Almonds
Side Dishes - Home Style Mashed
Potatoes
Side Dishes - Honey Baked Apples
Side Dishes - Marinated Grilled
Vegetables
Side Dishes - Old Fashioned Baked
Beans
Side Dishes - Oven Roasted Vegetables
Side Dishes - Rosemary Roasted
Potatoes
Side Dishes - Skillet Hash Brown
Potatoes
Side Dishes - Spinach Supreme

Side Dishes - Steamed Garden
Vegetables
Side Dishes - Sugar Snap Peas with Red
Peppers
Side Dishes - Whipped Redskin
Potatoes
Side Dishes - Yellow Squash with Sweet
Onions
Side Dishes - Zucchini with Yellow
Corn Medley

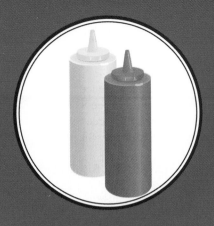

CONDIMENTS, SAUCES & DRESSINGS

Asian, Misc.

Bone Suckin' Sauce
Bone Suckin' Yaki

Dynasty
Chinese Style BBQ Sauce
Hoisin Sauce
Plum Sauce

Earth Family
Asian Sauce

Eden Foods
Mirin (Rice Cooking Wine)
Tekka (Miso Condiment)
Ume Plum Vinegar

Gold's
"Squeeze Me" Wasabi Sauce
Cantonese Style Sweet and Sour Duck
Sauce
Oriental Garlic Duck Sauce
Polynesian Duck Sauce
Szechuan Hot Duck Sauce

Jack Daniel's Sauces
EZ Marinader - Teriyaki Variety

Kraft
Sweet 'N Sour Sauce

Moore's
Moore's Teriyaki Marinade

Premier Japan
Organic Wheat-Free Hoisin
Organic Wheat-Free Teriyaki

Taste of Thai, A
Fish Sauce
Garlic Chili Pepper Sauce
Green Curry Paste

Panang Curry Paste
Peanut Satay Sauce
Peanut Sauce Mix
Red Curry Paste
Rice Noodles
Yellow Curry Paste
Yellow Curry Rice

Thai Kitchen
Fish Sauce
Green Curry Paste
Green Curry Simmer Sauce
Original Pad Thai Sauce
Panang Curry Simmer Sauce
Red Curry Paste
Red Curry Simmer Sauce
Yellow Curry Simmer Sauce

Trader Joe's
Sweet and Sour Sauce
Thai Curry Sauce - Red
Thai Curry Sauce - Yellow

Asian, Soy & Tamari Sauces

Eden Foods
Organic Tamari

Hy-Vee
Soy Sauce

Jade Dragon (Save-A-Lot)
Soy Sauce

Laura Lynn (Ingle's)
Soy Sauce (ONLY Red Label)

San-J
Organic Wheat Free Reduced Sodium
Tamari (Platinum Label)

Organic Wheat Free Tamari (Gold Label)

BARBEQUE SAUCE

Annie's Naturals ()
Annie's Organic Original BBQ Sauce
Organic Hot Chipotle BBQ Sauce
Organic Smokey Maple BBQ Sauce

Bone Suckin' Sauce
Bone Suckin' Sauce - Hiccuppin' Hot
Bone Suckin' Sauce - Hot
Bone Suckin' Sauce - Hot Thicker Style
Bone Suckin' Sauce - Regular
Bone Suckin' Sauce - Thicker Style

Cattlemen's Barbecue
Cattlemen's Barbecue Sauces (All BUT Honey Flavor and Southern Gold)

Fischer & Wieser
Elly May's Wild Mountain Honey BBQ Sauce
Plum Chipotle BBQ Sauce

Giant
BBQ Sauce - Hickory Smoke
BBQ Sauce - Honey
BBQ Sauce - Original

Gold's
Barbecue Sauce with Horseradish
New England Barbecue Sauce

Heinz ()
Chicken & Rib BBQ Sauce
Garlic BBQ Sauce
Honey Garlic BBQ Sauce
Original BBQ Sauce

Homestyle Meals
Original BBQ Sauce
Smoked Chipotle BBQ Sauce

Hy-Vee
Hickory BBQ Sauce
Honey Smoke BBQ Sauce
Original BBQ Sauce

Jack Daniel's Sauces ()
Hickory Brown Sugar BBQ Sauce
Honey Smokehouse BBQ Sauce
Original #7 BBQ Sauce
Spicy BBQ Sauce

Kraft Barbecue Sauce
Char-Grill Barbecue Sauce
Hickory Sauce Barbecue Sauce
Hickory Smoke Barbecue Sauce
Hickory Smoke Family Size Barbecue Sauce
Hickory Smoke Onion Bits Barbecue Sauce
Honey Barbecue Sauce
Honey Hickory Smoke Barbecue Sauce
Honey Mustard Barbecue Sauce
Honey Roasted Garlic Barbecue Sauce
Hot Barbecue Sauce
Light Original Barbecue Sauce
Mesquite Smoke Barbecue Sauce
Original Barbecue Sauce
Spicy Honey Barbecue Sauce
Sweet Recipes Honey Barbecue Sauce
Thick 'N Spicy Brown Sugar Barbecue Sauce
Thick 'N Spicy Brown Sugar Family Size Barbecue Sauce
Thick 'N Spicy Hickory Smoke Barbecue Sauce
Thick 'N Spicy Honey Barbecue Sauce
Thick 'N Spicy Original Barbecue Sauce

Midwest Country Fare (Hy-Vee)
Hickory BBQ Sauce
Honey BBQ Sauce
Original BBQ Sauce

Nathan's
Barbecue Sauce

Organicville
Organicville (All)

Publix ()
Hickory BBQ Sauce
Honey BBQ Sauce
Original BBQ Sauce

Select Brand (Safeway)
Hickory Smoked BBQ Sauce
Honey Mustard BBQ Sauce
Honey Smoked BBQ Sauce
Original BBQ Sauce

Stop & Shop
BBQ Sauce - Hickory Smoke
BBQ Sauce - Original

Sweet Baby Ray's ()
  Sweet Baby Rays Barbeque Sauce (All)
Trader Joe's ()
  BBQ Sauce
  BBQ Sauce - Kansas City
Ukrop's
  Dips/Spreads/Sauces - Honey BBQ
  Sauce
Walden Farms
  Walden Farms (All)

CHOCOLATE SYRUP

Albertsons
  Chocolate Syrup
Giant
  Chocolate Syrup
Hershey's
  Chocolate Syrup
Hy-Vee
  Chocolate Syrup
Manischewitz
  Chocolate Syrup
Meijer
  Syrup - Chocolate
Midwest Country Fare (Hy-Vee)
  Chocolate Flavored Syrup
Nesquik ()
  Syrup (All Flavors)
Publix ()
  Chocolate Syrup
Safeway
  Chocolate Syrup
Stop & Shop
  Chocolate Syrup
Trader Joe's ()
  Organic Chocolate Midnight Moo

CHUTNEYS

Native Forest () ()
  Organic Hot Mango Chutney
  Organic Mango Passion Chutney
  Organic Papaya Chutney
  Organic Pineapple Chutney

Trader Joe's ()
  Apple Cranberry Chutney
  Mango Ginger Chutney

COCKTAIL SAUCE

Cains
  Seafood Cocktail Sauce FS
Captains Choice (Safeway)
  Cocktail Sauce
Crosse & Blackwell
  Crosse & Blackwell (All BUT Branston
  Pickle Relish, Fish & Chip Vinegar,
  and Plum Pudding)
Del Monte ()
  Tomatoes & Tomato Products (All BUT
  Del Monte Spaghetti Sauce Flavored
  with Meat)
Giant
  Seafood Cocktail Sauce
Gold's
  Cocktail Sauce
Heinz ()
  Cocktail Sauce
Heluva Good
  Cocktail Sauce
Hy-Vee
  Cocktail Sauce For Seafood
Ken's Steak House ()
  Blue Label Cocktail Sauce
  Green Label Cocktail Sauce
Kraft
  Cocktail Sauce
  Hot & Spicy Cocktail Sauce
Safeway
  Cocktail Sauce
Stop & Shop
  Seafood Cocktail Sauce
Trader Joe's ()
  Seafood Cocktail Sauce
Ukrop's
  Dips/Spreads/Sauces - Cocktail Sauce

CROUTONS

Ener-G
Plain Croutons
Gluten-Free Pantry, The
Olive Oil & Garlic Croutons
Mariposa Baking Company 👤
Croutons

DESSERT SYRUPS, SAUCES & GLAZES

Eden Foods
Apple Cherry Sauce
Apple Cherry Sauce - Single Serve
Apple Cinnamon Sauce - Single Serve
Apple Strawberry Sauce
Apple Strawberry Sauce - Single Serve
Giant
Strawberry Syrup
Hy-Vee
Strawberry Syrup
Litehouse
Blueberry Glaze
Peach Glaze
Strawberry Glaze
Sugar Free Strawberry Glaze
Mrs. Richardson's Toppings
Mrs. Richardson's Toppings (All)
Robert Rothschild Farm
Butter Rum Dessert Sauce & Dip
Cherry Almond Gourmet Sauce
Cinnamon Bun Caramel Dessert Sauce
  & Dip
Old-Fashioned Caramel Sauce
Old-Fashioned Hot Fudge Sauce
Red Raspberry Gourmet Sauce
Santa Cruz Organic
Santa Cruz Organic (All)

DIP & DIP MIXES - SAVORY

EatSmart
Sweet Salsa Dip
Three Bean Dip
Emerald Valley Kitchen
Emerald Valley Kitchen (All)

Fantastic World Foods ()
Garlic Herb Dip
Onion & Mushroom Dip
Onion Soup & Dip
Vegetable Soup & Dip
Fritos ()
Bean Dip
Chili Cheese Dip
Hot Bean Dip
Jalapeno & Cheddar Flavored Cheese
  Dip
Mild Cheddar Flavor Cheese Dip
Giant
French Onion Dip
Ranch Dip
Refrigerated Veggie Dip
Salsa Dip
Guiltless Gourmet
Bean Dips (All) 👤
Heluva Good
Bacon Horseradish
Bodacious Onion
Buttermilk Ranch
Creamy Salsa
Dinosaur BBQ
French Onion
Jalapeno Cheddar
New England Clam
Ranch
Roasted Red Pepper
Herr's ()
Bean Dip
Jalapeno Cheddar Dip
Mild Cheddar Dip
Salsa and Cheese Dip
Hy-Vee
Bacon & Cheddar Sour Cream Dip
French Onion Sour Cream Dip
Ranch & Dill Sour Cream Dip
Salsa Sour Cream Dip
Toasted Onion Sour Cream Dip
Vegetable Party Sour Cream Dip
Kraft Dips 〰
Bacon & Cheddar
Creamy Ranch
Creamy Ranch 33% More

French Onion
French Onion 33% More
Green Onion
Guacamole Flavor

Laura Lynn (Ingle's)
Ranch Dip Mix
Refrigerated Dips (All Sizes)

Lay's ()
Creamy Ranch Dip
French Onion Dip
French Onion Flavored Dry Dip Mix
Green Onion Flavored Dry Dip Mix
Ranch Flavored Dry Dip Mix

Litehouse
Avocado Dip
Dilly Dip
Garden Ranch Dip
Lite Ranch Veggie Dip
Organic Ranch Dip
Ranch Dip
Ranch Veggie Dippers
Southwest Ranch Dip

Lucerne (Safeway)
Avocado Dip
Bacon Onion Dip
Clam Dip
French Onion Dip
Green Onion Dip
Guacamole Dip
Ranch Dip

Publix ()
French Onion Dip
Green Onion Dip
Guacamole Dip

Road's End Organics ⚗ ()
Mild Nacho Chreese Dip
Spicy Nacho Chreese Dip

Robert Rothschild Farm
Artichoke Dip
Blackberry Honey Mustard Pretzel Dip
Honey Chipotle Dip
Jalapeno Pepper Dip
Onion Blossom Horseradish Dip
Onion Dill Vegetable Dip
Raspberry Honey Mustard Pretzel Dip
Roasted Pineapple & Habanero Dip
Roasted Red Pepper and Onion Dip &

Relish
Sesame Honey Mustard Pretzel Dip
Southwest Dip
Sun-Dried Tomato Vegetable Dip
Sweet Heat Pretzel Dip
Toasted Garlic Horseradish Dip

Select Brand (Safeway)
Honey Mustard Gourmet Dipping Sauce

Simply Enjoy (Giant)
Smoked Salmon Dill Sandwich Spread

Stop & Shop
Refrigerated French Onion Dip
Refrigerated Ranch Dip
Refrigerated Veggie Dip

Tostitos ()
Creamy Southwestern Ranch Dip
Creamy Spinach Dip
Monterey Jack Queso
Reduced Fat Zesty Cheese Dip
Salsa Con Queso
Spicy Queso Supreme

Trader Joe's ()
Blue Cheese with Roasted Pecan Dip
    (Refrigerated)
Cilantro and Chive Yogurt Dip
    (Refrigerated)
Fat Free Spicy Black Bean Dip
Spinach Dip (Refrigerated)
Tuscan White Bean Dip (Refrigerated)

Ukrop's
Dips/Spreads/Sauces - Garlic Herb Dip
Dips/Spreads/Sauces - Honey Yogurt
    Poppy Seed Dip

Utz
Jalapeno/Cheddar Dip (Can)
Mild Cheddar Dip (Can)

Walden Farms
Walden Farms (All)

DIP & DIP MIXES - SWEET

Concord Foods
Chocolate Fudge Fruit Dips
Creamy Caramel Apple Dips
Fat Free Caramel Apple Dip
Organic Caramel Apple Dip

Litehouse
Chocolate Caramel
Chocolate Yogurt Fruit Dip
Low Fat Caramel Dip
Original Caramel
Strawberry Yogurt Fruit Dip
Strawberry Yogurt Fruit Dip - Single
    Serve
Vanilla Yogurt Fruit Dip - Single Serve
Robert Rothschild Farm
Chocolate Mint Dessert Sauce & Dip
Cinnamon Apple Caramel Fruit Dip
Raspberry Chocolate Pretzel Dip
Ukrop's
Dips/Spreads/Sauces - Fruit Dip

FRUIT BUTTERS & CURDS

Bramley's (Save-A-Lot)
Bramley's Apple Butter
Dickinson's
Dickinson's (All)
Eden Foods
Apple Butter
Apple Cherry Butter
Cherry Butter
Fischer & Wieser
Texas Pecan Apple Butter
Texas Pecan Peach Butter
Giant
Apple Butter
Knouse Foods
Apple Butter
Manischewitz
Apple Butter Spreads
Robert Rothschild Farm
Apricot Pumpkin Butter
Key Lime Curd Sauce
Lemon Curd
Pumpkin Curd
Santa Cruz Organic
Santa Cruz Organic (All)
Trader Joe's ()
Fruit Sauces (All)
Lemon Curd
Pumpkin Butter

GRAVY & GRAVY MIXES

Mayacamas
Brown Gravy
Chicken Gravy
Savory Herb Gravy
Turkey Gravy
OrgraN
OrgraN (All)
Pacific Natural Foods
Natural Beef Flavored
Natural Chicken
Natural Mushroom Gravy
Natural Turkey
Road's End Organics ()
Organic Golden Gravy Mix
Organic Savory Herb Gravy Mix
Organic Shiitake Gravy Mix

HORSERADISH

Boar's Head
Condiments (All)
Gold's
"Squeeze Me" Horseradish Sauce
Extra Hot Cream Style Horseradish
Red Horseradish
Sweet Horseradish
White Horseradish
Heinz ()
Horseradish Sauce
Heluva Good
Horseradish
Hy-Vee
Prepared Horseradish
Kaneku
Horseradish Powder
Kraft
Horseradish Sauce
Manischewitz
Horseradish (All)
Robert Rothschild Farm
Horseradish Sauce
Raspberry Cranberry Horseradish Sauce

HOT SAUCE

Bayou Heat (Save-A-Lot)
Bayou Heat Hot Sauce

Butcher's Cut (Safeway)
Jazz N Spicy Buffalo Wing Sauce

Cholula Hot Sauce
Cholula (All)

Emeril's
Kick It Up Green Pepper Sauce
Kick It Up Red Pepper Sauce
Wing Sauce

Fischer & Wieser
Mango Ginger Habanero Sauce
Original Roasted Raspberry Chipotle
Sauce, The
Papaya Lime Serrano Sauce
Pomegranate & Mango Chipotle Sauce

Frank's RedHot
Frank's Original RedHot Sauce
Frank's RedHot Buffalo Wing Sauce
Frank's RedHot Chile 'N Lime Hot
Sauce
Frank's Xtra RedHot Sauce

Giant
Chili Sauce
Hot Sauce

Heinz ()
Chili Sauce

Hy-Vee
Chili Sauce

Laura Lynn (Ingle's)
Chili Sauce

Meijer
Chili Sauce
Hot Dog Chili Sauce

Moore's 🦷 🦷
Moore's Buffalo Wing Sauce
Moore's Honey BBQ Wing Sauce

Nance's Mustards & Condiments
Chili Sauce
Wing Sauces

Robert Rothschild Farm
Hot Pepper Raspberry Chipotle Sauce

Stop & Shop
Chili Sauce

Tabasco 🦷
Tabasco Brand Chipotle Pepper Sauce
Tabasco Brand Garlic Basting Sauce
Tabasco Brand Garlic Pepper Sauce
Tabasco Brand Green Pepper Sauce
Tabasco Brand Habanero Pepper Sauce
Tabasco Brand New Orleans Style
Sauce
Tabasco Brand Pepper Sauce

Taco Bell 〰
Hot Sauce
Mild Hot Sauce

Taste of Thai, A
Sweet Red Chili Sauce

Texas Pete
Buffalo Chicken Wing Sauce
Hot Sauce
Pepper Sauce

Thai Kitchen
Roasted Red Chili Paste
Spicy Thai Chili Sauce
Sweet Red Chili Sauce

Trader Joe's ()
Sweet Chili Sauce (Refrigerated)

Trappey
Hot Sauces

TryMe
Cajun Sunshine
Tennessee Sunshine
TryMe Liquid Smoke
Yucatan Sunshine Habanero Sauce

Wingo (Save-A-Lot)
Wing Sauce

Wizard's, The 🦷 ()
Organic Hot Stuff

JAMS, JELLIES & PRESERVES

Albertsons
Jelly, Jams & Preserves

Bionaturae
Fruit Spreads

Bramley's (Save-A-Lot)
Bramley's Squeeze Jelly & Spread

Crofter's
Crofter's Food (All)

Crosse & Blackwell
Crosse & Blackwell (All BUT Branston Pickle Relish, Fish & Chip Vinegar, and Plum Pudding)

Dickinson's
Dickinson's (All)

Fischer & Wieser
Apricot Orange Marmalade
Cinnamon-Orange Tomato Preserves
Old Fashioned Peach Preserves
Rhubarb Strawberry Preserves
Texas Amaretto Peach Pecan Preserves
Texas Hot Red Jalapeno Jelly
Texas Jalapeach Preserves
Texas Mild Green Jalapeno Jelly
Whole Lemon Fig Marmalade

Four Monks
Jellies

Garner
Jams, Jellies & Preserves

Giant
Apple Jelly
Apricot Preserves
Apricot Spread
Blueberry Preserves
Cherry Preserves
Concord Grape Jelly
Currant Jelly
Grape Preserves
Mint Jelly
Orange Marmalade
Peach Preserves
Pineapple Preserves
Red Raspberry Preserves
Red Raspberry Spread
Seedless Blackberry Preserves
Squeezable Grape Jelly
Squeezable Strawberry Fruit Spread
Strawberry Jam
Strawberry Jelly
Strawberry Preserves
Strawberry Spread
Sugar Free Preserves - Apricot
Sugar Free Preserves - Blackberry
Sugar Free Preserves - Red Raspberry
Sugar Free Preserves - Strawberry

Goya ()
Fruit Preserves / Jelly

Hy-Vee
Apple Jelly
Apricot Preserves
Blackberry Jelly
Cherry Jelly
Cherry Preserves
Concord Grape Jelly
Concord Grape Preserves
Grape Jelly
Orange Marmalade
Peach Preserves
Plum Jelly
Red Raspberry Jelly
Red Raspberry Preserves
Strawberry Jelly
Strawberry Preserves

Ingles Markets
Apple Jelly
Apricot Preserves
Grape Jam
Grape Jelly
Orange Marmalade
Peach Preserves
Peanut Butter & Grape Jelly Spread
Peanut Butter & Strawberry Jelly Spread
Red Raspberry Preserves
Strawberry Preserves

Knouse Foods
Fruit Spread

Kroger ()
Jams
Jellies
Preserves

Mediterranean Organics
Mediterranean Organics (All)

Meijer
Apple Jelly
Fruit Spread - Apricot
Fruit Spread - Blackberry Seedless
Fruit Spread - Red Raspberry
Fruit Spread - Strawberry
Grape Jam
Grape Jelly
Preserves - Apricot

Preserves - Blackberry Seedless
Preserves - Marmalade Orange
Preserves - Peach
Preserves - Red Raspberry
Preserves - Red Raspberry w/Seeds
Preserves - Strawberry

Nature's Promise (Giant)

Organic Fruit Spread - Raspberry
Organic Fruit Spread - Strawberry
Organic Grape Jelly

Nature's Promise (Stop & Shop)

Organic Raspberry Fruit Spread
Organic Strawberry Fruit Spread

Polaner

All Fruit
Sugar Free Jams, Jellies & Preserves

Publix ()

Jams/Jellies/Preserves (All Flavors)

Robert Rothschild Farm

Caramelized Onion Balsamic Spread
Hot Pepper Berry Patch Preserves
Hot Pepper Peach Preserves
Hot Pepper Raspberry Preserves
Peach Pie Jam
Red Pepper Jelly
Red Raspberry Preserves
Seedless Raspberry Preserves
Strawberry Rhubarb Preserves
Triple Berry Preserves
Wild Maine Blueberry Preserves

Safeway

Jams
Jellies

Select Brand (Safeway)

Jams
Jellies

Simply Enjoy (Giant)

Balsamic Sweet Onion Preserves
Blueberry Preserves
Raspberry Champagne Peach Preserves
Red Pepper Jelly
Roasted Garlic and Onion Jam
Spiced Apple Preserves
Strawberry Preserves

Simply Enjoy (Stop & Shop)

Balsamic Sweet Onion Preserves
Blueberry Preserves

Raspberry Champagne Peach Preserves
Red Pepper Jelly
Roasted Garlic and Onion Jam
Spiced Apple Preserves
Strawberry Preserves

Smucker's

Jams, Jellies and Preserves (All)
Peanut Butter (All)

Stop & Shop

Apple Jelly
Apricot Preserves
Apricot Spread
Blueberry Spread
Concord Grape Jelly - Spreadable
Concord Grape Jelly - Squeezable
Currant Jelly
Grape Preserves
Mint Jelly
Orange Marmalade
Peach Preserves
Pineapple Preserves
Red Raspberry Preserves
Seedless Blackberry Preserves
Squeezable Grape Jelly
Strawberry Preserves
Strawberry Spread
Sugar Free Preserves - Apricot
Sugar Free Preserves - Blackberry
Sugar Free Preserves - Red Raspberry
Sugar Free Preserves - Strawberry

Trader Joe's ()

Jams, Jellies, and Preserves (All)

Walden Farms

Walden Farms (All)

Welch's

Welch's (All)

KETCHUP

Del Monte ()

Tomatoes & Tomato Products (All BUT Del Monte Spaghetti Sauce Flavored with Meat)

Gold's

Ketchup with Horseradish

Heinz ()

Easy Squeeze Ketchup

Hot & Spicy Kick'rs
Ketchup
No Sodium Added Ketchup
One Carb Ketchup
Organic Ketchup

Hy-Vee
Ketchup
Squeezable Thick & Rich Tomato
  Ketchup
Thick & Rich Tomato Ketchup

Manischewitz
Ketchup

Meijer
Ketchup
Ketchup Squeeze
Tomato Ketchup - Organic

Midwest Country Fare (Hy-Vee)
Ketchup

Organicville
Organicville (All)

Publix ()
Ketchup

Publix GreenWise Market ()
Organic Ketchup

Safeway
Ketchup

Streit's
Ketchup

Trader Joe's ()
Ketchup - Organic

Walden Farms
Walden Farms (All)

MARASCHINO CHERRIES

Hy-Vee
Green Maraschino Cherries
Red Maraschino Cherries
Red Maraschino Cherries with Stems

Meijer
Maraschino Cherry Red
Maraschino Cherry Red w/Stems

Midwest Country Fare (Hy-Vee)
Maraschino Cherries

Publix ()
Maraschino Cherries

Safeway
Maraschino Cherries

MARINADES & COOKING SAUCES

Annie's Naturals ()
Baja Lime Marinade
Roasted Garlic & Balsamic Marinade

Emeril's
Herbed Lemon Pepper Marinade
Hickory Maple Chipotle Marinade &
  Grilling Sauce
Lemon Rosemary & Gaaahlic Marinade
Orange Herb with Poppy Seed
  Marinade
Roasted Vegetable Marinade

Fischer & Wieser
Blueberry Chipotle Sauce
Charred Pineapple Bourbon Sauce
Granny's Peach 'n' Pepper Pourin'
  Sauce
Sweet & Savory Onion Glaze

Giant
Lemon Pepper Marinade

Gold's
Dip 'N Joy Saucy Chicken Sauce
Dip 'N Joy Saucy Rib Sauce

Goya ()
Mojo Chipotle
Mojo Criollo

Holland House
Cooking Wines (All)

Hy-Vee
Citrus Grill Marinade
Herb & Garlic Marinade
Lemon Pepper Marinade
Mesquite Marinade

Jack Daniel's Sauces ()
EZ Marinader - Garlic & Herb Variety

Mayacamas
Hollandaise Gourmet Sauce

Meijer
Marinade - Garlic & Herb
Marinade - Lemon Pepper
Marinade - Mesquite

Moore's

Moore's Original Marinade
Moore's Teriyaki Marinade

Newman's Own

Herb & Roasted Garlic Marinade
Lemon Pepper Marinade
Mesquite with Lime (Organic Line)

Olde Cape Cod

Cranberry Grilling Sauce
Honey Orange Grilling Sauce
Lemon Ginger Grilling Sauce
Sweet & Bold Grilling Sauce

Regina

Cooking Wines (All)

Robert Rothschild Farm

Anna Mae's Sweet Smoky Chipotle
Oven & Grill Sauce
Anna Mae's Sweet Smoky Oven & Grill
Sauce
Apricot Ginger Mustard
Apricot Mango Wasabi Sauce
Asian Sesame Oven & Grill Sauce
Blackberry Chipotle Oven & Grill

Sauce
Ginger Wasabi Sauce
Lemon Dill & Capers Sauce
Lemon Wasabi Sauce
Raspberry Pineapple Oven & Grill
Sauce

Santa Barbara Salsa

Pestos (All)

Select Brand (Safeway)

Cook'n Grill Plum Gourmet Dipping
Sauce

Trader Joe's

Balela (East Coast/Midwest)
(Refrigerated)
Cacciatore Simmer Sauce
Cuban Mojito Sauce
Curry Simmer Sauce
Korma Simmer Sauce
Mango Sauce
Masala Simmer Sauce
Piccata Simmer Sauce
Punjab Spinach Sauce
Spicy India Spread

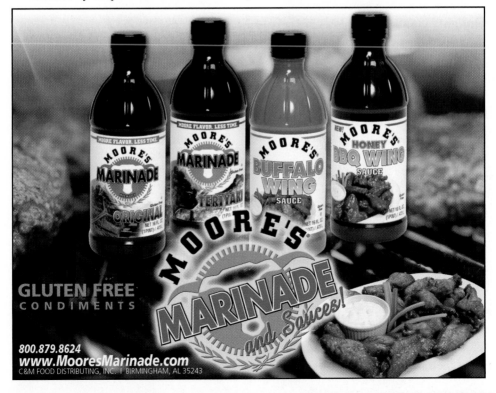

GLUTEN FREE
CONDIMENTS

800.879.8624
www.MooresMarinade.com
C&M FOOD DISTRIBUTING, INC. | BIRMINGHAM, AL 35243

ALWAYS READ LABELS

TryMe
- TryMe Tiger Sauce

Wild Thymes
- Wild Thymes (All BUT Toasted Sesame Wasabi Vinaigrette, Indonesian Peanut Sesame Dipping Sauce, Hawaiian Teriyaki Marinade and Korean Ginger Scallion Marinade.)

MAYONNAISE

Best Foods
- Best Foods (All)

Blue Plate
- Low Fat Mayonnaise
- Mayonnaise
- Sugar Free Mayonnaise

Boar's Head
- Condiments (All)

Cains
- All Natural Mayonnaise
- Fat Free Mayonnaise Dressing
- Light Reduced Calorie Mayonnaise
- Reduced Fat Mayonnaise Dressing

Enlighten (Safeway)
- Mayonnaise

French's
- GourMayo - Caesar Ranch
- GourMayo - Creamy Dijon
- GourMayo - Smoke Chipotle
- GourMayo - Sun Dried Tomato
- GourMayo - Wasabi Horseradish

Hellmann's
- Mayonnaise Products & Spreads (All)

Hy-Vee
- Mayonnaise
- Squeezable Mayonnaise

JFG Mayonnaise
- Mayonnaise
- Reduced Fat Mayonnaise
- Squeeze Mayonnaise

Kraft Mayonnaise ᘒ
- All-Out Squeeze! Light Mayo
- All-Out Squeeze! Real Mayo
- Fat Free Dressing Mayo
- Light Big Mouth Jar Mayo
- Light Mayonnaise
- Light Mayonnaise Big Mouth Jar
- Real Mayonnaise
- Real Mayonnaise Big Mouth Jar
- Real Mayonnaise Easy Squeeze
- Real Mayonnaise Hot 'N Spicy Super Easy Squeeze
- Real Mayonnaise Light Super Easy Squeeze
- Real Mayonnaise Super Easy Squeeze

Laura Lynn (Ingle's)
- Fat Free Mayonnaise
- Mayonnaise

Manischewitz
- Mayonnaise

Meijer
- Mayonnaise
- Mayonnaise Lite

Miracle Whip ᘒ
- All-Out Squeeze! Miracle Whip Dressing
- Dressing
- Easy Squeeze Dressing
- Free Nonfat Dressing
- Light Dressing
- Light Super Easy Squeeze Dressing
- Super Easy Squeeze Dressing

Portmann's (Save-A-Lot)
- Portmann's Mayonnaise

Publix ()
- Mayonnaise

Select Brand (Safeway)
- Mayonnaise - Fat Free, Reduced Fat, Regular & with Canola Oil

Streit's
- Mayonnaise

Trader Joe's ()
- Mayonnaise - Real
- Mayonnaise - Reduced Fat
- Mayonnaise Dressing - Eggless
- Wasabi Mayo

Vegenaise
- Expeller
- Grapeseed
- Organic
- Original

Walden Farms
Walden Farms (All)

MEXICAN, MISC.

Chi-Chi's ()
Taco Sauce

Del Pino's (Save-A-Lot)
Del Pino's Taco Sauce

Fischer & Wieser
Just Add Avocados Guacamole Starter

Hy-Vee
Medium Taco Sauce
Mild Enchilada Sauce
Mild Taco Sauce

Ingles Markets
Taco Sauce

Las Palmas
Crushed Tomatillos
Red Chile Sauce
Red Enchilada Sauce

Select Brand (Safeway)
Enchilada Sauce - Mild

Taco Bell
Medium Taco Sauce
Mild Taco Sauce

Trader Joe's ()
Guacamole (All Varieties; Refrigerated)

MUSTARD

Best Foods
Best Foods (All)

Boar's Head
Condiments (All)

Bone Suckin' Sauce
Bone Suckin' Mustard

Delouis Fils
Mustards

Eden Foods
Brown Mustard - Squeeze Bottle
Organic Brown Mustard
Organic Yellow Mustard
Organic Yellow Mustard - Squeeze
Bottle

Emeril's
Dijon Mustard
Kicked Up Horseradish Mustard
NY Deli Style Mustard
Smooth Honey Mustard

Fischer & Wieser
Honey Horseradish Mustard
Smokey Mesquite Mustard
Sweet, Sour & Smokey Mustard Sauce

French's
Honey Mustard
Prepared Mustards

Giant
Creamy Dijon Mustard
Dijon Mustard
Honey Mustard
Old Grainy Mustard
Raspberry Grainy Mustard
Tarragon Dijon Mustard
Yellow Mustard

Gold's
"Squeeze Me" Deli Mustard
"Squeeze Me" Dijon Mustard
"Squeeze Me" Honey Mustard
"Squeeze Me" Mustard w/Horseradish
"Squeeze Me" Mello Yellow Mustard
Dijon Mustard
Honey Mustard Sauce
Mustard with Horseradish

Grey Poupon
Country Dijon Mustard
Deli Mustard
Dijon Mustard
Harvest Coarse Ground Mustard
Hearty Spicy Brown Mustard
Honey Mustard
Savory Honey Mustard
Spicy Brown Mustard

Heinz ()
Mustard (All Varieties)

Hy-Vee
Dijon Mustard
Honey Mustard
Mustard
Spicy Brown Mustard

Laura Lynn (Ingle's)
Mustards

Meijer
- Mustard - Dijon Squeeze
- Mustard - Honey Squeeze
- Mustard - Horseradish Squeeze
- Mustard - Hot & Spicy
- Mustard - Salad
- Mustard - Salad Squeeze
- Mustard - Spicy Brown Squeeze

Midwest Country Fare (Hy-Vee)
- Mustard

Nathan's
- Original Coney Island Style Deli Mustard
- Original Coney Island Style Deli Mustard (Squeeze)

Olde Cape Cod
- Mustards

Publix ()
- Classic Yellow Mustard
- Deli Style Mustard
- Dijon Mustard
- Honey Mustard
- Spicy Brown Mustard

Raley's ()
- Deli Mustard with Horseradish
- Dijon Mustard
- Spicy Brown Mustard
- Yellow Mustard

Robert Rothschild Farm
- Anna Mae's Smoky Mustard
- Champagne Garlic Mustard
- Horseradish Mustard
- Raspberry Honey Mustard
- Raspberry Wasabi Mustard

Sabrett
- Mustard

Safeway
- Mustard (including Stone Ground Horseradish)

Select Brand (Safeway)
- Mustard - Classic/Country Dijon
- Mustard - Spicy Brown
- Mustard - Stone Ground Horseradish

Stop & Shop
- Creamy Dijon Mustard
- Deli Mustard

- Dijon Mustard
- Honey Mustard
- Old Grainy Mustard
- Raspberry Grainy Mustard
- Spicy Brown Mustard
- Tarragon Dijon Mustard
- Yellow Mustard

Texas Pete
- Honey Mustard Sauce (Ensure "Best By" 11/2006 and Later)

Trader Joe's ()
- Mustard - Dijon
- Mustard - Organic Yellow

NUT BUTTERS

Adams Peanut Butter
- Adams Peanut Butter (All)

Albertsons
- Peanut Butter

Arrowhead Mills
- Creamy Almond Butter
- Creamy Cashew Butter
- Creamy Peanut Butter
- Crunchy Almond Butter
- Crunchy Cashew Butter
- Crunchy Peanut Butter
- Honey Sweet Creamy Peanut Butter
- Honey Sweet Crunchy Peanut Butter
- Sesame Tahini

Giant
- Peanut Butter - All Natural
- Peanut Butter - Creamy
- Peanut Butter - Crunchy
- Peanut Butter - No Added Salt
- Peanut Butter - Reduced Fat
- Peanut Butter - Regular

Hy-Vee
- Creamy Peanut Butter
- Crunchy Peanut Butter
- Reduced Fat Peanut Butter

Jif
- Jif (All)

Kettle Brand
- Nut Butters (All)

Kroger ()
Creamy Peanut Butter
Crunchy Peanut Butter
Natural Creamy Peanut Butter
Natural Crunchy Peanut Butter
Reduced Fat Creamy Peanut Butter
Reduced Fat Crunchy Peanut Butter

Laura Scudder's Peanut Butter
Laura Scudder's Peanut Butter (All)

MaraNatha
Nut Butters (All)

Meijer
Peanut Butter - Creamy
Peanut Butter - Crunchy
Peanut Butter - Natural Creamy
Peanut Butter - Natural Crunchy

Midwest Country Fare (Hy-Vee)
Creamy Peanut Butter
Crunchy Peanut Butter

Nature's Promise (Giant)
Cashew Butter
Organic Almond Butter - Crunchy
Organic Almond Butter - Salted
Organic Almond Butter - Smooth
Organic Almond Butter - Unsalted
Organic Peanut Butter - Crunchy
Organic Peanut Butter - Salted
Organic Peanut Butter - Smooth
Organic Peanut Butter - Unsalted

Nature's Promise (Stop & Shop)
Cashew Butter
Organic Almond Butter - Smooth &
Unsalted
Organic Peanut Butter (All Varieties)

Panner (Save-A-Lot)
Panner Peanut Butter

Publix ()
Creamy Peanut Butter
Crunchy Peanut Butter
Old Fashioned Creamy Peanut Butter
Old Fashioned Crunchy Peanut Butter
Reduced Fat Spread Creamy Peanut
Butter
Reduced Fat Spread Crunchy Peanut
Butter

Safeway
Peanut Butter - Regular & Reduced Fat
Creamy and Crunchy

Santa Cruz Organic
Santa Cruz Organic (All)

Skippy
Skippy

Stop & Shop
All Natural Smooth Peanut Butter -
Regular, No Added Salt & Reduced
Fat
Peanut Butter - Crunchy, Creamy &
Smooth

Trader Joe's ()
Nut Butters (All)
Soybean Butter - Creamy
Soybean Butter - Crunchy
Sunflower Seed Butter

Walden Farms
Walden Farms (All)

OLIVES

Albertsons
Olives

B&G Foods
Black Olives
Green Olives

DeLallo
Jumbo Calamata Olives
Olive Medley
Olives Gigante
Organic Extra Large Pitted Calamata
Olives, Seasoned
Organic Olives Jubilee
Pitted Calamata Olives, Seasoned

Di Lusso ()
Green Ionian Olives
Mediterranean Mixed Olives

Giant
Queen Olives - Plain
Queen Olives - Stuffed
Stuffed Manzanilla Olives
Stuffed Queen Olives

Hy-Vee
Chopped Ripe Olives

Large Ripe Black Olives
Manzanilla Olives
Medium Ripe Black Olives
Queen Olives
Sliced Ripe Black Olives
Sliced Salad Olives

Ingles Markets
Olives - Green & Ripe (All)

Kroger ()
Black Olives - Not Stuffed
Green Olives - Not Stuffed
Green Olives - Pimento Stuffed

Mediterranean Organics
Mediterranean Organics (All)

Meijer
Olives - Manz Stuffed Placed
Olives - Manz Stuffed Thrown
Olives - Manz Stuffed Tree
Olives - Queen Stuffed Placed
Olives - Queen Whole Thrown
Olives - Ripe Large
Olives - Ripe Medium
Olives - Ripe Pitted (Jumbo)
Olives - Ripe Pitted (Small)
Olives - Ripe Sliced
Olives - Salad
Olives - Salad Sliced

Midwest Country Fare (Hy-Vee)
Large Ripe Black Olives
Sliced Ripe Black Olives

Peloponnese ()
Kalamata Olives

Publix ()
Colossal Olives
Green Olives (All Sizes & Styles)
Large Olives
Ripe Olives
Small Olives

Raley's ()
Colossal Ripe Pitted Olives
Pimiento Stuffed Manzanilla Olives
Pimiento Stuffed Queen Olives
Pitted Green Medium Olives
Pitted Wedge Olives
Ripe Jumbo Pitted Olives
Ripe Pitted Chopped Olives

Ripe Pitted Extra Large Olives
Ripe Pitted Large Olives
Ripe Pitted Medium Olives
Ripe Pitted Sliced Olives
Ripe Pitted Small Olives
Ripe Sliced Pitted Olives
Sliced Olives with Pimiento

Safeway
Black Olives
Manzanilla Olives

Stop & Shop
Manzanilla Olives - Stuffed & Sliced
Pitted Black Ripe Olives - Jumbo,
Large, Medium & Small (Chopped,
Whole & Sliced)
Stuffed Queen Olives

Trader Joe's ()
Colossal Olives Stuffed with Garlic
Cloves
Colossal Olives Stuffed with Jalapeno
Peppers
Mingling Olives
Mixed Olive Bruschetta
Pitted Kalamata Olives (Deli)
Pitted Moroccan Oil Cured Olives
Stuffed Queen Sevillano Olives

PASTA & PIZZA SAUCE

Amy's Kitchen
Organic Family Marinara Pasta Sauce
Organic Family Marinara Pasta Sauce -
Low Sodium
Organic Garlic Mushroom Pasta Sauce
Organic Roasted Garlic Pasta Sauce
Organic Tomato Basil Pasta Sauce
Organic Tomato Basil Pasta Sauce -
Light in Sodium
Puttanesca Sauce

Bove's of Vermont
Sauces

Classico ()
Alfredo Sauces (All Varieties)
Bruschetta (All Varieties)
Pesto Sauces (All Varieties)
Red Sauces   (All Varieties)

Contadina ()
Tomatoes & Tomato Products (All BUT Contadina Tomato Paste with Italian Herbs)

Cucina Antica
Tomato Sauces (All BUT La Vodka Sauce)

Del Monte ()
Tomatoes & Tomato Products (All BUT Del Monte Spaghetti Sauce Flavored with Meat)

Eden Foods
Pizza Pasta Sauce
Spaghetti Sauce
Spaghetti Sauce - No Salt Added

Emeril's
Home Style Marinara Pasta Sauce
Kicked Up Tomato Pasta Sauce
Mushroom & Onion Pasta Sauce
Puttanesca Pasta Sauce
Roasted Gaahlic Pasta Sauce
Roasted Red Pepper Pasta Sauce
Sicilian Gravy Pasta Sauce
Vodka Pasta Sauce

Francesco Rinaldi
Garden Style Sauces (All)
Hearty Sauces (All)
Organic Sauces (All)
Traditional Sauces (All)

Furmano's
Furmano's (All)

Health Market (Hy-Vee)
Tomato Basil Sauce

Hy-Vee
3 Cheese Spaghetti Sauce
Garden Spaghetti Sauce
Mushroom Spaghetti Sauce
Pizza Sauce
Spaghetti Sauce with Meat
Traditional Spaghetti Sauce

Manischewitz
Pasta Sauce (All)
Tomato & Mushroom Sauce

Mayacamas
Alfredo Pasta Sauce
Chicken Fettuccine Pasta Sauce

Cream Pesto Pasta Sauce
Creamy Clam Pasta Sauce
Peppered Lemon Pasta Sauce
Pesto Pasta Sauce

Meijer
Pasta Sauce - Four Cheese-Select
Pasta Sauce - Marinara-Select
Pasta Sauce - Mush & Olive-Select
Pasta Sauce - Onion & Garlic-Select
Pizza Sauce
Spaghetti Extra Chunk Garden Combo
Spaghetti Sauce Extra Chunk 3 Cheese
Spaghetti Sauce Extra Chunk Garlic & Cheese
Spaghetti Sauce Extra Chunk Mushroom/Green Pepper
Spaghetti Sauce Plain
Spaghetti Sauce w/Meat
Spaghetti Sauce w/Mushroom

Midwest Country Fare (Hy-Vee)
All Natural Garlic & Onion Spaghetti
Four Cheese Spaghetti Sauce
Garden Vegetable Spaghetti Sauce
Garlic & Herb Spaghetti Sauce
Meat Flavor Spaghetti Sauce
Mushroom Spaghetti Sauce
Traditional Spaghetti Sauce

Mom's
Artichoke Heart & Asiago Cheese Pasta Sauce
Garlic & Basil Spaghetti Sauce
Martini Pasta Sauce
Organic Roasted Pepper Pasta Sauce
Organic Traditional Pasta Sauce
Puttanesca
Special Marinara
Spicy Arrabbiata

Nature's Promise (Giant)
Organic Pasta Sauce - Garden Vegetable
Organic Pasta Sauce - Original
Organic Pasta Sauce - Parmesan

Nature's Promise (Stop & Shop)
Organic Pasta Sauce - Garden Vegetable
Organic Pasta Sauce - Parmesan
Organic Pasta Sauce - Plain

Newman's Own
Bombolina (Basil)

Cabernet Marinara
Diavolo (Spicy Simmer Sauce)
Five Cheese
Italian Sausage & Peppers
Marinara (Venetian)
Marinara with Mushrooms
Organic Marinara Sauce
Organic Tomato Basil Sauce
Organic Traditional Herb Sauce
Pesto & Tomato
Roasted Garlic & Peppers
Sockarooni - Mushrooms, Onions &
   Peppers
Sweet Onion & Roasted Garlic
Tomato & Roasted Garlic
Vodka Sauce

OrgraN
OrgraN (All)

Pastapali (Save-A-Lot)
Pastapali Pasta Sauces

Prego
Mushroom
Organic Sauces (All)
Three Cheese Sauce
Traditional Sauce

Robert Rothschild Farm
Artichoke Pasta Sauce
Roasted Portabella & Roma Tomato
   Pasta Sauce
Vodka Pasta Sauce

Saclà
Antipasto Clasico - Mixed Mushrooms
Classic Sauces - Arrabbiata
Classic Sauces - Marinara
Classic Sauces - Napoletana
Concentrated Pasta Sauces - Arrabbiata
Concentrated Pasta Sauces - Classic
   Basil Pesto
Concentrated Pasta Sauces - Olive &
   Tomato
Concentrated Pasta Sauces - Pepper &
   Eggplant
Concentrated Pasta Sauces - Sun-Dried
   Tomato & Garlic
Concentrated Pasta Sauces - Sun-Dried
   Tomato Pesto

Safeway
Meat Spaghetti Sauce
Mushroom Spaghetti Sauce
Traditional Spaghetti Sauce

Santa Barbara Salsa
Bruschetta (All)

Sauces 'n Love
Sauces 'n Love (All)

Select Brand (Safeway)
Classic Pesto Pasta Sauce (Refrigerated)
Creamy Parmesan Basil Pasta Sauce
   (Refrigerated)
Garden Vegetable & Herb Pasta Sauce
   (Refrigerated)
Light Alfredo Pasta Sauce
   (Refrigerated)
Mushroom/Onion Pasta Sauce
   (Refrigerated)
Pasta/Marinara Sauce (All VERDI BUT
   Vodka)
Pizza Sauce
Roasted Garlic & Mushroom Pasta
   Sauce (Refrigerated)

Simply Enjoy (Giant)
Fra Diavolo Sauce
Marinara Sauce
Roasted Garlic Sauce
Sicilian Eggplant Sauce
Tomato Basil Sauce
Vodka Sauce

Simply Enjoy (Stop & Shop)
Fra Diavolo Sauce
Marinara Sauce
Roasted Garlic Sauce
Sicilian Eggplant Sauce
Tomato Basil Sauce
Vodka Sauce

Trader Joe's ()
Aglio Olio Pesto Sauce
Bruschetta
Bruschetta (Refrigerated)
Creamy Prosciutto Pasta Sauce
Grilled Vegetable Bruschetta
Italian Sausage Pasta Sauce
Marinara Sauce
Organic Marinara Sauce
Organic Marinara Sauce - No Salt

Added
Organic Spaghetti Sauce
Organic Tomato Basil Marinara
Organic Vodka Sauce
Pesto Alla Genovese Basil Pesto
Pizza Sauce - Fat Free
Roasted Garlic Marinara
Rustico Pasta Sauce
Sun Dried Tomato Bruschetta
Three Cheese Pasta Sauce
Tomato Basil Marinara
Tomato Basil Pasta Sauce (Refrigerated)
Tuscan Marinara Sauce - Low Fat
Vodka Marinara

Ukrop's
Dips/Spreads/Sauces - Bruschetta
Dips/Spreads/Sauces - Marinara Sauce
Dips/Spreads/Sauces - Pizza Sauce

Walden Farms
Walden Farms (All)

PEPPERS

B&G Foods
Peppers

Di Lusso ()
Roasted Red Peppers

Goya ()
Red Pimientos

Heinz ()
Peppers (All Varieties)

Hy-Vee
Green Salad Pepperoncini
Hot Banana Peppers
Mild Banana Peppers

Mediterranean Organics
Mediterranean Organics (All)

Meijer
Hot Pepper Rings
Mild Pepper Rings
Pepper Ring - Banana Hot
Pepper Rings - Banana Mild
Pepperoncini

Mount Olive Pickle Company
Mt. Olive's Products (Ensure "Best If
Used by Date" of July 2008 or later

for: 12 oz Hot Dog Relish, 16 oz No
Sugar Added Sweet Gherkins & 16 oz
Sweet India Relish)

Peloponnese ()
Roasted Sweet Peppers

Saclà
Antipasto Clasico - Peperonata

Trader Joe's ()
Fire Roasted Red Peppers - Regular
Fire Roasted Red Peppers - Sweet &
Yellow
Marinated Red Peppers

Trappey
Peppers

Vlasic
Vlasic (All)

PICKLES

Albertsons
Pickles

B&G Foods
Pickles

Claussen Ꮧ
Bread 'N Butter Chips
Burger Slices - Pickles Kosher Dill
Deli Style Kosher Dill Halves
Deli Style Kosher Dill Spears
Hearty Garlic Deli Style Wholes
Sweet Gherkins

Easton (Save-A-Lot)
Easton Pickles

Gedney
Pickle Products (All)

Hans Jurgen
Pickles (All)

Heinz ()
Pickles (All Varieties)

Hermann Pickles
Hermann Pickles (All)

Hy-Vee
Bread & Butter Sandwich Slices
Bread & Butter Sweet Chunk Pickles
Bread & Butter Sweet Slices
Dill Kosher Sandwich Slices
Fresh Pack Kosher Baby Dills

Hamburger Dill Slices
Kosher Baby Dills
Kosher Cocktail Dills
Kosher Dill Pickles
Kosher Dill Spears
Polish Dill Pickles
Polish Dill Spears
Refrigerated Kosher Dill Halves
Refrigerated Kosher Dill Sandwich
  Slices
Refrigerated Kosher Dill Spears
Refrigerated Kosher Dill Whole Pickles
Special Recipe Baby Dills
Special Recipe Bread & Butter Slices
Special Recipe Hot & Spicy Zingers
Special Recipe Hot & Sweet Zinger
  Chunks
Special Recipe Jalapeno Baby Dills
Special Recipe Sweet Garden Crunch
Sweet Gherkins
Whole Dill Pickles
Whole Sweet Pickles
Zesty Kosher Dill Spears
Zesty Sweet Chunks

Ingles Markets
Pickles (All)

Meijer
Bread & Butter Chips - Sugar Free
Bread & Butter Chips, FP
Dill Spears - Zesty, FP
Halves - Kosher Dill (Refrigerated)
Kosher Baby Dills, FP
Kosher Dills, FP
Pickle - Bread & Butter Chips-FP
Pickle - Dill Hamburger Slices-PROC
Pickle - Dill Kosher Baby-FP
Pickle - Dill Kosher Spears-FP
Pickle - Dill Kosher Whole-FP
Pickle - Dill Kosher Whole-PROC
Pickle - Dill Polish Spears-FP
Pickle - Dill Polish-FP
Pickle - Dill Whole-FP
Pickle - No Garlic Dill Spears
Pickle - Sweet Gherkin Whole - PROC
Pickle - Sweet Midgets Whole-PROC
Pickle - Sweet Whole - PROC
Pickles - Whole - Refrigerated

Sandwich Slice - Bread & Butter
Sandwich Slice - Kosher Dill
Sandwich Slice - Kosher Dill Zesty
Slickles Sandwich Slice - Kosher Dill
Slickles Sandwich Slice - Polish Dill
Sweet Pickles - Sugar Free
Sweet Relish - Sugar Free
Wholes - Kosher Dill (Refrigerated)

Midwest Country Fare (Hy-Vee)
Dill Pickles
Hamburger Dill Pickle Slices
Kosher Dill Pickles
Whole Sweet Pickles

Mount Olive Pickle Company
Mt. Olive's Products (Ensure "Best If
  Used by Date" of July 2008 or later
  for: 12 oz Hot Dog Relish, 16 oz No
  Sugar Added Sweet Gherkins & 16 oz
  Sweet India Relish)

Publix ()
Pickles (All Varieties)

Raley's ()
Baby Whole Kosher Dill Pickles
Bread and Butter Pickles
Dill Pickles
Kosher Dill Spears
Kosher Whole Dill Pickles
Sandwich Slice Kosher Dills
Sandwich Slice Tangy Bread and Butter
Sweet Whole Pickles
Zesty Whole Dill Pickles

Safeway
Pickles (All)

Trader Joe's ()
Organic Kosher Sandwich Pickles
Organic Sweet Butter Pickles
Pickles (All; Deli)

Vlasic
Vlasic (All)

RELISH

Albertsons
Relish

B&G Foods
Relishes

Cains
Retail Relishes (All)

Claussen ✍
Sweet Squeeze Pickle Relish

Crosse & Blackwell
Crosse & Blackwell (All BUT Branston
Pickle Relish, Fish & Chip Vinegar,
and Plum Pudding)

Dickinson's
Dickinson's (All)

Giant
Relish - Dill
Relish - Sweet

Gold's
"Squeeze Me" Hot Dog Relish

Heinz ()
Relish (All Varieties)

Hy-Vee
Dill Relish
Squeeze Sweet Relish
Sweet Relish

Meijer
Relish - Dill
Relish - Sweet

Midwest Country Fare (Hy-Vee)
Sweet Pickle Relish

Mount Olive Pickle Company
Mt. Olive's Products (Ensure "Best If
Used by Date" of July 2008 or later
for: 12 oz Hot Dog Relish, 16 oz No
Sugar Added Sweet Gherkins & 16 oz
Sweet India Relish)

Nance's Mustards & Condiments
Corn Relish

Raley's ()
Tangy Sweet Relish

Trader Joe's ()
India Relish

Vlasic
Vlasic (All)

SALAD DRESSING & MIXES

Annie's Naturals ()
Artichoke Parmesan Dressing
Balsamic - Organic Dressing
Balsamic Vinaigrette Dressing
Buttermilk - Organic Dressing
Caesar - Organic Dressing
Cowgirl Ranch - Organic Dressing
Cowgirl Ranch Dressing
French - Organic Dressing
Green Garlic - Organic Dressing
Green Goddess - Organic Dressing
Lemon & Chive Dressing
Light Italian Dressing
Low Fat Honey Mustard Vinaigrette
Dressing
Low Fat Raspberry Vinaigrette Dressing
Mango Fat-Free Dressing
Maple Ginger Dressing - Organic
Dressing
Oil & Vinegar - Organic Dressing
Papaya Poppy Seed - Organic Dressing
Raspberry & Balsamic Fat Free
Dressing
Red Wine & Olive Oil - Organic
Dressing
Roasted Garlic - Organic Dressing
Roasted Red Pepper Vinaigrette
Dressing
Sesame Ginger with Chamomile -
Organic Dressing
Strawberry & Balsamic Fat-Free
Dressing
Tuscany Italian Dressing

Bolthouse Farms
Chunky Blue Cheese
Classic Ranch
Thousand Island

Brianna Fine Salad Dressings
Brianna's (All BUT Asiago Caesar,
Chipotle Cheddar, Ginger Mandarin,
Lemon Tarragon, Monterey Ranch &
Thousand Island)

Cains
Bell Pepper Italian (Pouch)
Caesar (Pouch)
Chipotle Ranch Dressing
Country Blue Cheese (Pouch)
Country Peppercorn & Parm (Pouch)
Country Thousand Island (Pouch)
County Ranch (Pouch)

Creamy French (Pouch)
Creamy Garlic Italian (Pouch)
Creamy Italian Dressing
Fat Free Italian Dressing
Fat Free Raspberry Vinaigrette Dressing
French Dressing
Golden Italian (Pouch)
Greek Deluxe (Pouch)
Italian Dressing
Italian Light Cains (Pouch)
Light Caesar (Pouch)
Light Caesar Dressing
Light French Dressing
Light Italian Dressing
Light Raspberry Vinaigrette Dressing
Lite Ranch Cains (Pouch)
Low Fat Caesar (Pouch)
Mayo Cains with EDTA (Pouch)
Peppercorn Dressing
Peppercorn Parmesan Dressing
Raspberry Vinaigrette (Pouch)
Robust Italian Dressing
White Balsamic & Honey Vinaigrette
   Dressing

Caroline's
Sweet Blue Onion
Sweet Celery Dressing
Sweet French Onion
Sweet Orange Dressing
Sweet Razzmataz

Drew's All Natural
Buttermilk Ranch
Garlic Italian
Honey Dijon
Kalamata Olive & Caper
Poppy Seed
Raspberry
Roasted Garlic & Peppercorn
Romano Caesar
Rosemary Balsamic
Smoked Tomato

Durkee
Buttermilk Ranch Dressing

Emeril's
Balsamic Vinaigrette
Blush Wine Vinaigrette
Caesar Dressing

Dijon Vinaigrette
Honey Mustard Dressing
House Herb Vinaigrette Dressing
Italian Vinaigrette
Kicked Up French Dressing
Raspberry Balsamic Vinaigrette

Enlighten (Safeway)
Balsamic & Red Wine Vinaigrette
Garden Italian Dressing
Honey Mustard Dressing
Roasted Sweet Pepper & Garlic
   Vinaigrette Dressing

Fischer & Wieser
Citrus, Herb & Truffle Oil Vinaigrette
Creamy Garlic & Chile Dressing
Original Roasted Raspberry Chipotle
   Vinaigrette
Southwestern Herb & Tomato
   Vinaigrette
Spicy Lime & Coriander Dressing
Sweet Corn & Shallot Dressing

Follow Your Heart
Caesar Dressing
Caesar with Parmesan Dressing
Creamy Garlic Dressing
Honey Mustard Dressing
Lemon Herb Dressing
Low Fat Ranch Dressing
Organic Balsamic Vinaigrette Dressing
Organic Chipotle Lime Ranch Dressing
Organic Chunky Bleu Cheese Dressing
Organic Creamy Caesar Dressing
Organic Creamy Miso Ginger Dressing
Organic Creamy Ranch Dressing
Organic Italian Vinaigrette Dressing
Sesame Dijon Dressing
Sesame Miso Dressing
Spicy Southwest Ranch Dressing
Thousand Island Dressing

Giant
Balsamic Vinaigrette
Blue Cheese
Caesar
French - Creamy
French - Regular
French - Spicy Sweet
Italian - Creamy

Italian - Fat Free
Italian - Lite
Italian - Regular
Ranch - Fat Free
Ranch - Lite
Ranch - Regular
Raspberry Vinaigrette - Reduced Fat
Raspberry Vinaigrette - Regular
Thousand Island

Good Seasons
Cheese Garlic Salad Dressing Mix
Classic Balsamic Vinaigrette with Extra
  Virgin Olive Dressing
Garlic & Herb Salad Dressing Mix
Italian Cruet Kit
Italian Salad Dressing Mix
Italian Vinaigrette with Extra Virgin
  Olive Oil Dressing
Light Greek Vinaigrette with Oregano
  & Athenos Feta Dressing
Light Honey Dijon with Grey Poupon
  Mustard Dressing
Mild Italian Salad Dressing Mix
Red Raspberry Vinaigrette with
  Poppyseed Dressing
Sun Dried Tomato Vinaigrette with
  Roasted Red Pepper Dressing
Zesty Italian Salad Dressing Mix

Health Market (Hy-Vee)
Organic Creamy Caesar Dressing
Organic Honey Mustard Dressing
Organic Raspberry Vinaigrette

Henri's
Salad Dressings (All)

Hy-Vee
Chunky Blue Cheese Salad Dressing
French Dressing
Italian Dressing
Light French Salad Dressing
Light Italian Dressing
Light Italian Salad Dressing
Light Ranch Dressing
Light Thousand Island Dressing
Lite Salad Dressing
Ranch Dressing
Salad Dressing
Squeezable Salad Dressing

Thousand Island Dressing
Zesty Italian Dressing

Ingles Markets
Spoonable Salad Dressing

JFG Mayonnaise
Salad Dressing

Ken's Steak House ()
3 Cheese Italian
Balsamic & Basil
Balsamic Vinaigrette Lite Accent
  Dressing
Buffalo Wing Sauce Marinade
Buttermilk Ranch
Caesar
Christos' Yasou Greek
Chunky Blue Cheese
Country French w/Vermont Honey
Creamy Caesar
Creamy French
Creamy Italian
Creamy Parmesan w/Cracked
  Peppercorn
Creamy Tomato Bacon
Fat Free Italian
Fat Free Raspberry Pecan
Fat Free Sun Dried Tomato
Greek
Herb & Garlic Marinade
Honey Mustard
Honey Mustard Vinaigrette Lite Accent
  Dressing
Italian
Italian Vinaigrette Lite Accent Dressing
Italian w/Aged Romano
Lite Balsamic & Basil
Lite Caesar
Lite Chunky Blue Cheese
Lite Country French w/Vermont Honey
Lite Creamy Caesar
Lite Creamy French
Lite Creamy Italian
Lite Creamy Parmesan w/Cracked
  Peppercorn
Lite Honey Mustard
Lite Italian
Lite Northern Italian
Lite Olive Oil Vinaigrette

Lite Ranch
Lite Raspberry Pomegranate
Lite Raspberry Walnut
Lite Red Wine Vinaigrette
Lite Russian
Lite Sun Dried Tomato Vinaigrette
Lite Sweet Vidalia Onion
New & Improved Ranch
Raspberry Walnut Vinaigrette Lite
   Accent Dressing
Red Wine Vinegar & Olive Oil
Russian
Sweet Vidalia Onion
Thousand Island
Zesty Italian

Kraft ⌒
Coleslaw Maker
Tuna Salad Maker Super Easy Squeeze

Kraft Salad Dressing ⌒
Creamy Italian
French Style Fat Free
Honey Dijon
Honey Dijon Fat Free
Italian Fat Free
Light Done - Right Creamy French
Light Done - Right Red Wine
   Vinaigrette
Ranch Garlic
Special Collection - Caesar Vinaigrette
   with Parmesan
Special Collection - Classic Italian
   Vinaigrette
Special Collection - Greek Vinaigrette
Special Collection - Parmesan Romano
Special Collection - Sun Dried Tomato
Special Collection - Sweet Honey
   Catalina
Special Collection - Tangy Tomato
   Bacon
Thousand Island with Bacon

La Martinique
Balsamic Vinaigrette
Blue Cheese Vinaigrette
Original Poppy Seed
True French Vinaigrette

Laura Lynn (Ingle's)
1000 Island Dressing

Buttermilk Dressing
California French Dressing
California Honey French Dressing
Chunky Blue Cheese Dressing
Creamy Cucumber Dressing
Creamy Italian Dressing
Fat Free Italian Dressing
Fat Free Ranch Dressing
French Dressing
Garlic Ranch Dressing
Italian Dressing
Lite Ranch Dressing
Peppercorn Ranch Dressing
Poppyseed Dressing
Ranch Dressing
Ranch Dressing Mix
Red Wine Vinegar & Oil Dressing
Salad Dressing
Zesty Italian

Lily's Gourmet Dressings ()
Balsamic Vinaigrette
Northern Italian
Poppyseed
Raspberry Walnut Vinaigrette

Litehouse
100 Calorie Reduced Sugar
Bacon Bleu Cheese
Balsamic Vinaigrette
Big Bleu
Bleu Cheese Crumbles
Bleu Cheese Vinaigrette
Caesar Dressing
Caesar Sensation
Chunky Bleu Cheese
Chunky Garlic Caesar
Classic Feta
Coleslaw
Creamy Garlic
Greek Feta
Harvest Cranberry Vinaigrette
Homestyle Ranch
Honey Mustard
Huckleberry Vinaigrette
Jalapeno Ranch Dressing
Lite 1000 Island
Lite Bleu Cheese
Lite Honey Dijon Vinaigrette

Lite Ranch
Organic Balsamic Vinaigrette
Organic Caesar
Organic Ranch
Organic Raspberry Lime Vinaigrette
Original Bleu Cheese
Pomegranate Blueberry Vinaigrette
Poppyseed
Poppyseed Dressing
Ranch
Raspberry Walnut Vinaigrette
Red Wine Olive Oil Vinaigrette
Rustic Ranch
Salsa Ranch
Spinach Salad
Thousand Island

Manischewitz
Fat Free Italian Dressing
Garlic Ranch Salad Dressing

Midwest Country Fare (Hy-Vee)
Ranch Dressing

Nature's Promise (Stop & Shop)
Ranch

Newman's Own
Balsamic Dressing Spray Mist
Balsamic Vinaigrette
Caesar
Creamy Caesar
Creamy Italian (Parmesanio Italiano)
Italian Dressing Spray Mist
Light Balsamic Vinaigrette
Light Caesar Dressing
Light Cranberry & Walnut
Light Honey Mustard
Light Italian
Light Lime Vinaigrette
Light Raspberry & Walnut
Light Red Wine & Vinegar
Light Sun Dried Tomato
Olive Oil & Vinegar
Organic Creamy Caesar Dressing
Organic Light Balsamic Vinaigrette
 Dressing
Organic Tuscan Italian Dressing
Parmesan & Roasted Garlic
Ranch Dressing
Red Wine & Vinegar

Southwest
Three Cheese Balsamic Vinaigrette
Two Thousand Island

Olde Cape Cod
Blue Cheese & Chive
Chipotle Ranch
Garlic & Herb
Honey Dijon
Lite Raspberry Vinaigrette
Lite Sweet & Sour Poppyseed
Sundried Tomato Lite

Organicville
Organicville (All)

Publix ()
Balsamic Vinaigrette
Caesar
California French
Chunky Blue Cheese
Creamy Parmesan
Fat Free Italian
Fat Free Thousand Island
Italian
Lite Caesar
Lite Honey Dijon
Lite Ranch
Lite Raspberry Walnut
Ranch
Thousand Island
Zesty Italian

Robert Rothschild Farm
Peanut Ginger Dressing and Marinade
Raspberry Dressing
Raspberry Wasabi Dressing

Safeway
Creamy Italian Dressing
Fat Free 1000 Island Dressing
Italian Dressing Mix
Light Ranch Dressing
Light Zesty Italian Salad Dressing
Ranch Dressing Mix
Ranch with Bacon Dressing
Regular 1000 Island Dressing
Regular Ranch Dressing
Regular Zesty Italian Dressing

Select Brand (Safeway)
Balsamic & Olive Oil Vinaigrette
Basil Ranch Salad Dressing

Blue Cheese Salad Dressing
Cranberry/Orange Salad Dressing
Creamy Goat Cheese/Dried Tomato
   Salad Dressing
Harvest Vegetable Salad Dressing
Italian Salad Dressing Mix
Ranch Salad Dressing
Raspberry Cranberry Vinaigrette
Raspberry Vinaigrette
Red Wine Balsamic
Roasted Red Pepper & Garlic
   Vinaigrette
Tuscan Basil Herb Salad Dressing

Seven Seas Salad Dressing ⌒
Green Goddess Dressing
Red Wine Vinaigrette Dressing
Viva Italian Dressing

South Beach Living ⌒
Balsamic with Extra Virgin Olive Oil
Italian with Extra Virgin Olive Oil
Ranch

Stop & Shop
Balsamic Vinaigrette
Blue Cheese
Caesar
French - Creamy
French - Regular
Italian - Creamy
Italian - Fat Free
Italian - Lite
Ranch - Fat Free
Ranch - Regular
Raspberry Vinaigrette
Thousand Island

Taste of Thai, A
Peanut Salad Dressing Mix

Trader Joe's ()
Balsamic Vinaigrette - Fat Free
Balsamic Vinaigrette - Organic
Balsamic Vinaigrette - Regular
Country Italian Style Dressing
   (Refrigerated)
Italian Vinaigrette Salad Dressing
   (Refrigerated)
Low Fat Parmesan Ranch Dressing
   (Refrigerated)
Organic Red Wine & Olive Oil

Vinaigrette (Refrigerated)
Organic Red Wine and Olive Oil
   Vinaigrette
Pear Champagne Vinaigrette
   (Refrigerated)
Raspberry Lowfat Salad Dressing
Romano Caesar Dressing
Tuscano Italian Dressing with Balsamic
   Vinegar

Walden Farms
Walden Farms (All)

Wild Thymes
Wild Thymes (All BUT Toasted Sesame
   Wasabi Vinaigrette, Indonesian Peanut
   Sesame Dipping Sauce, Hawaiian
   Teriyaki Marinade and Korean Ginger
   Scallion Marinade.)

SALSA

Albertsons
Salsa

Amy's Kitchen
Fire Roasted Vegetable Salsa
Organic Black Bean & Corn Salsa
Organic Medium Salsa
Organic Mild Salsa
Organic Spicy Chipotle Salsa

Bachman
Mild and Medium Salsa
Salsa Con Queso

Bone Suckin' Sauce ⎍
Bone Suckin' Salsa - Hot
Bone Suckin' Salsa - Regular

Drew's All Natural
Organic Black Bean, Cilantro & Corn
   Salsa
Organic Chipotle Lime Medium Salsa
Organic Double Fire Roasted Medium
   Salsa
Organic Hot Salsa
Organic Medium Salsa
Organic Mild Salsa

EatSmart
Fire Roasted Salsa
Salsa Con Queso

Emerald Valley Kitchen
Emerald Valley Kitchen (All)

Emeril's
Gaaahlic Lovers Medium Salsa
Kicked Up Chunky Hot Salsa
Original Recipe Medium Salsa
Southwest Style Medium Salsa

Fischer & Wieser
Das Peach Haus Peach Salsa
Salsa A La Charra
Salsa Verde Ranchera

Giant
Salsa - Hot
Salsa - Medium
Salsa - Mild

Gold's
Extra Chunky Salsa-Hot
Extra Chunky Salsa-Mild

Goya ()
Salsas - Pico De Gallo
Salsas - Taquera
Salsas - Verde

Grand Selections (Hy-Vee)
Medium Black Bean & Corn Salsa
Mild Black Bean & Corn Salsa

Green Mountain Gringo
Salsas

Guiltless Gourmet
Salsas (All)

Health Market (Hy-Vee)
Organic Medium Salsa
Organic Mild Salsa
Organic Pineapple Salsa

Herr's ()
Medium Chunky Salsa
Mild Chunky Salsa

Hy-Vee
Thick & Chunky Hot Salsa
Thick & Chunky Medium Salsa
Thick & Chunky Mild Salsa

Kroger ()
Thick & Chunky Salsa - Hot
Thick & Chunky Salsa - Medium
Thick & Chunky Salsa - Mild
Traditional Salsa - Hot
Traditional Salsa - Medium

Traditional Salsa - Mild

Laura Lynn (Ingle's)
Salsa (All)

Meijer
Salsa - Hot
Salsa - Medium
Salsa - Mild
Salsa - Restaurant Style Hot
Salsa - Restaurant Style Medium
Salsa - Restaurant Style Mild
Salsa - Santa Fe Style Medium
Salsa - Santa Fe Style Mild
Salsa - Santa Fe Style Mild
Salsa - Thick & Chunky Hot
Salsa - Thick & Chunky Medium
Salsa - Thick & Chunky Mild

Nathan's
Salsa - Hot
Salsa - Mild

Nature's Promise (Giant)
Chipotle Organic Salsa - Medium
Chipotle Organic Salsa - Mild

Nature's Promise (Stop & Shop)
Chipotle Organic Salsa
Organic Salsa - Medium
Organic Salsa - Mild

Newman's Own
Black Bean & Corn Salsa
Garden Salsa
Hot Salsa
Mango Salsa
Medium Salsa
Mild Salsa
Organic Chunky Medium Salsa
Organic Cilantro Medium Salsa
Peach Salsa
Pineapple Salsa
Roasted Garlic Salsa
Tequila Lime Salsa

Pace
Thick & Chunky Flavored Salsas (All)
Thick & Chunky Salsas (All)

Publix ()
All Natural - Hot Salsa
All Natural - Medium Salsa
All Natural - Mild Salsa
Southwestern Black Bean and Corn

Salsa
Thick & Chunky - Hot Salsa
Thick & Chunky - Medium Salsa
Thick & Chunky - Mild Salsa
Publix GreenWise Market ()
Organic Salsa - Medium
Organic Salsa - Mild
Robert Rothschild Farm
Cilantro Lime Salsa
Ginger Peach Salsa
Mango Salsa
Raspberry Chipotle Salsa
Raspberry Original Salsa
Safeway
Salsa Con Queso
Santa Barbara Salsa
Salsas (All)
Select Brand (Safeway)
Fiesta Fajita Salsa
Salsa (All Varieties)
Senora (Save-A-Lot)
Senora Verde Salsa
Simply Enjoy (Giant)
Black Bean and Corn Salsa
Peach Mango Salsa
Pineapple Chipotle Salsa
Tequila Lime Salsa
Simply Enjoy (Stop & Shop)
Black Bean and Corn Salsa
Peach Mango Salsa
Pineapple Chipotle Salsa
Tequila Lime Salsa
Stop & Shop
Salsa - Hot
Salsa - Medium
Salsa - Mild
Taco Bell
Home Originals - Medium Salsa Con
Queso
Home Originals - Mild Salsa Con
Queso
Thick 'N Chunky Medium Salsa
Thick 'N Chunky Mild Salsa
TGI Friday's (Heinz) ()
Salsa (All Varieties)

Timpone's Organic
Salsa Muy Rica
Tostitos ()
All Natural Hot Chunky Salsa
All Natural Hot Salsa
All Natural Medium Black Bean &
Corn Salsa
All Natural Medium Chunky Salsa
All Natural Medium Pineapple & Peach
Salsa
All Natural Medium Salsa
All Natural Mild Chunky Salsa
All Natural Mild Salsa
Restaurant Style Salsa
Trader Joe's ()
3 Pepper Salsa
Black Bean & Roasted Corn Salsa
Chunky Salsa
Corn and Chili Salsa
Double Roasted Salsa
Fire Roasted Tomato Salsa
Fresh Salsa (All Varieties; Refrigerated)
Hot and Smoky Chipotle Salsa
Pineapple Salsa
Salsa - Autentica
Salsa - Verde
Spicy, Smoky, Peach Salsa
Ukrop's
Dips/Spreads/Sauces - Pico De Gallo
Dips/Spreads/Sauces - Salsa
Dips/Spreads/Sauces - Tropical Salsa
Utz
Mt. Misery Mike's Salsa Jug
Sweet Salsa

SAUERKRAUT

B&G Foods
Sauerkraut
Claussen
Premium Crisp Sauerkraut
Eden Foods
Sauerkraut
Giant
Sauerkraut (Canned)

Hy-Vee
Shredded Kraut
Ingles Markets
Sauerkraut
Meijer
Sauerkraut
Sabrett
Sauerkraut
Safeway
Sauerkraut
Stop & Shop
Sauerkraut

SLOPPY JOE SAUCE

Heinz ()
Sloppy Joe Sauce
Hy-Vee
Sloppy Joe Sauce
Ingles Markets
Sloppy Joe Sauce
Meijer
Sloppy Joe Sauce
Safeway
Sloppy Joe

STEAK SAUCE

A.1. &
Bold & Spicy with Tabasco
Carb Well
New York Steakhouse
Roasted Garlic
Smoky Mesquite
Steak House Chicago
Steak House Cracked Peppercorn
Steak House New Orleans Cajun
Steak House Sweet Hickory with Bull's
Eye BBQ Sauce
Steak Sauce
Steakhouse Jamaican Jerk
Teriyaki
Thick & Hearty
Crosse & Blackwell
Crosse & Blackwell (All BUT Branston
Pickle Relish, Fish & Chip Vinegar,

and Plum Pudding)
Fischer & Wieser
Jethro's Heapin' Helping Steak Sauce
Steak & Grilling Sauce
Gold's
Steak Sauce w/Horseradish
Hargis House (Save-A-Lot)
Steak Sauce
Heinz ()
Traditional Steak Sauce
Hy-Vee
Classic Steak Sauce
Ingles Markets
Elmer Ingle 1922 Sauce
Steak Sauce
Steak Seasoning
Jack Daniel's Sauces ()
Steak Sauce - Both Varieties
Laura Lynn (Ingle's)
Steak Sauce
Lea & Perrins ()
Traditional Steak Sauce
Meijer
Steak Sauce
Nathan's
Steak Sauce
Select Brand (Safeway)
Steak Sauce
Tabasco 𝓤
Tabasco Brand Caribbean Style Steak
Sauce
TryMe
Bullfighter Steak & Burger Sauce

SYRUP, PANCAKE & MAPLE

Cary's
Syrups (All)
Eggo
Kellogg's Eggo Syrup
Grand Selections (Hy-Vee)
100% Pure Maple Syrup
Hungry Jack
Syrups (All)

Hy-Vee
Butter Flavor Syrup
Lite Syrup
Pancake & Waffle Syrup
Laura Lynn (Ingle's)
Butter Pancake & Waffle Syrup
Lite Pancake & Waffle Syrup
Pancake & Waffle Syrup
Log Cabin
Butter Flavored Syrup
Lite Syrup
Original Syrup
Sugar Free Syrup
Manischewitz
Pancake Syrup
Maple Ridge (Save-A-Lot)
Buttery Syrup
Meijer
Syrup - Lite Butter
Syrup Butter Flavored
Syrup Lite
Syrup Regular
Michele's
Michele's (All)
Midwest Country Fare (Hy-Vee)
Pancake & Waffle Syrup
Mrs. Butterworth's
Mrs. Butterworth's (All)
Publix ()
Butter Flavor Pancake Syrup
Lite Butter Flavor Pancake Syrup
Lite Maple Flavor Pancake Syrup
Maple Flavor Pancake Syrup
Raley's ()
100% Pure Maple Syrup - Dark Amber
Robert Rothschild Farm
Maple Praline Gourmet Syrup
Roasted Pecan Gourmet Syrup
Safeway
Syrup - Butter Light, Light, Old
Fashioned & Original and Pure Maple
Select Brand (Safeway)
Blueberry Syrup
Pure Maple Syrup
Trader Joe's ()
Maple Syrup (All)

Vermont Maid
Syrup - Sugar Free
Syrup - Sugar Free Butter
Walden Farms
Walden Farms (All)
Wholesome Sweeteners
Organic Pancake & Waffle Syrup

Tartar Sauce

Best Foods
Best Foods (All)
Cains
Tartar Sauce
Crosse & Blackwell
Crosse & Blackwell (All BUT Branston
Pickle Relish, Fish & Chip Vinegar,
and Plum Pudding)
Gold's
"Squeeze Me" Tartar Sauce
Kraft
Fat Free Tartar Sauce
Hot & Spicy Tartar Sauce
Lemon & Herb Tartar Sauce
Tartar Sauce
Laura Lynn (Ingle's)
Squeeze Tarter Sauce

Vinegar

Barengo
Balsamic Vinegar (All)
Bionaturae
Vinegar
Di Lusso ()
Red Wine Vinegar
Eden Foods
Organic Apple Cider Vinegar
Organic Brown Rice Vinegar
Red Wine Vinegar
Giant
Cider Vinegar
Red Wine Vinegar
White Distilled Vinegar
Goya ()
Cider Vinegar

Grand Selections (Hy-Vee)
Balsamic Vinegar of Modena
Red Wine Vinegar
White Wine Vinegar

Heinz ()
Apple Cider Flavored Vinegar
Apple Cider Vinegar
Distilled White Vinegar
Garlic Wine Vinegar
Red Wine Vinegar

Holland House
Premium Vinegars (All BUT malt
vinegar)

Hy-Vee
Apple Cider Flavored Distilled Vinegar
White Distilled Vinegar

Knouse Foods
Apple Cider Vinegar
White Distilled Vinegar

Lorenzi
Balsamic Vinegar

Manischewitz
Apple Cider Vinegar
White Vinegar

Marukan
Genuine Brewed Rice Vinegar
Seasoned Gourmet Rice Vinegar
Dressing

Meijer
Vinegar
Vinegar - Balsamic 12 Yr Aged
Vinegar - Balsamic 4 Yr Old Aged
Vinegar - Cider
Vinegar - Red Wine
Vinegar - White
Vinegar - White Wine

Nakano
Natural & Seasoned Rice Vinegars

Newman's Own Organics
Balsamic Vinegar

Publix ()
Red Wine Vinegar
White Distilled Vinegar

Rapunzel
Balsamic Vinegar ()
White Balsamic Vinegar ()

Regina
Vinegar (All)

Select Brand (Safeway)
Vinegar (All BUT Malt Vinegar)

Simply Enjoy (Giant)
Balsamic Vinegar of Modena
White Balsamic Vinegar

Simply Enjoy (Stop & Shop)
Balsamic Vinegar of Modena
White Balsamic Vinegar

Stop & Shop
Cider Vinegar
White Vinegar
Wine Vinegar

Trader Joe's ()
Orange Muscat Champagne Vinegar

Westcott (Save-A-Lot)
White Vinegar

WORCESTERSHIRE SAUCE

French's
Worcestershire Sauce

Hargis House (Save-A-Lot)
Worcestershire Sauce

Hy-Vee
Worcestershire Sauce

Laura Lynn (Ingle's)
Worcestershire Sauce

Lea & Perrins ()
Worcestershire Sauce

Meijer
Worcestershire Sauce

Safeway
Worcestershire Sauce

TryMe
Wine & Pepper Worcestershire

Wizard's, The 🍴 ()
Organic Wheat-Free Vegan
Worcestershire

MISCELLANEOUS

Best Foods
Best Foods (All)

Blue Plate
Sandwich Spread

Boar's Head
Condiments (All)

Chugwater Chili
Chugwater Chili (All)

Crosse & Blackwell
Crosse & Blackwell (All BUT Branston Pickle Relish, Fish & Chip Vinegar, and Plum Pudding)

Dickinson's
Dickinson's (All)

Goya ()
Achiotina (Annatto in Lard)

Hy-Vee
Sandwich Spread

JFG Mayonnaise
Sandwich Spread

Manischewitz
Tehina (Ready to Serve)

Mediterranean Organics
Mediterranean Organics (All)

Mount Olive Pickle Company
Mt. Olive's Products (Ensure "Best If Used by Date" of July 2008 or later for: 12 oz Hot Dog Relish, 16 oz No Sugar Added Sweet Gherkins & 16 oz Sweet India Relish)

Para MiCasa (Giant)
Minced Garlic in Water

Robert Rothschild Farm
Raspberry Seafood Sauce

Sabrett
Onions in Sauce

Select Brand (Safeway)
Capers

Simply Enjoy (Stop & Shop)
Smoked Salmon Dill Sandwich Spread

Texas Pete
Seafood Sauce

Trader Joe's ()
Artichoke Antipasto
Artichoke Red Pepper Tapenade
Eggplant Garlic Spread
Nonpareil Capers
Olive Green Tapenade

Red Pepper Spread with Garlic and Eggplant

TryMe
Oyster & Shrimp Sauce

Walden Farms
Walden Farms (All)

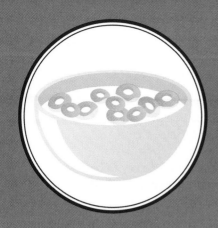

CEREAL & BREAD

BREAD

Ener-G

Broken Melba Toast
Brown Rice English Muffins with Sweet Potato
Brown Rice Hamburger Buns
Brown Rice Loaf
Corn Loaf
Egg Free Raisin Loaf
English Muffins
Four Flour Loaf
Hi Fiber Loaf
Light Brown Rice Loaf
Light Tapioca Loaf
Light White Rice Flax Loaf
Light White Rice Loaf
Papas Loaf
Raisin Loaf with Egg
Rice Starch Loaf
Seattle Brown Loaf
Seattle Hamburger Buns
Seattle Hot Dog Buns
Tapioca Dinner Rolls
Tapioca Hamburger Buns
Tapioca Hot Dog Buns
Tapioca Loaf (thin sliced)
White Rice Flax Loaf
White Rice Hamburger Buns
White Rice Loaf
Yeast Free Brown Rice Loaf
Yeast Free Sweet Loaf
Yeast Free White Rice Loaf

Enjoy Life Foods

Cinnamon Raisin Bagels
Classic Original Bagels

Food for Life

Fruit & Seed Medley Bread
Multi Grain Bread
Wheat & Gluten Free Raisin Pecan Bread
Wheat & Gluten Free Rice Almond Bread
Wheat & Gluten Free Rice Pecan Bread
Wheat & Gluten Free White Rice Bread
White Rice Bread
Whole Grain Bhutanese Red Rice Bread
Whole Grain Brown Rice Bread
Whole Grain Brown Rice Bread

Foods By George

English Muffins - Cinnamon Currant
English Muffins - No-Rye Rye
English Muffins - Plain

Glutino

Premium Baguettes
Premium Brown Rice Bread Homestyle
Premium Brown Rice With Inulin
Premium Cinnamon & Raisin Bread
Premium Corn Bread
Premium Fiber Bread
Premium Flax Seed Bread

Lydia's Organics

Lydia's Organics (All)

Mariposa Baking Company

Bagels

Trader Joe's

Gluten Free Bagels (Midwest)
Gluten Free French Rolls (East Coast/ Midwest)
Rye-Less "Rye" Bread (Midwest)

BREAKFAST CEREALS

Arrowhead Mills
  Maple Buckwheat Flakes
  Rice & Shine Cereal
  Sweetened Rice Flakes
Bamm-Bamm Berry Pebbles 🌀
  Bamm-Bamm Berry Pebbles
Cocoa Pebbles 🌀
  Cocoa Pebbles
Enjoy Life Foods ☒ ☒
  Cinnamon Crunch Granola
  Cranapple Crunch Granola
  Very Berry Crunch Granola
Envirokidz () ☒
  Amazon Frosted Flakes
  Gorilla Munch
  Koala Crisp
  Leapin Lemurs Peanut Butter &
    Chocolate Cereal
  Peanut Butter Panda Puffs
Erewhon
  Aztec Crunchy Corn & Amaranth
  Corn Flakes
  Crispy Brown Rice - Gluten Free
  Crispy Brown Rice with Mixed Berries
  Rice Twice
Fruity Pebbles 🌀
  Fruity Pebbles
Glutino ☒
  Cereal - Apple
  Cereal - Honey Nut
Lydia's Organics
  Lydia's Organics (All)
Malt-O-Meal ()
  Fruity Dyno-Bites
Nature's Path () ☒
  Crispy Rice
  Fruit Juice Cornflakes
  Honey'd Cornflakes
  Mesa Sunrise Flakes
New Morning
  Cocoa Crispy Rice
Newman's Own
  Sweet Enough Honey Nut O's

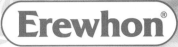

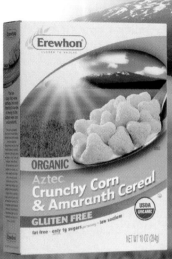

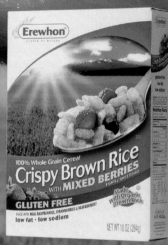

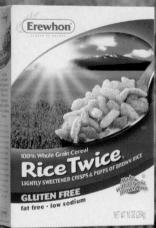

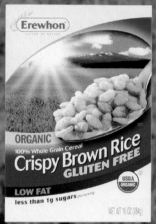

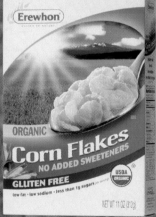

Eat our gluten-free cereal because you want to, not because you have to.

All of our cereals are made from the purest, finest, natural ingredients – organically grown whenever possible. Available wherever natural foods are sold. For nutritional information visit www.usmillsllc.com.

Nu-World Amaranth
Amaranth Berry Delicious Puffed
Cereal
Amaranth Cinnamon Delight Puffed
Cereal
Amaranth O's Original
Amaranth O's Peach
Amaranth Original Puffed Cereal
Amaranth Snaps - Cinnamon
Amaranth Snaps - Cocoa
Amaranth Snaps - Original

OrgraN
OrgraN (All)

Perky's 100% Natural
Nutty Flax
Nutty Rice
Perky O's - Apple Cinnamon
Perky O's - Frosted
Perky O's - Original

Rice Chex 🍴 🍴
Rice Chex (only newer formulations -
look for the phrase "Gluten-Free" on
the box OR check for a "better if used
by date" of 1/12/09 or later)

Safeway
Cocoa Astros Cereal ( )

Fruity Nuggets Cereal ( )

Puffed Corn Cereal ( )

Seitenbacher
Gluten-Free Muesli

Trader Joe's ( )
Golden Roasted Flaxseed with
Blueberries
Golden Roasted Whole Flaxseed

GRANOLA

Bakery on Main
Apple Raisin Walnut Gluten-Free
Granola
Cranberry Orange Cashew Gluten-Free
Granola
Extreme Fruit & Nut Gluten-Free
Granola
Nutty Cranberry Maple Gluten-Free
Granola

Rainforest Gluten-Free Granola

Trader Joe's ( )
Gluten Free Granola

HOT CEREALS

AltiPlano Gold 🍴
Instant Hot Cereals

Arrowhead Mills
Yellow Corn Grits

Bob's Red Mill 🍴
Brown Rice Farina
GF Mighty Tasty Hot Cereal
Organic Brown Rice Farina
Organic Creamy Buckwheat Cereal
Soy Grits

Cream of Rice
Cream of Rice Cereal

Erewhon
Brown Rice Cream

Lundberg Family Farms
Hot Cereal - Purely Organic

Meijer
Grits Buttered Flavored Instant
Grits Quick

OrgraN
OrgraN (All)

Trader Joe's ( )
Organic Southern Style Grits

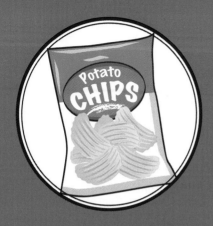

SNACKS & CONVENIENCE FOODS

APPLESAUCE

Albertsons
Applesauce

Applesnax
Applesnax Products (All)

Eden Foods
Apple Sauce
Apple Sauce - Single Serve

Giant
Applesauce - Chunky
Applesauce - Cinnamon
Applesauce - Mixed Berry
Applesauce - Natural
Applesauce - Strawberry

Hy-Vee
Applesauce
Cinnamon Applesauce
Natural Applesauce
Natural Style Applesauce

Knouse Foods
Apple-Cherry Sauce
Apple-Grape Sauce
Apple-Green Apple Sauce
Apple-Orange-Mango Sauce
Apple-Peach Sauce
Apple-Raspberry Sauce
Apple-Strawberry Sauce
Chunky Apple Sauce
Cinnamon Apple Sauce
Golden Delicious Apple Sauce
Granny Smith Apple Sauce
McIntosh Apple Sauce
Red Delicious Apple Sauce
Sweetened Apple Sauce

Unsweetened Apple Sauce

Kroger ()
Applesauce - Flavored
Applesauce - Plain

Meijer
Applesauce
Applesauce - Organic Cinnamon
Applesauce - Organic Sweetened
Applesauce - Original
Applesauce Chunky
Applesauce Cinnamon
Applesauce Cinnamon (Single Serve)
Applesauce Mixed Berry (Single Serve)
Applesauce Natural
Applesauce Natural (Single Serve)
Applesauce Organic Unsweetened
Applesauce Regular (Single Serve)
Applesauce Strawberry (Single Serve)

Midwest Country Fare (Hy-Vee)
Applesauce with Cinnamon
Applesauce with Peaches
Applesauce with Raspberries
Applesauce with Strawberries
Home Style Applesauce
Natural Applesauce

Mott's Applesauce
Mott's Applesauce (All)

Publix ()
Applesauce - Chunky
Applesauce - Cinnamon
Applesauce - Old Fashioned
Applesauce - Unsweetened

Safeway
Applesauce - Cups, Natural &
Sweetened

Stop & Shop
Applesauce - Chunky
Applesauce - Cinnamon
Applesauce - Mixed Berry
Applesauce - Natural
Applesauce - Regular
Applesauce - Strawberry

Tree Top
Apple Sauce

BAKED GOODS

Ener-G
Chocolate Iced Doughnuts (seasonal)
Cinnamon Rolls
Doughnut Holes (plain)
Doughnuts (plain)
Poundcake

Foods By George
Blueberry Muffins
Corn Muffins
Crumb Cake
Pound Cake

Mariposa Baking Company 😋
Coconut Lemon Squares
Sour Cream Coffeecake

Publix ()
New York Style Cheesecake, 6 Inch
Round (Plain)

Trader Joe's ()
Flourless Chocolate Cake

BARS

Arico Natural Foods Company
Cookie Bars (All)

Attune ()
Chocolate Probiotic Wellness Bar -
Chocolate Crisp
Chocolate Probiotic Wellness Bar -
Dark Chocolate
Chocolate Probiotic Wellness Bar -
Mint Chocolate
White Chocolate Probiotic Wellness Bar
- Blueberry Vanilla

Bakery on Main
Cranberry Maple Nut Gluten-Free
Granola Bar
Extreme Trail Mix Gluten-Free Granola
Bar
Peanut Butter Chocolate Chip Gluten-
Free Granola Bar

Betty Lou's
Organic Chocolate Tangerine Bar
Organic Krispy Bites
Organic Nutty Delight Bar

BoomiBar 😋
Almond Protein Plus
Apricot Cashew
Cashew Almond
Cashew Protein Plus
Cranberry Apple
Fruit and Nut
Healthy Hazel
Macadamia Paradise
Maple Pecan
Perfect Pumpkin
Pineapple Ginger
Pistachio Pineapple
Walnut Date

BumbleBar 😋
BumbleBar (All)

EAS
AdvantEdge Carb Control Bars -
Blueberry
AdvantEdge Carb Control Bars -
Chocolate Cream Pie
AdvantEdge Carb Control Bars - Peanut
Butter
AdvantEdge Carb Control RTD -
Chocolate Fudge
AdvantEdge Carb Control RTD -
Coffeehouse Café Caramel
AdvantEdge Carb Control RTD - Rich
Dark Chocolate
AdvantEdge Carb Control RTD -
Strawberry Cream
AdvantEdge Carb Control RTD -
Vanilla Cream
AdvantEdge Complete Nutrition Bar -
Chocolate Carmel
AdvantEdge Complete Nutrition Bar -

Double Chocolate
AdvantEdge Complete Nutrition Bar - Peanut Carmel
AdvantEdge Complete Nutrition RTD - Chocolate Fudge
AdvantEdge Complete Nutrition RTD - French Vanilla
Myoplex "Mass" Bar - Chocolate Chunk
Myoplex Carb Control Bar - Chocolate Chip Brownie
Myoplex Carb Control Bar - Peanut Butter

Ener-G
Chocolate Chip Snack Bars

Enjoy Life Foods
Caramel Apple Snack Bars
Cocoa Loco Snack Bars
Sunbutter Crunch Snack Bars
Very Berry Snack Bars

Envirokidz
Crispy Rice Bars - Berry
Crispy Rice Bars - Chocolate
Crispy Rice Bars - Peanut Butter

Frankly Natural Bakers
Gluten-Free Apricot Energy Bar
Gluten-Free Date Nut Energy Bar
Gluten-Free Raisin Energy Bar
Gluten-Free Tropical Energy Bar

Gertrude & Bronner's Magic ALPSNACK
Alpsnack (All)

Glucerna
Caramel Nut Glucerna Snack Bar ()

Glutino
Breakfast Bars Apple
Breakfast Bars Blueberry
Breakfast Bars Chocolate
Breakfast Bars Cranberry
Organic Bar - Choco & Peanut Butter
Organic Bar - Chocolate-Banana
Organic Bar - Wildberry

Gomacro
Gluten-Free Cashew Butter Bar
Gluten-Free Peanut Protein Bar
Gluten-Free Tahini Date Bar

Jŏcalat
Lärabar Jŏcalat (All)

Lärabar
Lärabar (All)

Lydia's Organics
Lydia's Organics (All)

Manischewitz
Raspberry Jell Bars

Meijer
Xtreme Snack Bars

Nutiva
Nutiva (All)

Omega Smart Bar
Omega Smart Bar (All)

Organic Food Bar
Organic Food Bar (All BUT Cherry Pie and Apple Pie)

OrgraN
OrgraN (All)

Planters
Original Peanut Bar

Planters Carb Well
Caramel Chocolate Crunch Crunchy Nut Bar
Peanut Butter Crunch Crunchy Nut Bar

PranaBar
Organic Apricot Goji
Organic Apricot Pumpkin
Organic Cashew Almond
Organic Cinnamon Apple
Organic Coconut Acai
Organic Pear Ginseng

Publix ()
Peanut Butter Bars

PureFit
PureFit (All)

Raw Revolution
Raw Revolution Bars (All)

Seitenbacher
Banana Cranberry Bar
Choco Apricot Bar
Energy Bar
Fitness Bar
Natural Cereal Bar
Natural Energizer Bar
Natural Sports Bar

Xtra Fiber Bar

South Beach Living 🖉
Caramel Peanut Crisp (Meal Replacement Bar)
Chocolate Caramel (Meal Replacement Bar)
Chocolate Crisp (Meal Replacement Bar)
Chocolate High Protein Cereal Bar
Chocolate Peanut Butter (Meal Replacement Bar)
Chocolate Raspberry Snack Bars
Cinnamon & Crème (Meal Replacement Bar)
Cinnamon Crème (Meal Replacement Bar)
Cinnamon Raisin High Protein Cereal Bar
Peanut Butter Snack Bars
Vanilla Crème (Meal Replacement Bar)

SoyJoy ()
SoyJoy Bars

thinkProducts 🏅
thinkProducts (All)

Trader Joe's ()
Fiberful Fruit Bar

ZonePerfect ()
Banana Nut Bar
Blueberry Bar
Chocolate Almond Raisin Bar
Chocolate Caramel Cluster Bar
Chocolate Coconut Crunch Bar
Chocolate Peanut Butter Bar
Chocolate Raspberry Bar
Double Dark Chocolate Bar
Fudge Graham Bar
Orange Cranberry Bar
Peanut Toffee Bar

BEEF JERKY & OTHER MEAT SNACKS

Hy-Vee
Original Beef Jerky
Lowrey's
Spicy Sticks

Oberto
Natural Style Beef Jerky - Hickory
Natural Style Beef Jerky - Jamaica Me
Natural Style Beef Jerky - Original
Natural Style Beef Jerky - Peppered
Smoked Beef Sticks

Old Wisconsin 🏅 ()
Gravity Feed
Snack Bites - Beef
Snack Bites - Pepperoni
Snack Bites - Turkey
Snack Sticks - Beef
Snack Sticks - Pepperoni
Snack Sticks - Spicy Beef
Snack Sticks - Turkey
Snacker Stackers - Beef
Snacker Stackers - Pepperoni

Rustler's ()
Beef Jerky
Spicy Flavor Beef Stick

Safeway
Original Beef Jerky
Peppered Beef Jerky

Shelton's
Beef Jerky
Beef Sticks
Hot Turkey Jerky
Pepperoni Turkey Stick
Regular Turkey Jerky
Regular Turkey Stick

Wellshire Farms
Matt's Select Pepperoni Sticks - Original
Turkey Tom Toms
Turkey Tom Toms - Hot & Spicy

Wild Ride Beef Jerky
Buckin' Barbecue
Gallopin' Pepper
Jumpin' Hot & Spicy

BROWNIES

Ener-G
Brownies
Foods By George
Brownies
Mini Brownies

Frankly Natural Bakers

Gluten-Free Carob Almondine Brownie
Gluten-Free Cherry Berry Brownie
Gluten-Free Java Jive Brownie
Gluten-Free Misty Mint Brownie
Gluten-Free Wacky Walnut Brownie

French Meadow Bakery

All Natural Gluten-Free Fudge Brownie

Gluten-Free & Fabulous

Brownie Bites

Mariposa Baking Company

Mocha Truffle Brownies
Triple Chocolate Truffle Brownies
Walnut Truffle Brownies

CANDY & CHOCOLATE

Alse Tois 🍷

Chocolate Raspberry Pecan Brittle

Alter Eco Fair Trade

Chocolate Bars (All)

Altoids

Altoids
Altoids Chocolate Dipped Mints ()

Andes

Andes

Annabelle's ()

The Big Hunk
The Skinny Hunk

Atomic FireBall 🍷

Atomic Fireball (All)

Baby Bottle Pop

Baby Bottle Pop

Baby Ruth ()

Baby Ruth
Baby Ruth Crème Egg (Seasonal,
Easter)

Before & After Candy

Before & After Candy (All)

Betty Lou's

Chocolate Walnut Balls
Coconut Macadamia Balls
Peanut Butter Balls

Bit-O-Honey ()

Bit-O-Honey

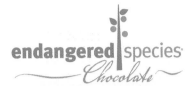

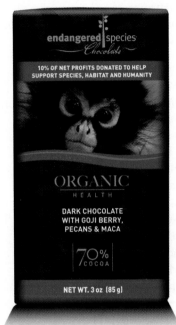

endangered species
Chocolate

10% OF NET PROFITS DONATED TO HELP
SUPPORT SPECIES, HABITAT AND HUMANITY

ORGANIC
H E A L T H

DARK CHOCOLATE
WITH GOJI BERRY,
PECANS & MACA

70% COCOA

NET WT. 3 oz (85 g)

Savor chocolate.
Save our planet.

Making chocolate is monkey business.
And dolphin business. And tree
business. New **organic flavors**, same
commitment to the planet.

Certified
GF
Gluten-Free

shop online at
ChocolateBar.com
or call **800.293.0160**

ALWAYS READ LABELS

Black Forest Gummies ☷
  Black Forest Gummies

Boston Baked Beans ☷
  Boston Baked Beans

Bottle Caps ()
  Bottle Caps

Butterfinger ()
  Butterfinger (BUT NOT Butterfinger
    Crisp & Butterfinger Stixx)
  Butterfinger Crème Eggs (Seasonal,
    Easter)
  Butterfinger Nesteggs (Seasonal, Easter)
  Nestle Milk Chocolate with Butterfinger
    Hearts (Seasonal, Valentines)
  Nestle Milk Chocolate with Butterfinger
    Tigger (Seasonal, Valentines)

Candy Carnival
  Candy Carnival

Caramel Apple Pops
  Caramel Apple Pops

Cella Cherries
  Cella Cherries

Charleston Chew
  Charleston Chew

Charms Blow Pops
  Charms Blow Pops

Charms Flat Pops
  Charms Flat Pops

Child's Play
  Child's Play

Chocolove
  Organic Bars (61% & 73% cocoa
    content)

Clark Bar
  Clark Bars

Concord Foods
  Candy Apple Kit
  Caramel Apple Kit
  Caramel Apple Wrap

Cry Baby
  Cry Baby

Dagoba
  Dagoba (All)

Dots
  Dots

Dove
  Dove Chocolate Products (All BUT
    Dove Jewel Roll Ups)

Endangered Species Chocolate ☷ ☷
  70% Cranberry/Almonds Bag Wolf
  70% Mint Bag Rainforest
  Assorted 70% Bag Sea Turtle/Grizzly
  Assorted 72% & 88% Bag Chimpanzee/
    Panther
  Bat Bar
  Black Panther Bar
  Black Rhino Bar
  Bug Bites Dark Treats
  Bug Bites Milk Treats
  Butterfly Bar
  Cheetah Bar
  Chimp Mints Treats
  Chimpanzee Bar
  Chocolate Covered Peanut Brittle -
    All-Natural Dark Chocolate Covered
    Peanut Butter Brittle
  Crane Bar
  Dolphin Bar
  Giraffe Bar
  Grizzly Bar
  Halloween Dark Treats
  Halloween Milk Treats
  Hoppy Dark Treats
  Hoppy Milk Treats
  Koala Bar
  Lion Bar
  Love Dark Treats
  Love Milk Treats
  Organic 70% Bag Butterfly
  Otter Bar
  Rainforest Bar
  Sea Turtle Bar
  Spider Monkey Bar
  Tiger Bar
  Toucan Bar
  Tree Frog Bar
  Winter Holiday Dark Treats
  Winter Holiday Milk Treats
  Wolf Bar
  Zebra Bar

Enjoy Life Foods 🍴 🍴

- boom CHOCO boom Dairy-Free Rice Milk Chocolatey Bar
- boom CHOCO boom Dairy-Free Rice Milk with Crispy Rice Chocolatey Bar
- boom CHOCO boom Dark Chocolate Bar

Fannie May

- Apricot Bon Bon
- Apricot Cream
- Candy Bars (All)
- Chocolate & Pastel Meltaways
- Chocolate Toffee
- Chocolate Wafers
- Citrus Peel
- Dark Filbert Cluster
- English Toffee
- Hostess Mints
- Irish Toffee
- Ivory & Chocolate Bark
- Milk & Dark Almond Clusters
- Milk & Dark Walnut Clusters
- Milk Peanut Butter Crunch Bar
- Pastel Toffee
- Pastel Wafers
- Peanut Cluster
- Solid Chocolate Novelties (All)

Fluffy Stuff Cotton Candy

- Fluffy Stuff

Frooties

- Frooties

Giant

- Assorted Fruit Filled Candy
- Assorted Star Drops
- Assorted Starlights
- Blue Gummi Sharks
- Butter Toffee
- Butterscotch Disks
- Canada Wintergreen
- Candy Corn
- Candy Necklaces
- Cinnamon Starlights
- Circus Peanuts
- Gum Balls
- Gum Drops
- Gummi Bears
- Jelly Beans
- Kiddie Mix
- Lemon Drops
- Neon Sour Crawlers
- Orange Slices
- Pastel Mints
- Peach Rings
- Red Ju Ju Coins
- Red Ju Ju Fish
- Root Beer Barrels
- Royal Mix
- Silver Mints
- Smarties
- Soft Peppermints
- Sour Balls
- Sour Gummi Worms
- Spearmint Leaves
- Spearmint Starlights
- Spice Drops
- Starlight Mints
- Strawberry Buds
- Watermelon Hard Candy

Glutino 🍴

- Dark Chocolate Bar
- Milk Chocolate Bar
- Peanut Butter Chocolate Bar

Gobstoppers ()

- Candy Canes (Seasonal, Christmas)
- Chewy
- Eggbreakers (Seasonal, Easter)
- Heartbreakers (Seasonal, Valentines)
- Original
- Snowballs (Seasonal, Christmas)

Golightly

- Golightly (All)

Goobers ()

- Goobers

Guittard

- Guittard (All)

Haviland

- Peppermint Patties
- Thin Mints
- Wintergreen Patties

Hershey's

- Milk Chocolate Bar with Almonds
- Plain Milk Chocolate Kisses
- Plain Milk Chocolate Milk Chocolate Bar

Hint Mint
  Mints (All)
Hy-Vee
  Assorted Gum Balls
  Butterscotch Buttons
  Chocolate Caramel Clusters
  Chocolate Covered Raisins
  Chocolate Peanut Clusters
  Chocolate Stars
  Cinnamon Imperials
  Circus Peanuts
  Double Dipped Chocolate Covered
    Peanuts
  Dum Dum Suckers
  Gum Drops
  Gummi Bears
  Gummi Peach Rings
  Gummi Sour Squiggles
  Gummi Squiggles
  Lemon Drops
  Milk Chocolate Peanut Butter Cups
  Milk Kraft Caramels
  Orange Slices
  Smarties
  Spice Drops
  Starlight Kisses
  Tootsie Flavored Rolls
  Tootsie Pops
  Wax Bottles
JawBusters 𝖸
  JawBusters
Jelly Belly
  Jelly Beans (All)
  Sport Beans
Jolly Rancher
  Hard Candies
  Lollipops
Junior Mints
  Junior Mints
Kroger ()
  Hard Candy
  Jellied Candy
Laffy Taffy ()
  Laffy Taffy
  Laffy Taffy Fruitarts Chews
  Laffy Taffy Rope

Lemonhead & Friends 𝖸
  Lemonhead & Friends
Let's Do…Organic 𝖸 ()
  Organic Classic Gummi Bears
  Organic Fruity Gummi Feet
  Organic Jelly Gummi Bears
  Organic Super Sour Gummi Bears
Lifesavers
  Lifesavers Products
Lik-M-Aid Fun Dip ()
  Lik-M-Aid Fun Dip
Luna
  Sport Moons
M&M's
  M&M's (All)
Manischewitz
  Caramel Cashew Patties
  Chocolate Frolic Bears
  Chocolate Lollycones
  Fruit Slices
  Hazelnut Truffles
  Mallo Cups
  Mini Sour Fruit Slices
  Peppermint Patties
  Swiss Chocolate Mints
  Viennese Crunch
Mary Janes
  Mary Jane Peanut Butter Kisses
  Mary Janes
Meijer
  Peanuts - Butter Toffee
Milky Way
  Milky Way Products (All BUT Milky
    Way Bar)
Munch Bar
  Munch Bar
Necco
  Banana Split Chews
  Canada Mint & Wintergreen Lozenges
  Candy Eggs (Easter)
  Candy Stix
  Mint Julep Chews
  Squirrel Nut Caramels
  Squirrel Nut Zippers
  Talking Pumpkins (Halloween)
  Ultramints

Wafers

Nerds ()
Nerds
Nerds Gumballs
Nerds Rope

Nestlé ()
Caramel Nesteggs (Seasonal, Easter)
Milk Chocolate Hearts (Seasonal, Valentines)
Milk Chocolate Nesteggs (Seasonal, Easter)

Nestlé Milk Chocolate ()
Nestlé Milk Chocolate

Nestlé Toll House ()
Gems (Seasonal, Christmas)

Nestlé Treasures ()
Nestlé Treasures (includes Treasures Bars)

Newman's Own Organics
Chocolate Bars (All BUT Crisp Rice) ()
Chocolate Cups (All) ()
Mint Rolls
Mints in Tins

Nik-L-Nip
Nik-L-Nip

Nips ()
Regular
Sugar Free

Oh Henry! ()
Oh Henry!

Old Dominion Peanut Company
Burnt Sugar Pecans
Butter Peanut Crunch
Butter Toffee Peanuts
Cashew Brittle
Dipped Butter Toffee Peanuts
Dipped Peanut Brittle
Double Dip Peanuts
Honey Toasted Cashews
Peanut Brittle
Peanut Candy
Peco Flakes
Single Dip Peanuts

OrgraN
OrgraN (All)

Original Bazooka Bubble Gum
Original Bazooka Bubble Gum

Planters 🖉
Almonds, Cashews & Mixed Nuts in Milk Chocolate
Chocolate Covered Cashews
Chocolate Lovers Milk Chocolate Cashews
Rich Roasted Whole Peanuts in Milk Chocolate

Pangburn's
Pangburn's (All BUT S'mores and Cookies & Cream Rabbits [Seasonal, Easter])

Pearson's
Pearson's (All)

PEZ 🍴
PEZ

Pixy Stix ()
Pixy Stix

Publix ()
Butterscotch Discs
Chocolate Covered Peanut Brittle
Double Dipped Chocolate Covered Peanuts
Gummi Worms
Lollipops
Party Time Mix
Pixy Stick Candy
Smarties Candy
Sour Worms
Spearmint Starlight Mints
Starlight Mints Candy
Strawberry Bon Bons

Push Pop
Push Pop

Queen Anne Candy
Cherries
Twist Wrapped Products

Raisinets ()
Raisinets

Rapunzel
Chocolate Hazelnut Butter ()
Dark Chocolate 55% ()
Dark Chocolate 70% ()

Dark Chocolate w/Almonds 55% ( )
Dark Chocolate w/Hazelnuts 55% ( )
Dark Espresso Chocolate 55% ( )
Lady Truffles w/NutTruffle Crm ( )
Milk Chocolate ( )
Milk Chocolate w/Hazelnuts ( )
Milk Chocolate w/Nut Truffle Crème ( )

Red Bird
Red Bird Brand (All)

Red Hots ⅄
Red Hots

Reed's
Reed's (All)

Ring Pop
Ring Pop

Runts ( )
Chewy
Hearts (Seasonal, Valentines)
Original

Russell Stover
Russell Stover (All BUT S'mores and
Cookies & Cream Rabbits [Seasonal,
Easter])

Safeway
Candy Corn
Cinnamon Imperials
Dessert Mints
Gummi Bears
Gummi Worms - Regular
Gummi Worms - Sour
Jelly Eggs - Classic Jelly Beans
Lemon Drops
Spice Drops
Star Light Mints

Select Brand (Safeway)
Butterscotch Truffles
Chocolate/Raspberry Truffles
Milk Chocolate Truffles
Mocha Truffles

Shockers ( )
Shockers

Simply Enjoy (Giant)
Dark Chocolate Amaretto Coated
Cranberries
Dark Chocolate Cappuccino Crunch
Bits
Dark Chocolate Caramel Squares
Dark Chocolate Covered Cherries
Dark Chocolate Covered Coffee Beans
Dark Chocolate Covered Cranberries
Dark Chocolate Covered Kona Almond
Coffee Beans
Dark Chocolate Covered Strawberries
Dark Chocolate Raspberry Sticks
Milk Chocolate Butter Toffee Squares
Milk Chocolate Coated Cashews
Milk Chocolate Cocoa Almonds
Milk Chocolate Covered Cashews
Milk Chocolate Covered Cherries
Milk Chocolate Covered Peanuts
Milk Chocolate Covered Raisins
Milk Chocolate Pecan Caramel Patties
White Chocolate Coated Coffee
Nuggets
Whole Chocolate Covered Raspberries
Yogurt Coated Cranberries

Simply Enjoy (Stop & Shop)
Dark Chocolate Amaretto Coated
Cranberries
Dark Chocolate Cappuccino Crunch
Bits
Dark Chocolate Caramel Squares
Dark Chocolate Covered Cherries
Dark Chocolate Covered Coffee Beans
Dark Chocolate Covered Cranberries
Dark Chocolate Covered Kona Almond
Coffee Beans
Dark Chocolate Covered Strawberries
Dark Chocolate Raspberry Sticks
Milk Chocolate Butter Toffee Squares
Milk Chocolate Coated Cashews
Milk Chocolate Cocoa Almonds
Milk Chocolate Covered Cashews
Milk Chocolate Covered Cherries
Milk Chocolate Covered Peanuts
Milk Chocolate Covered Raisins
Milk Chocolate Pecan Caramel Patties
White Chocolate Coated Coffee
Nuggets
Whole Chocolate Covered Raspberries
Yogurt Coated Cranberries

Skittles
  Skittles Bite-Sized Candies (All)

Skybar
  Skybars

Snickers
  Snickers
  Snickers Dark Bars

Sno-Caps ()
  Sno-Caps

Sour Patch Kids ☊
  Sour Patch Kids (All)

South Beach Living ᏉᏊ
  Dark Chocolate Covered Soynuts
    (Snack Pack Delights)

Spangler Candy Company
  Candy Canes
  Circus Marshmallow Peanuts
  Dum Dum Candy Canes
  Dum Dum Chewy Canes
  Dum Dum Chewy Pops
  Dum Dums
  Jelly Belly Candy Canes
  Marshmallow Treats
  Saf-T-Pops

Spree ()
  Candy Canes (Seasonal, Christmas)
  Spree

Starburst
  Starburst (All)

Stop & Shop
  Assorted Fruit Filled Candy
  Assorted Star Drops
  Assorted Starlights
  Blue Gummi Sharks
  Butter Toffee
  Butterscotch Disks
  Canada Wintergreen
  Candy Corn
  Candy Necklaces
  Cinnamon Starlights
  Circus Peanuts
  Gum Balls
  Gum Drops
  Gummi Bears
  Jelly Beans
  Kiddie Mix

Lemon Drops
Neon Sour Crawlers
Orange Slices
Pastel Mints
Peach Rings
Pina Colada Coated Cashews
Red Ju Ju Coins
Red Ju Ju Fish
Root Beer Barrels
Royal Mix
Silver Mints
Smarties
Soft Peppermints
Sour Balls
Sour Gummi Worms
Spearmint Leaves
Spearmint Starlights
Spice Drops
Starlight Mints
Strawberry Buds
Watermelon Hard Candy

Sugar Babies
  Sugar Babies

Sugar Daddy Pops
  Sugar Daddy Pops

SweeTARTS ()
  SweeTARTS
  SweeTARTS Lollipops (Seasonal,
    Valentines)

Sweethearts
  Sweethearts Conversation Hearts
    (Valentines Only)

Terrys ᏉᏊ
  Orange Dark Chocolate
  Orange Milk Chocolate
  Pure Milk Chocolate

Toblerone ᏉᏊ
  Minis - Swiss Chocolate with Honey &
    Almond Nougat
  Minis - White Confection with Honey
    & Almond Nougat
  Swiss Bittersweet with Honey &
    Almond Nougat
  Swiss Milk Chocolate with Honey &
    Almond Nougat
  Swiss White Confection with Honey &
    Almond Nougat

Truffle Peaks

Too Tarts
Too Tarts

Tootsie Pops
Tootsie Pops

Tootsie Rolls
Tootsie Rolls

Trader Joe's ()
Black Licorice Scottie Dogs
Candy Coated Peanuts
Chocolate Covered Blueberries
Chocolate Covered Orange and
    Raspberry Sticks
Chocolate Espresso Beans
Chocolate Fondue
Chocolate Sunflower Seed Drops
Chocolate Truffle
Dark Chocolate Almonds Sea Salt and
    Sugar
Dark Chocolate Covered Almonds
Dark Chocolate Covered Caramels
Dark Chocolate Covered Cherries
Dark Chocolate Covered Espresso
    Beans
Dark Chocolate Covered Raisins
Dark Chocolate Covered Toffee
Dark Chocolate Mint Creams
English Toffee
Fair Trade Dark Chocolate Truffles
Figments
Gourmet Chocolate Fudge with Walnuts
Imported Belgian Chocolate Sea Shells
Milk and Dark Chocolate Covered
    Almonds
Milk and Dark Chocolate Covered
    Cashews
Milk Chocolate Clouds
Milk Chocolate Covered Banana Chips
Milk Chocolate Covered Cranberries
Milk Chocolate Covered Peanut Butter
    Cups
Milk Chocolate Covered Peanuts
Milk Chocolate Covered Raisins
Mini Fruit Slices
Mini Milk Chocolate Peanut Butter
    Cups
Organic Chocolate Truffle Bars - Dark

Organic Chocolate Truffle Bars - Milk
Organic Pops
Peanut Butter Clusters
Peanut Butter Cups
Pecans Praline
Peppermint Marshmallows
Soft Peanut Toffee
Swiss 71% Dark Chocolate Bar
Swiss Milk Chocolate Bar
Yogurt Covered Raisins

Tropical Source
Bars

VerMints
VerMints (All)

Vertigo
Vertigo

Wack-O-Wax
Wack-O-Wax

Whitman's
Whitman's (All BUT S'mores and
    Cookies & Cream Rabbits [Easter])

Wonka ()
Chocolate Candy Canes (Seasonal,
    Christmas)
Large Golden Egg - Milk Chocolate
    Hollow Egg with SweeTARTS Inside
    (Seasonal, Easter)
Mix-Ups

Zip-A-DEE Pops
Zip-A-Dee-Pops

CHEESE PUFFS & CURLS

Bachman
Baked Jax Cheese Twists ()
Crunchy Jax Cheese Twists

Baked! Cheetos ()
Crunchy Cheese Flavored Snacks
Flamin' Hot Cheese Flavored Snacks

Cheetos ()
Cheddar Jalapeno Cheese Flavored
    Snacks
Chile Limon Flavored Snacks
Crunchy Cheese Flavored Snacks
Fantastixx! Chili Cheese Flavored
    Baked Corn/Potato Snack

Flamin' Hot Cheese Flavored Snacks
Flamin' Hot Limon Cheese Flavored
    Snacks
Jumbo Puffs Cheese Flavored Snacks
Jumbo Puffs Flamin' Hot Cheese
    Flavored Snacks
Mix & Move Cheese Flavored Snacks
Natural White Cheddar Puffs Cheese
    Flavored Snacks
Puffs Cheese Flavored Snacks
Reduced Fat Cheese Flavored Snacks
Twisted Cheese Flavored Snacks
Xxtra Flamin' Hot Cheese Flavored
    Snacks

EatSmart
Cheddairs

Golden Flake ()
Cheese Curls
Cheese Puff Corn
Cheese Puffs
Puff Corn

Herr's ()
Cheese Curls
Crunchy Cheese Sticks
Honey Cheese Curls

Laura Lynn (Ingle's)
Baked Cheese Curls
Cheese Krunchy

Meijer
Cheese Pops
Cheese Puffs
Cheezy Treats
White Cheddar Puffs

Michael Season's
Lite Cheddar Cheese Curls
Lite Cheddar Cheese Puffs
Ultimate Cheddar Cheese Curls
Ultimate Cheddar Cheese Puffs
Ultimate White Cheese Puffs

Old Dutch Foods
Bac'N Puffs - Regular (non-flavored)

Publix ()
Crunchy Cheese Curls
Crunchy Cheese Curls (Deli)
Crunchy Cheese Puffs
Jumbo Cheese Puffs (Deli)

Robert's American Gourmet ()
Snacks (All BUT CHAOS, Honey
    Wheat Pretzels, Veggie Tubes and
    Tubes)

Safeway
Cheese Curls
Puffed Cheese Snacks

Snyder's of Hanover
Cheese Twists
Multigrain Aged Cheddar Cheese Puff
Multigrain White Cheese Puff

Stop & Shop
Crunchy Cheese Corn Snacks
Puff Cheese Corn Snacks

Trader Joe's ()
Jalapeño Cheese Crunchies
Reduced Fat Cheese Crunchies

Utz
Cheese Ball Barrel
Cheese Balls
Cheese Curls
Crunchy Cheese Curls
White Cheddar Cheese Curls

CHIPS & CRISPS, OTHER

Arico Natural Foods Company
Cassava Chips (All)

Bachman
Corn Chips
Sweet Chile Lime Chipitos
Thai Barbeque Tortilla Chipitos

Baji's Products
Mango Chutney Papadums
Tangy Cilantro Papadums
Traditional Tandoori Papadums

Chester's ()
Flamin' Hot Flavored Fries

EatSmart
Cheddar Jalapeno Veggie Crisps
Garlic, Parmesan & Olive Oil Soy
    Crisps
Sundried Tomato Pesto Veggie Crisps
Tomato, Romano & Olive Oil Soy
    Crisps
Veggie Chips

Eden Foods
Brown Rice Chips

Fritos ( )
Flavor Twists Honey BBQ Flavored Corn Chips
Original Corn Chips
Scoops! Corn Chips
Tangy Roasted Corn Flavored Corn Chips

Funyuns ( )
Onion Flavored Rings

Giant
Crunchy Cheese Corn Snacks
Puff Cheese Corn Snacks

Golden Flake ( )
Chili Cheese Corn Chips
Regular & King Size Corn Chips

Goya ( )
Garlic Plantain Chips
No Salt Plantain Chips
Plantain Chips
Plantain Chips - Loose
Plantain Strips

Herr's ( )
Veggie Crisps

Kitchen Table Bakers
Wafer Crisps (All)

Laura Lynn (Ingle's)
Regular Corn Chips

Lundberg Family Farms
Rice Chips - Fiesta Lime
Rice Chips - Honey Dijon
Rice Chips - Nacho Cheese
Rice Chips - Pico De Gallo
Rice Chips - Santa Fe Barbecue
Rice Chips - Sea Salt
Rice Chips - Sesame & Seaweed
Rice Chips - Wasabi

Michael Season's
Soy Protein Chip - Original ( )

Mr. Krispers
Mr. Krispers (All)

Nature's Promise (Giant)
Soy Crisps - BBQ
Soy Crisps - Ranch

Nature's Promise (Stop & Shop)
Soy Crisps - BBQ
Soy Crisps - Ranch

Newman's Own Organics
Barbeque Soy Crisps ( )
Cinnamon Sugar Soy Crisps ( )
Lightly Salted Soy Crisps ( )
White Cheddar Soy Crisps ( )

Publix ( )
Corn Chips - King Size

Robert's American Gourmet ( )
Snacks (All BUT CHAOS, Honey Wheat Pretzels, Veggie Tubes and Tubes)

Safeway
Golden Chips (Casa del Pueblo)

Stacy's
Simply Cheese Soy Thin Crisps
Sticky Bun Soy Thin Crisps
Sweet BBQ Soy Thin Crisps

Stop & Shop
BBQ Rice Crisps
Cheddar Rice Crisps
Ranch Rice Crisps

Trader Joe's ( )
Rice Sticks
Roasted Plantain Chips
Sea Salt & Pepper Rice Crisps
Sour Cream & Onion Rice Crisps
Soy Crisps - BBQ
Soy Crisps - Olive Oil
Soy Crisps - White Cheddar
Terra Exotic Vegetable Chips
Vegetable Root Chips
Veggie Chips

Utz
BBQ Corn Chips
Regular Corn Chips

CHIPS & CRISPS, POTATO

Bachman
Golden Crisps
Golden Ridges
Golden Wavy

Baked! Lay's ()
Cheddar & Sour Cream Flavored Potato Crisps
Original Potato Crisps
Sour Cream & Onion Artificially Flavored Potato Crisps

Baked! Ruffles ()
Cheddar & Sour Cream Flavored Potato Crisps
Original Potato Crisps

EatSmart
French Onion Potato Chips
Sweet BBQ Potato Chips

French's
Potato Sticks - Barbecue Flavor
Potato Sticks - Cheezy Cheddar
Potato Sticks - Original Flavor

Giant
Plain Potato Chips
Salt and Vinegar Potato Chips
Sour Cream and Onion Chips
Wavy Cut Potato Chips

Golden Flake ()
BBQ Potato Chips
Cheddar & Sour Cream Dip Style Chips
Dill Pickle Potato Chips
Dip Style Potato Chips
Hot Potato Chips
Mesquite Dip Style Potato Chips
Mrs. B's Cajun Hot Potato Chips
Mrs. B's Regular Potato Chips
Regular Potato Chips
Sweet Heat Potato Chips
Vinegar & Salt Potato Chips

Herr's ()
Cheddar & Sour Cream Potato Chips
Crisp N' Tasty Potato Chips
Honey BBQ Potato Chips
Jalapeno Kettle Potato Chips
Lightly Salted Potato Chips
Potato Sticks
Russett Kettle Potato Chips
Salt & Pepper Potato Chips
Salt & Vinegar Potato Chips

J Higgs (Save-A-Lot)
Regular Potato Chips

Kettle Brand
Potato Chips (All BUT Cheddar Beer)

Kroger ()
Plain Potato Chips

Laura Lynn (Ingle's)
Regular Potato Chips
Ripple Potato Chips
Sour Cream & Onion Potato Chips
Wavy Potato Chips

Lay's ()
Cheddar & Sour Cream Artificially Flavored Potato Chips
Chile Limon Potato Chips
Classic Potato Chips
Deli Style Original Potato Chips
Dill Pickle Flavored Potato Chips
Hot & Spicy Barbecue Flavored Potato Chips
Kettle Cooked Jalapeno Flavored Extra Crunchy Potato Chips
Kettle Cooked Mesquite BBQ Flavored Extra Crunchy Potato Chips
Kettle Cooked Original Potato Chips
Kettle Cooked Reduced Fat Original Flavored Potato Chips
Kettle Cooked Southwestern Ranch Flavored Potato Chips
Kettle Cooked Sweet Chili & Sour Cream Flavored Potato Chips
Light Original Potato Chips
Lightly Salted Potato Chips
Limon Tangy Lime Flavored Potato Chips
Natural Country BBQ Thick Cut Potato Chips
Natural Sea Salt Thick Cut Potato Chips
Salt & Vinegar Artificially Flavored Potato Chips
Sour Cream & Onion Artificially Flavored Potato Chips
Wavy Au Gratin Flavored Potato Chips
Wavy Hickory BBQ Flavored Potato Chips
Wavy Ranch Flavored Potato Chips
Wavy Regular Potato Chips

Lay's Stax
Cheddar Flavored Potato Crisps

Hot'N Spicy Barbecue Flavored Potato Crisps

Jalapeno Cheddar Flavored Potato Crisps

Mesquite Barbecue Flavored Potato Crisps

Original Flavored Potato Crisps

Pizza Flavored Potato Crisps

Ranch Flavored Potato Crisps

Salt & Vinegar Flavored Potato Crisps

Sour Cream & Onion Flavored Potato Crisps

Spicy Buffalo Wings Flavored Potato Crisps

Manischewitz
Potato Chips (All Varieties)

Maui Style ()
Regular Potato Chips

Salt & Vinegar Flavored Potato Chips

Meijer
Potato Sticks

Michael Season's
Lite Baked Potato Crisps - BBQ

Lite Baked Potato Crisps - Lightly Salted

Lite Baked Potato Crisps - Sour Cream & Onion

Reduced Fat Kettle Style Potato Chip - Lightly Salted

Reduced Fat Kettle Style Potato Chip - Sea Salt & Balsamic Vinegar

Reduced Fat Kettle Style Potato Chip - Sea Salt & Cracked Pepper

Reduced Fat Lightly Salted Chips

Reduced Fat Potato Honey Barbecue Chips ()

Reduced Fat Potato Ripple Chips

Reduced Fat Potato Salt & Pepper Chips

Reduced Fat Potato Unsalted Chips

Reduced Fat Potato Yogurt & Green Onion Chips ()

Miss Vickie's ()
Jalapeno Flavored Potato Chips

Lime & Black Pepper Potato Chips

Mesquite BBQ Flavored Potato Chips

Original Potato Chips

Munchos ()
Regular Potato Crisps

O'Keely's ()
Cheddar & Bacon Potato Skins Flavored Potato Crisps

Old Dutch Foods
Original Dutch Crunch Potato Chips (non-flavored)

Original Regular Potato Chips (non-flavored)

Original Rip-l Potato Chips (non-flavored)

Original Ripples Potato Chips (non-flavored)

Pringles
Fat Free Original Pringles

Fat Free Sour Cream & Onion Pringles

Publix ()
Potato Chips - Dip Style

Potato Chips - Original Thins

Potato Chips - Salt & Vinegar

Raley's ()
Hamburger Chips

Ruffles ()
Authentic Barbecue Flavored Potato Chips

Cheddar & Sour Cream Flavored Potato Chips

Light Cheddar & Sour Cream Flavored Potato Chips

Light Original Potato Chips

Natural Reduced Fat Regular Sea Salted Potato Chips

Reduced Fat Potato Chips

Regular Potato Chips

Sour Cream & Onion Flavored Potato Chips

Sabritas ()
Adobadas Tomato & Chile Flavored Potato Chips

Snyder's of Hanover
BBQ Potato Chips

Hot Buffalo Wing Potato Chips

Jalapeno Potato Chips

Kosher Dill Potato Chips

Regular Potato Chips, Not Seasoned

Ripple Potato Chips - Not Seasoned
Salt and Vinegar Potato Chips
Sour Cream and Onion Potato Chips

Stop & Shop

Kettle Cooked Potato Chips
Plain Potato Chips
Rippled Potato Chips
Salt & Vinegar Potato Chips
Sour Cream & Onion Chips
Wavy Cut Potato Chips

Trader Joe's ()

Baked Potato Slims - Lightly Salted
BBQ Chips
Blue Potato Chips
Buttermilk Garlic Mash Potato Chips
Popped Potato Chips - Barbecue
Popped Potato Chips - Salted
Potato Chips
Red Bliss Potato Chips
Reduced Guilt Potato Chips
Sweet Potato Chips

Utz

BBQ Potato Chips
Carolina BBQ Potato Chips
Cheddar & Sour Cream Potato Chips
Grandma Utz BBQ Kettle Potato Chips
Grandma Utz Regular Kettle Potato
  Chips
Homestyle Regular Kettle Potato Chips
Kettle Classic Dark Russet Potato Chips
Kettle Classic Jalapeno Potato Chips
Kettle Classic Potato Chips
Kettle Classic Smokin' Sweet Potato
  Chips
Kettle Classic Sour Cream & Chive
  Potato Chips
Kettle Classic Sweet Potato Chips
Mystic Dark Russet Kettle Potato Chips
Mystic Regular Kettle Potato Chips
Mystic Sea Salt & Vinegar Kettle Potato
  Chips
Natural Dark Russet Kettle Potato Chips
Natural Gourmet Medley Kettle Potato
  Chips
Natural Lightly Salted Kettle Potato
  Chips
Natural Sea Salt & Vinegar Kettle

Potato Chips
No Salt Potato Chips
Red Hot Potato Chips
Reduced Fat Regular Potato Chips
Reduced Fat Ripple Potato Chips
Regular Potato Chips
Ripple Potato Chips
Salt & Pepper Potato Chips
Salt & Vinegar Potato Chips
Sour Cream & Onion Potato Chips
Wavy Potato Chips

CHIPS, TORTILLA

Bachman

Black Bean Salsa Tortilla Chipitos
Deli Style Tortilla Chips
Durangos White Corn Tortilla Chips
Restaurant Style Tortilla Chips

Baked! Tostitos ()

Scoops! Tortilla Chips

Chi-Chi's ()

Chips (All Varieties)

Doritos ()

Black Pepper Jack Cheese Flavored
  Tortilla Chips
Blazin' Buffalo & Ranch Flavored
  Tortilla Chips
Collisions Hot Wings and Blue Cheese
  Flavored Tortilla Chips
Collisions Zesty Taco and Chipotle
  Ranch Flavored Tortilla Chips
Cool Ranch Flavored Tortilla Chips
Fiery Habanero Flavored Tortilla Chips
Light Nacho Cheesier Flavored Tortilla
  Chips
Natural White Nacho Cheese Tortilla
  Chips
Poppin' Jalapeno Flavored Tortilla Chips
Reduced Fat Cool Ranch Flavored
  Tortilla Chips
Salsa Verde Flavored Tortilla Chips
Sizzlin' Picante Flavored Tortilla Chips
Smokin' Cheddar BBQ Flavored
  Tortilla Chips
Spicy Nacho Flavored Tortilla Chips
Taco Flavored Tortilla Chips

Toasted Corn Tortilla Chips

Giant
Nacho Tortilla Chips
White Restaurant Tortilla Chips - Regular
White Restaurant Tortilla Chips - Rounds

Golden Flake ()
Nacho Tortilla Chips
Spicy Hot Nacho Tortilla Chips

Green Mountain Gringo
Tortilla Strips

Guiltless Gourmet
Tortilla Chips (All) ()

Health Market (Hy-Vee)
Organic Blue Corn Tortilla Chips
Organic White Corn Tortilla Chips
Organic Yellow Corn Tortilla Chips

Herr's ()
Corn/Tortilla Chips (All)

Kettle Brand
Tortilla Chips (All BUT Multi-Grain)

Kroger ()
Plain Tortilla Chips

Laura Lynn (Ingle's)
Mini Corn Tortilla Chips
Nacho Tortilla Chips
Ranch Tortilla Chips
White Corn Tortilla Chips

Michael Season's
Organic Corn Tortilla Chips - Blue
Organic Corn Tortilla Chips - White
Organic Corn Tortilla Chips - Yellow

Mission Foods 💧
Corn Tortilla Chips

Publix ()
White Corn Tortilla Chips - Restaurant Style
Yellow Corn Tortilla Chips - Round Style

R.W. Garcia
Berry Tortilla Chips
Blue Corn Tortilla Chips
Blue Corn with Flaxseed Tortilla Chips
Extra Thin Tortilla Chips
Flaxseed with Soy Tortilla Chips

Organic Veggie Tortilla Chips
Salsa Fresca Tortilla Chips
Spice Flaxseed with Soy Tortilla Chips
Stone Ground Yellow Corn Tortilla Chips
Thai Sweet and Spicy Tortilla Chips

Safeway
Tortilla Strips (Casa del Pueblo)
White Corn Tortilla Chips

Santitas ()
White Corn Restaurant Style Tortilla Chips
Yellow Corn Tortilla Chips

Snyder's of Hanover
Restaurant Style Tortilla Chips
White Corn Tortilla Chips
Yellow Corn Tortilla Chips

Stop & Shop
Nacho Tortilla Chips
White Restaurant Tortilla Chips - Regular & Round
Yellow Round Tortilla Chips

Tostitos ()
100% White Corn Restaurant Style Tortilla Chips
Bite Size Gold Tortilla Chips
Bite Size Rounds Tortilla Chips
Crispy Rounds Tortilla Chips
Light Restaurant Style Tortilla Chips
Natural Blue Corn Restaurant Style Tortilla Chips
Natural Yellow Corn Restaurant Style Tortilla Chips
Restaurant Style with A Hint of Lime Flavor Tortilla Chips
Scoops! Tortilla Chips

Trader Joe's ()
Blue Corn Tortilla Chips - Salted
Blue Corn Tortilla Chips - Unsalted
Organic Baked Blue Corn Tortilla Chips - Salted
Organic Blue Corn Tortilla Chips
Organic White Corn Tortilla Chips - Salted
Organic White Corn Tortilla Chips - Unsalted
Organic Yellow Corn Tortilla Chips -

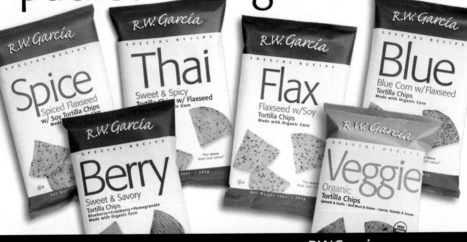

Gluten Free and packed with great taste!

Available at fine retailers near you or online at RWGarcia.com

Round
Restaurant Style Tortilla Chips
Salsa Tortilla Chips
Soy and Flaxseed Tortilla Chips -
   Regular
Soy and Flaxseed Tortilla Chips - Spicy
Spiced Tortilla Chips
Tortilla Longboard Chips
Veggie Flaxseed Tortilla Chips
White Corn Tortilla Chips - Restaurant
   Style
White Corn Tortilla Strips - Salted

Utz
Baked Tortilla Chips
Cheesier Nacho Tortilla Chips
Creamy Ranch Tortilla Chips
Restaurant Style Tortilla Chips
White Round Tortilla Chips

COOKIES

Andean Dream
Quinoa Cookies

Arico Natural Foods Company
Cookie Pouches (All)

Cherrybrook Kitchen
Gluten-Free Dreams - Mini Chocolate
   Chip Cookies
Gluten-Free Dreams - Mini Vanilla
   Graham Cookies

Ener-G
Chocolate Chip Biscotti Cookies
Chocolate Chip Potato Cookies
Chocolate Cookies
Chocolate Sandwich Cookies
Chocolate Vanilla Cream Cookies
Cinnamon Cookies
Ginger Cookies
Lemon Sandwich Cookies
Vanilla Chocolate Sandwich Cookies
Vanilla Cookies
Vanilla Cream Cookies
Vanilla Lemon Cream Cookies
White Chocolate Chip Cookies

Enjoy Life Foods
Chewy Chocolate Chip Cookies

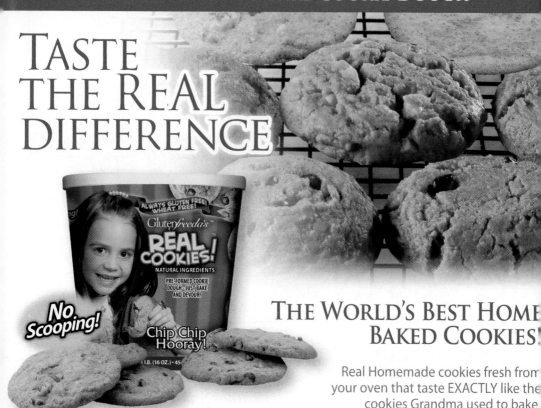

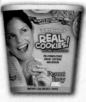
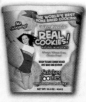
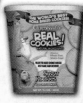

Chewy Chocolate Chip: Cookie Pack
Double Chocolate Brownie Cookies
Gingerbread Spice Cookies
Happy Apple Cookies
Lively Lemon Cookies
No-oats "Oatmeal" Cookies
Snickerdoodle Cookies
Snickerdoodle: Cookie Pack

Envirokidz
Vanilla Animal Cookies

French Meadow Bakery
All Natural Gluten-Free Chocolate Chip Cookies

Gluten-Free & Fabulous
Butterscotch Cookie Bites
Chocolate Chip Cookie Bites
Shortbread Cookie Bites

Glutino
Cookies - Chocolate Dreams
Cookies - Shortcake Dreams
Cookies - Vanilla Dreams
Cookies - Zebra Dreams

Ian's Natural Foods
Wheat Free Gluten Free Chocolate Chip Cookie Buttons
Wheat Free Gluten Free Crunchy Cinnamon Cookie Buttons

Manischewitz
Banana Split Macaroons
Cappuccino Chip Macaroons
Chocolate Chip Macaroons
Chocolate Chunk Cherry Macaroons
Chocolate Macaroons
Cinnamon Raisin Macaroons
Coconut Macaroons
Coffee Flavored Macaroons
Dark Chocolate Covered Macaroons
Fudgey Nut Brownie Macaroons
Honey Nut Macaroons
Maple Pecan Macaroons
Meringues (All)
Rocky Road Macaroons
Tender Coconut Patties
Toffee Crunch Macaroons
Ultimate Triple Chocolate Macaroons

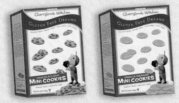

Mariposa Baking Company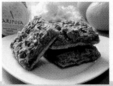
- Almond Biscotti
- Anise Almond Biscotti
- Biscotti Crumbs
- Biscotti Ends & Pieces
- Cinnamon Toast Biscotti
- Ginger Spice Biscotti
- Orange Walnut Biscotti
- Rustic Raisin Biscotti

Mi-Del Cookies
- Gluten-Free Arrowroot Animal Cookies
- Gluten-Free Chocolate Chip Cookies
- Gluten-Free Chocolate Sandwiches
- Gluten-Free Cinnamon Snaps
- Gluten-Free Ginger Snaps
- Gluten-Free Pecan Cookies
- Gluten-Free Royal Vanilla Sandwich Cookies

Nana's
- No Gluten Cookie - Chocolate
- No Gluten Cookie - Chocolate Crunch
- No Gluten Cookie - Ginger
- No Gluten Cookie - Lemon
- No Gluten Cookie Bars - Berry Vanilla
- No Gluten Cookie Bars - Chocolate Munch
- No Gluten Cookie Bars - Nana Banana
- No Gluten Nana's Cookie Bites

OrgraN
- OrgraN (All)

Pamela's Products
- Almond Anise Biscotti
- Butter Shortbread
- Chocolate Chip Walnut Cookies
- Chocolate Chunk Pecan Shortbread Organic Cookies
- Chocolate Walnut Biscotti
- Chunky Chocolate Chip Cookies
- Dark Chocolate-Chocolate Chunk Organic Cookies
- Espresso Chocolate Chunk Organic Cookies
- Ginger Cookies with Almonds
- Lemon Almond Biscotti
- Lemon Shortbread Cookies
- Old Fashioned Raisin Walnut Organic Cookies

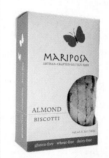

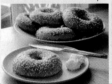
- Peanut Butter Chocolate Chip Organic Cookies
- Peanut Butter Cookies
- Pecan Shortbread Cookies
- Shortbread Swirl Cookies
- Simplebites - Chocolate Chip Mini Cookies
- Simplebites - Extreme Chocolate
- Simplebites - Mini Ginger Snapz
- Spicy Ginger Organic Cookies with Crystallized Ginger

Trader Joe's
- Flourless Chocolate Walnut Cookies
- Gluten Free Ginger Snaps
- Meringue Cookies (All)

CRACKERS

Blue Diamond Growers
- Nut-Thins Crackers (All)

Brown Rice Snaps
- Black Sesame (with Organic Brown Rice)

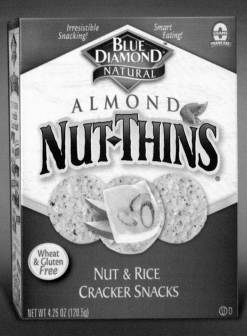

WHAT MORE COULD YOU WANT FROM A DELICIOUS TASTING CRACKER? OK THEY'RE GLUTEN FREE.

12 CRACKERS = 100 CALORIES

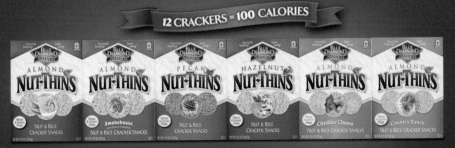

Indulge in a scrumptious line of crackers that are sure to satisfy. In fact, the only things missing are wheat, gluten,* trans fat and artificial ingredients. Try all 6 irresistible flavors with your favorite topping or all by themselves.

 Strong supporter of the Celiac Foundation

Cheddar (with Organic Brown Rice)
Onion Garlic
Salsa (with Organic Brown Rice)
Tamari Seaweed
Tamari Sesame
Toasted Onion (with Organic Brown Rice)
Unsalted Plain (with Organic Brown Rice)
Unsalted Sesame
Vegetable (with Organic Brown Rice)

Crunchmaster
Crunchmaster (All)

Eden Foods
Brown Rice Crackers
Nori Maki Rice Crackers

Ener-G
Cinnamon Crackers
Ener-G Gourmet Crackers
Gourmet Onion Crackers
Seattle Crackers

Gluten-Free & Fabulous
Sweet Savory Bites

Glutino
Breadsticks Pizza
Breadsticks Sesame
Crackers
Crackers - Cheddar
Crackers - Multigrain
Crackers - Original
Crackers - Vegetable

Hol-Grain
Brown Rice Crackers - Lightly Salted
Brown Rice Crackers - No Salt
Brown Rice Crackers - Onion & Garlic Flavor
Brown Rice Crackers - Organic Lightly Salted
Brown Rice Crackers - Sesame Lightly Salted

Lydia's Organics
Lydia's Organics (All)

Mary's Gone Crackers
Seed Cracker - Black Pepper
Seed Cracker - Caraway
Seed Cracker - Herb
Seed Cracker - Onion

Seed Cracker - Original
Sticks & Twigs - Chipotle Tomato
Sticks & Twigs - Curry
Sticks & Twigs - Sea Salt

Nu-World Amaranth
Amaranth Bar-B-Q Sweet & Sassy Snackers
Amaranth Chili-Lime Snackers
Amaranth French Onion Snackers
Amaranth Non-Dairy Cheddar Mini-Ridge
Amaranth Rosemary Basil Mini-Ridges

OrgraN
OrgraN (All)

Trader Joe's ()
Savory Thins - Minis
Savory Thins - Multiseed with Soy Sauce
Savory Thins - Original

DRIED FRUIT

Albertsons
Raisins

Craisins
Cherry
Orange
Original

Crunchies
100% Organic Bananas
100% Organic Mangoes
100% Organic Mixed Fruit
100% Organic Strawberries
Blueberries
Mangoes
Mixed Fruit
Pineapple
Raspberries
Strawberries
Strawberry/Banana
Tropical Fruit
Very Berry

Eden Foods
Dried Montmorency Tart Cherries
Organic Dried Cranberries
Organic Dried Wild Blueberries
Organic Wild Berry Mix

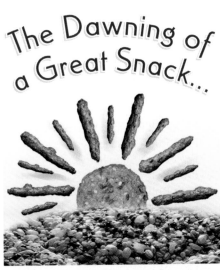

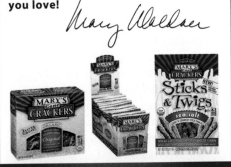
Hy-Vee
California Sun Dried Raisins
Dried Apples
Dried Apricots
Dried Blueberries
Dried Cherries
Dried Cranberries
Dried Mixed Berries
Dried Mixed Fruit
Dried Pineapple

Just Tomatoes
Just Tomatoes (All)

L'Esprit de Campagne ♆
Dried Apples
Dried Cherries
Dried Cranberries

Mariani
Dried Fruits (All BUT Vanilla and Chocolate Yogurt Raisins)

Meijer
Prunes - Pitted Canister
Prunes - Pitted-Rte Carton
Raisins (Canister)
Raisins - Seedless
Raisins - Seedless (Carton)

Newman's Own Organics
Dried Fruit - Apples
Dried Fruit - Apricots and Berry Blend
Dried Fruit - Cranberries and Pitted Prunes
Dried Fruit - Raisins

Publix ()
Dinosaurs Dry Fruit
Raisins
Rescue Heroes Dry Fruit
Sharks Dry Fruit
Snoopy Dry Fruit
Veggie Tales Dry Fruit

Safeway
Dried Fruit - Apples
Dried Fruit - Apricots
Dried Fruit - Cherries
Dried Fruit - Peaches
Dried Fruit - Prunes
Raisins

Sensible Foods
Sensible Foods (All)

Trader Joe's ()
Dried Fruit (All BUT Black Currants)
Welch's
Welch's (All)

Fruit Cups

Del Monte ()
Fruit Chillers (Metal & Plastic) (All)
Fruit Snack Cups (Metal & Plastic)
(All)
Hy-Vee
Diced Peaches Fruit Cups
Mandarin Orange Fruit Cups
Mixed Fruit - Fruit Cups
Pineapple Tidbit Fruit Cup
Tropical Fruit Cups
Kroger ()
Fruit - Cups

Fruit Snacks

Clif
Clif Kid Twisted Fruit
Fruit Flips (Save-A-Lot)
Fruit Rollups
Fruit Snacks
Giant
Build A Bear Fruit Snacks
Curious George Fruit Snacks
Dinosaur Fruit Snacks
Justice League Fruit Snacks
Peanuts Fruit Flavored Snacks
Sharks Fruit Snacks
Underwater World Fruit Snacks
Veggie Tales Fruit Snacks
Hy-Vee
Dinosaurs Fruit Snacks
Fruit Snacks (Variety Pack)
Sharks Fruit Snacks
Snoopy Fruit Snacks
Strawberry Fruit Rolls
Veggie Tales Fruit Snacks
Kellogg's
Fruit Flavored Snacks
Yogos

Kroger ()
Fruit Snacks
Laura Lynn (Ingle's)
Aliens Fruit Snacks
Animal Fruit Snacks
Creepy Fruit Snacks
Dinosaur Fruit Snacks
Meijer
Fruit Roll - Justice League Berry
Fruit Roll - Rescue Heroes
Fruit Roll - Strawberry
Fruit Roll - Strawberry Garfield
Fruit Roll - Wildberry Rush
Fruit Snack - Sharks
Fruit Snack - Veggie Tales
Fruit Snack - Dinosaurs
Fruit Snacks - Curious George
Fruit Snacks - Justice League
Fruit Snacks - Justice League Big Box
Fruit Snacks - Peanuts
Fruit Snacks - Rescue Heroes (Big Box)
Fruit Snacks - Variety Pack
Fruit Snacks - Variety Pack-Big Boy
Mixed Fruit Snacks
Safeway
Fruit Snacks (All)
Stop & Shop
Build A Bear Fruit Snacks
Curious George Fruit Snacks
Dinosaur Fruit Snacks
Justice League Fruit Snacks
Peanuts Fruit Flavored Snacks
Sharks Fruit Snacks
Tom & Jerry Fruit Snacks
Underwater World Fruit Snacks
Variety Pack Fruit Snacks
Veggie Tales Fruit Snacks
Stretch Island Fruit Company
Stretch Island Fruit Company (All)
Trader Joe's ()
Fruit Leathers (All)
Welch's
Welch's (All)

Gelatin Snacks & Mixes

Albertsons
Gelatin Fruit Cups

Flan Rico
Assorted Gelatin Snack
Parfait Gelatin Treat
Parfait Gelatin Treat # 3
Rainbow Gelatin
Rainbow Gelatin (Giant)
Vanilla Gelatin Treat

Gela (Save-A-Lot)
Gelatin & Instant Puddings

Giant
Cherry Gelatin Mix
Orange Gelatin Mix
Raspberry Gelatin Mix
Refrigerated Gelatin Fun Pack
Refrigerated Rainbow Fruit Gelatin
Refrigerated Rainbow Parfait
Refrigerated Sugar Free Gelatin - Black
Cherry
Refrigerated Sugar Free Gelatin -
Cherry
Refrigerated Sugar Free Gelatin -
Strawberry
Refrigerated Sugar Free Gelatin Fun
Pack

Hy-Vee
Cherry Gelatin
Cranberry Gelatin
Lemon Gelatin
Lime Gelatin
Orange Gelatin
Raspberry Gelatin
Strawberry Gelatin
Sugar Free Cherry Gelatin
Sugar Free Cranberry Gelatin
Sugar Free Lime Gelatin
Sugar Free Orange Gelatin
Sugar Free Raspberry Gelatin
Sugar Free Strawberry Gelatin

Jell-O
Black Cherry Sugar Free Low Calorie
Gelatin Dessert
Cherry Sugar Free Low Calorie Gelatin
Dessert
Cranberry Sugar Free Low Calorie
Gelatin Dessert
Lemon Sugar Free Low Calorie Gelatin
Dessert
Lime Sugar Free Low Calorie Gelatin
Dessert
Mixed Fruit Sugar Free Low Calorie
Gelatin Dessert
Orange Sugar Free Low Calorie Gelatin
Dessert
Peach Sugar Free Low Calorie Gelatin
Dessert
Raspberry Sugar Free Low Calorie
Gelatin Dessert
Strawberry Banana Sugar Free Low
Calorie Gelatin Dessert
Strawberry Kiwi Sugar Free Low
Calorie Gelatin Dessert
Strawberry Sugar Free Low Calorie
Gelatin Dessert
Tropical Blends Strawberry Kiwi Sugar
Free Low Calorie Gelatin Dessert
Berry Blue Gelatin Dessert
Black Cherry Gelatin Dessert
Cherry & Black Cherry Sugar Free
Gelatin Snacks
Cherry Gelatin Dessert
Cranberry Gelatin Dessert
Grape Gelatin Dessert
Island Pineapple Gelatin Dessert
Lemon Gelatin Dessert
Lime & Orange Variety Pack Sugar
Free Gelatin Snacks
Lime Gelatin Dessert
Margarita Limited Edition Gelatin
Dessert
Orange Gelatin Dessert
Peach & Watermelon Sugar Free
Gelatin Snacks
Peach Gelatin Dessert
Pear Chunks in Cherry Pomegranate
Gelatin Snacks
Pina Colada Limited Edition Gelatin
Dessert
Raspberry & Orange Sugar Free Gelatin
Snacks
Raspberry Gelatin Dessert
Real Chunks of Pineapple in Tropical

Fusion - Sugar Free Gelatin Snacks
Strawberry & Orange Gelatin Snacks
Strawberry & Orange Variety Pack
Sugar Free Gelatin Snacks
Strawberry & Raspberry Gelatin Snacks
Strawberry Banana Gelatin Dessert
Strawberry Daiquiri Limited Edition
Gelatin Dessert
Strawberry Gelatin Dessert
Strawberry Gelatin Snacks
Strawberry Kiwi Gelatin Dessert
Strawberry Sugar Free Gelatin Snacks
Strawberry-Kiwi & Tropical Berry
Sugar Free Gelatin Snacks
Watermelon Gelatin Dessert
Wild Strawberry Gelatin Dessert
X-Treme Cherry & Blue Raspberry Gel
Cups
X-Treme Watermelon & Green Apple
Gel Cups

Kool-Aid ⌐

Cherry Tropical Punch Gel Snacks
Groovalicious Grape Gel Snacks
Ice Blue Raspberry Gel Snacks
Oh Yeah Orange Gel Snacks
Soarin' Strawberry Gel Snacks

Kroger ()

Gelatin - Flavored
Gelatin - Plain
Gelatin - Snack Cups

Laura Lynn (Ingle's)

Gelatins RTE Dairy (All)

Meijer

Gelatin Dessert - Berry Blue
Gelatin Dessert - Cherry
Gelatin Dessert - Cherry Sugar Free
Gelatin Dessert - Cranberry
Gelatin Dessert - Cranberry Sugar Free
Gelatin Dessert - Grape
Gelatin Dessert - Lime
Gelatin Dessert - Lime Sugar Free
Gelatin Dessert - Orange
Gelatin Dessert - Orange Sugar Free
Gelatin Dessert - Raspberry
Gelatin Dessert - Raspberry Sugar Free
Gelatin Dessert - Strawberry
Gelatin Dessert - Strawberry Sugar Free

Gelatin Dessert - Strawberry Wild
Gelatin Dessert - Unflavored

Publix ()

Mandarin Oranges in Gel
Sugar Free Black Cherry & Cherry
Gelatin
Sugar Free Raspberry & Orange Gelatin
Sugar Free Strawberry Gelatin

Safeway

Gelatin Mix (All Flavors)
Instant Gelatins - Regular
Instant Gelatins - Sugar Free
Pineapple Lime Gel Cups

Stop & Shop

Cherry Gelatin Mix
Cranberry Gelatin Mix
Orange Gelatin Mix
Raspberry Gelatin Mix
Refrigerated Gelatin Fun Pack
Refrigerated Rainbow Fruit Gelatin
Refrigerated Rainbow Parfait
Refrigerated Sugar Free Gelatin Fun
Pack

GUM

5

5 Products (All)

Big Red

Big Red Gum

Doublemint

Doublemint Gum

Dubble Bubble

Dubble Bubble

Eclipse

Eclipse Gum

Extra

Extra Gum

Freedent

Freedent Gum

Hy-Vee

Dubble Bubble Gum

Juicy Fruit

Juicy Fruit Gum

Orbit

Orbit Gum

Orbit White Gum

Publix ()
Super Bubble Bubble Gum

Stride
Forever Fruit
Spearmint
Sweet Cinnamon
Sweet Peppermint
Winterblue

Trident
Trident (All Flavors)
Trident White (All Flavors)

Winterfresh
Winterfresh Gum

Wrigley
Wrigley's Spearmint Gum

NUTS & NUT MIXES

Albertsons
Peanuts, Dry Roast

Arrowhead Mills
Sesame Seeds
Sesame Seeds Whole

Carole's Soycrunch
Cinnamon Raisin
Coconut
Original
Sesame
Toffee

Earth Family
Organic Peanuts with Sea Salt

Eden Foods
All Mixed Up
All Mixed Up Too
Organic Pumpkin Seeds - Roasted & Salted
Organic Tamari Roasted Almonds
Organic Tamari Roasted Spicy Pumpkin Seeds

Fannie May
Assorted Nuts
Cashews

Fire Dancer
Fire Dancer Jalapeno Seasoned Peanuts

Frito Lay ()
Cashews
Deluxe Mixed Nuts
Flamin' Hot Flavored Sunflower Seeds
Honey Roasted Cashews
Honey Roasted Peanuts
Hot Peanuts
Praline Pecans
Ranch Sunflower Seeds
Salted Almonds
Salted Peanuts
Smoked Almonds
Sunflower Seed Kernels
Sunflower Seeds

Giant
Pina Colada Coated Cashews
Pistachios

Harrison Select Brand (Save-A-Lot)
Dry Roasted Peanuts

Hy-Vee
Black Walnuts
English Walnut Pieces
English Walnuts
Natural Almonds
Natural Sliced Almonds
Pecan Pieces
Pecans
Raw Spanish Peanuts
Salted Blanched Peanuts
Salted Spanish Peanuts
Slivered Almonds

Laura Lynn (Ingle's)
Cashew Halves
Deluxe Mixed Nuts
Dry Roast Nuts
Honey Roast Peanuts
Light Salt Cashews
Light Salt Dry Roast Nuts
Light Salt Mixed Nuts
Light Salt Peanuts
Mixed Nuts
Party Peanuts
Roasted Almonds
Smoked Almonds
Spanish Peanuts
Sunflower Seeds
Unsalted Dry Roast Nuts

Whole Cashews

Lydia's Organics

Lydia's Organics (All)

Manitoba Harvest ᛏ

Manitoba Harvest (All)

Meijer

Almonds - Blanched (Sliced)
Almonds - Blanched (Slivered)
Almonds - Natural (Sliced)
Almonds - Slivered
Almonds - Whole
Cashew Halves w/Pieces
Cashew Halves w/Pieces Lightly Salted
Cashews Whole
Nut Topping
Nuts - Blanched Peanuts
Nuts - Blanched Peanuts Slightly Salted
Nuts - Deluxe Mixed
Nuts - Mixed
Nuts - Mixed Lightly Salted
Peanuts - Dry Roasted
Peanuts - Dry Roasted Lightly Salted
Peanuts - Dry Roasted Unsalted
Peanuts - Honey Roasted
Peanuts - Hot & Spicy
Peanuts - Spanish
Pecan Chips
Pecan Halves
Pine Nuts
Sunflower Seeds
Sunflower Seeds Salted in Shell
Walnut Chips
Walnuts Black
Walnuts Halves & Pieces

Nut Harvest ()

Natural Honey Roasted Peanuts
Natural Lightly Roasted Almonds
Natural Nut & Fruit Mix
Natural Sea Salted Peanuts
Natural Sea Salted Whole Cashews

Planters ⌒

Pecan Halves
Cashews with Almonds & Pecans Select
Chopped Hazelnuts
Chopped Macadamias
Cocktail Peanuts
Deluxe Cashews, Almonds, Brazils,

Hazelnuts & Pecans
Deluxe Lightly Salted Mixed Nuts
Dry Roasted Cashews
Dry Roasted Lightly Salted Peanuts
Dry Roasted Peanuts
Dry Roasted Pistachios
Dry Roasted Sunflower Kernels
Dry Roasted Unsalted Peanuts
GoNuts - Lightly Salted Heart-Healthy
  Mix
Halves & Pieces - Cashews
Halves & Pieces - Lightly Salted
  Cashews
Halves & Pieces - Salted Cashews
Heat Peanuts
Honey & Dry Roasted Peanuts
Honey Peanuts & Cashews Sweet
  Roasts
Honey Roasted Big Bag Peanuts
Honey Roasted Cashews
Honey Roasted Mixed Nuts
Honey Roasted Peanuts
Jumbo Cashews
Lightly Salted Cocktail Peanuts
Lightly Salted Dry Roasted Peanuts
Lightly Salted Mixed Nuts
Macadamia Cashew Mix & Almonds
  Select
Macadamias
Mixed Nuts
Nut-Rition Almonds Lightly Salted
Nut-Rition Heart Healthy Mix
Nut-Rition Mix - Lightly Salted
Nut-Rition Smoked Almonds Lightly
  Salted
Party Pack Cocktail Peanuts
Party Pack Unsalted Cocktail Peanuts
Party Size Cocktail Peanuts
Pecan Halves
Pecan Lovers Mix with Cashews &
  Pistachios
Pecan Pieces
Pepitas Made with Pistachios, Peanuts
  & Almonds
Pine Nuts
Pistachio Lovers Mix with Cashews &
  Almonds
Raw Spanish Peanuts

Recipe Ready Almonds
Recipe Ready Black Walnuts
Recipe Ready Pecan Chips
Recipe Ready Pecan Halves
Recipe Ready Pecan Pieces
Recipe Ready Walnut Pieces
Recipe Ready Walnuts
Redskin Spanish Peanuts
Roasted & Salted Big Bag Sunflower
  Seeds
Roasted & Salted Sunflower Seeds
Roasted Salted Pepitas
Salted Big Bag Peanuts
Salted Cashews
Salted Peanuts
Sliced Almonds
Slivered Almonds
Smoked Almonds
Stadium Roasted In-Shell Salted
  Peanuts
Sunflower Kernels
Sunflower Kernels Big Bag
Sweet N' Crunchy Peanuts
Unsalted Cocktail Peanuts
Unsalted Mixed Nuts
Walnuts
Whole Cashews
Whole Honey Roasted Cashews
Whole Lightly Salted Cashews
Wicked Hot Chipotle Pepitas

Publix ()

Almonds - Natural Whole
Almonds - Salted
Almonds - Sliced
Cashews - Dry Roasted
Cashews - Halves & Pieces
Cashews - Lightly Salted (Halves &
  Pieces)
Cashews - Whole
Mixed Nuts
Mixed Nuts- Deluxe
Mixed Nuts- Dry Roasted
Mixed Nuts- Lightly Salted
Peanuts - Dry Roasted, Lightly Salted
Peanuts - Dry Roasted, Salted
Peanuts - Dry Roasted, Unsalted
Peanuts - Oil Roasted, Honey Roasted

Peanuts - Salted Party
Pecans
Pistachios
Sunflower Seeds
Walnuts

Sabritas ()

Picante Peanuts
Salt & Lime Peanuts

Safeway

Cashews - Halves & Pieces
Cashews - Whole
Dry Roasted Peanuts
Roasted/Salted Spanish Peanuts
Sunflower Seeds - Kernels

Seapoint Farms

Seapoint Farms

Select Brand (Safeway)

Baking Nuts - Almonds

Sensible Foods

Sensible Foods (All)

Trader Joe's ()

Almond Clusters
Almond Nut Meal
Almonds, Cranberries, Pistachio,
  Almond, and Cherry Mix
Cinnamon Almonds
Cocoa Almonds
Dry Roasted Edamame
Macadamia Nut Clusters
Marcona Almonds (All)
Nutty American Trek Mix
Pistachio, Almond & Cherry Mix
Pumpkin Seeds and Pepitas
Raw and Roasted Nuts (All)
Sunflower Seeds
Sweet & Spicy Peanuts
Very Crunchy Slightly Sweet Candied
  Mixed Nuts

Wine Nuts ☖

Chardonnay Wine Nus
Choco~Late Wine Nuts
Lemoncella Wine Nuts
Margarita Mix Wine Nuts
Merlot Wine Nuts

PICANTE SAUCE

Hy-Vee
Hot Picante Sauce
Medium Picante Sauce
Mild Picante Sauce

Kroger ()
Picante Sauce Salsa - Hot
Picante Sauce Salsa - Medium
Picante Sauce Salsa - Mild

Laura Lynn (Ingle's)
Picante (All)

Pace
Organic Picante - Medium
Organic Picante - Mild
Picante Sauces (All)

Tostitos ()
All Natural Medium Picante Sauce
All Natural Mild Picante Sauce

POPCORN

Arrowhead Mills
Whole Yellow Popcorn

Bachman
Asiago Peppercorn Popcorn
Buffalo Wing Popcorn
Cheese Popcorn
Garlic and Herb Popcorn
Lite Popcorn
Premium White Cheddar Popcorn
Regular Popcorn
White Cheddar Popcorn

Chester's ()
Butter Flavored Puffcorn Snacks
Cheddar Cheese Flavored Popcorn
Cheese Flavored Puffcorn Snacks

Cracker Jack ()
Original Caramel Coated Popcorn &
Peanuts

Eden Foods
Organic Popcorn

Giant
Microwave Popcorn - 94% Fat Free
Butter
Microwave Popcorn - Butter Flavored
- Light
Microwave Popcorn - Butter Flavored -
Regular
Microwave Popcorn - Kettle Corn
Microwave Popcorn - Movie Theatre
Butter Flavored
Microwave Popcorn - Natural Light
Microwave Popcorn - Sweet & Buttery
White Cheddar Popcorn
Yellow Popcorn

Herr's ()
Light Popcorn
Original Popcorn
White Cheddar Ranch Popcorn

Hy-Vee
94% Fat Free Butter Microwave
Popcorn
Butter Microwave Popcorn
Extra Butter Lite Microwave Popcorn
Extra Butter Microwave Popcorn
Kettle Microwave Popcorn
Light Butter Microwave Popcorn
Natural Flavor Microwave Popcorn
White Popcorn
Yellow Popcorn

Jolly Time
American's Best 94% Fat Free Butter
Flavor
Blast O Butter
Blast O Butter Light
Butter-Licious
Butter-Licious Light
Crispy 'N White
Crispy 'N White Light
Healthy Pop 94% Fat Free Butter Flavor
Healthy Pop 94% Fat Free Caramel
Apple
Healthy Pop 94% Fat Free Kettle Corn
Kernel Corn - American's Best White
Kernel Corn - American's Best Yellow
Kernel Corn - White Pop Corn
Kernel Corn - Yellow Pop Corn
KettleMania
Mallow Magic
Sassy Salsa
Sea Salt & Cracked Pepper
The Big Cheez

White & Buttery

Kroger ( )
Plain Popcorn Kernels

Laura Lynn (Ingle's)
Popcorn (All)

LesserEvil
LesserEvil Snacks

Meijer
Caramel Corn
Cheese Popcorn
Chicago Style Popcorn
Popcorn
Popcorn - Micro Kettle Sweet & Salty
Popcorn - Microwave 94% Fat Free
Popcorn - Microwave Butter
Popcorn - Microwave Butter 75% Ft Fr
Popcorn - Microwave Butter GP
Popcorn - Microwave Extra Butter
Popcorn - Microwave Extra Butter GP
Popcorn - Microwave Extra Butter Lite
Popcorn - Microwave Hot N' Spicy
Popcorn - Microwave Natural Lite
Popcorn - White
Popcorn - Yellow
Purple Cow Butter Popcorn
White Cheddar Popcorn

Newman's Own
Microwave Popcorn - 94% Fat Free
Microwave Popcorn - Butter
Microwave Popcorn - Butter Boom
Microwave Popcorn - Light Butter
Microwave Popcorn - Natural
Microwave Popcorn - Natural 100
  Calorie Mini Bags
Microwave Popcorn - Tender White
  Kernel
Microwave Popcorn - White Cheddar
  Cheese
Popcorn - Jars (Regular Pop)

Newman's Own Organics
Butter Flavored Pop's Corn ( )
Light Butter Pop's Corn ( )
No Butter/No Salt Pop's Corn ( )

Old Dutch Foods
Premium Gourmet White Popcorn (non-
  flavored)

Puffcorn - (non-flavored; ensure
  package reads "Made in The USA")

Oogie's
Oogie's Snacks (All)

Publix ( )
Popcorn (Deli)

Robert's American Gourmet ( )
Snacks (All BUT CHAOS, Honey
  Wheat Pretzels, Veggie Tubes and
  Tubes)

Safeway
Microwave Popcorn (All Varieties)
Popcorn - Light Butter Microwave
Popcorn - Yellow & Kettle

Smartfood ( )
Reduced Fat White Cheddar Cheese
  Flavored Popcorn
White Cheddar Cheese Flavored
  Popcorn

Snyder's of Hanover
Butter Popcorn

Stop & Shop
Microwave Popcorn - 94% Fat Free
  Butter
Microwave Popcorn - Butter Flavored
Microwave Popcorn - Butter Light
Microwave Popcorn - Kettle Corn
Microwave Popcorn - Movie Theatre
  Butter Flavored
Microwave Popcorn - Natural Light
Microwave Popcorn - Sweet & Buttery
Yellow Popcorn

Trader Joe's ( )
Buccaneer Joes White Cheddar Corn
  Puffs
Chocolate Drizzled Peppermint Caramel
  Corn
Cranberry Nut Clusters Popcorn
Fat Free Caramel Popcorn
Gourmet White Popcorn
Lite Popcorn 50% Less Salt
White Cheddar Popcorn

Utz
Butter Popcorn
Cheese Popcorn
Hulless Caramel Puff'n Corn

Hulless Cheese Puff'n Corn
Hulless Original Puff'n Corn
White Cheddar Popcorn

PORK SKINS & RINDS

Baken-Ets ()
Fried Pork Skins
Hot 'N Spicy Flavored Pork Skins
Salt & Vinegar Fried Pork Skins

Golden Flake ()
Hot Pork Skins
Pork Skins and Pork Cracklins
Sweet Heat Pork Skins
Vinegar & Salt Pork Cracklins
Vinegar & Salt Pork Skins

Herr's ()
BBQ Flavored Pork Rinds
Original Pork Rinds

PRETZELS

Ener-G
Crisp Pretzels
Sesame Pretzel Rings
Wylde Poppyseed Pretzels
Wylde Pretzels
Wylde Sesame Pretzels

Glutino ⛎
Pretzels - Family Bag
Pretzels - Sesame Rings
Pretzels - Snack Pack
Pretzels - Sticks
Pretzels - Sticks Family Bag
Pretzels - Twists
Pretzels - Unsalted

PUDDING & PUDDING MIXES

Concord Foods
Banana Cream Pie Mix
Banana Crème Pudding & Pie Filling

Flan Rico
12 Pack Assorted Tray # 1
12 Pack Assorted Tray # 6
24 Pack Assorted Tray # 5
Caramel Cream

Caramel Flan Ring Molds
Caramel Rice Pudding
Creamy Flan Pudding
Parfait Treat
Parfait Treat (Giant)
Parfait Treat Ring Molds
Rain/Van Combo Pack # 4
Rainbow Triple Treat
Rainbow Triple Treat # 2
Rainbow Vanilla Combo Pack
Rice Pudding
Rice Pudding Ring Molds
Vanilla Milk Base

Gela (Save-A-Lot)
Gelatin & Instant Puddings

Giant
Butterscotch Pudding Mix
Chocolate Fudge Pudding Snack Cups
Chocolate Instant Pudding and Pie
    Filling
Chocolate Pudding Snack Cups - Fat
    Free
Chocolate Pudding Snack Cups -
    Regular
Refrigerated Chocolate Pudding - Fat
    Free
Refrigerated Chocolate Pudding -
    Regular
Refrigerated Chocolate/Vanilla Pudding
    - Fat Free
Refrigerated Chocolate/Vanilla Pudding
    - Regular
Rice Pudding
Tapioca Pudding Mix
Vanilla Pudding Snack Cups

Handi-Snacks Pudding ᑲ
Banana Pudding
Banana Split Pudding Doubles
Butterscotch Pudding
Chocolate Chip Cookie Pudding
    Doubles
Chocolate Pudding
Chocolate Vanilla Pudding Doubles
Fudge Rocky Road Pudding Doubles
Rice Pudding
Vanilla Pudding

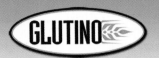

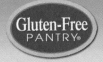

www.glutino.com
www.glutenfreepantry.com
1.800.363.3438

Committed to helping people who have Celiac disease and other food intolerances since 1983.

Candy Bars

Crackers

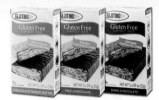

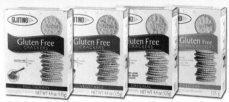

Pretzels

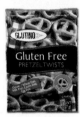

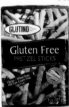

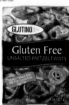

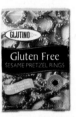

Hy-Vee

Butterscotch Pudding Cups
Chocolate Fudge Pudding Cups
Chocolate Pudding Cups
Cooked Chocolate Pudding
Cooked Vanilla Pudding
Fat Free Chocolate Pudding Cups
Instant Butterscotch Pudding
Instant Chocolate Pudding
Instant Fat Free/Sugar Free Chocolate
  Pudding
Instant Fat Free/Sugar Free Vanilla
  Pudding
Instant Lemon Pudding
Instant Pistachio Pudding
Instant Vanilla Pudding
Tapioca Pudding Cups
Vanilla Pudding Cups

Jell-O

Americana Fat Free Rice Pudding
Banana Cream Cook & Serve Pudding
  & Pie Filling
Banana Cream Instant Pudding & Pie
  Filling

Banana Cream Instant Sugar Free & Fat
  Free Pudding & Pie Filling
Butterscotch Cook & Serve Pudding &
  Pie Filling
Butterscotch Instant Pudding & Pie
  Filling
Butterscotch Instant Sugar Free & Fat
  Free Pudding & Pie Filling
Cheesecake Instant Pudding & Pie
  Filling
Cheesecake Instant Sugar Free & Fat
  Free Pudding & Pie Filling
Chocolate Cook & Serve Pudding & Pie
  Filling
Chocolate Cook & Serve Sugar Free
  Pudding & Pie Filling
Chocolate Fat Free Pudding Snacks
Chocolate Fudge Cook & Serve
  Pudding & Pie Filling
Chocolate Fudge Instant Pudding & Pie
  Filling
Chocolate Fudge Instant Sugar Free &
  Fat Free Pudding & Pie Filling
Chocolate Fudge Sundaes Pudding

ALWAYS READ LABELS

Snacks
Chocolate Instant Pudding & Pie Filling
Chocolate Instant Sugar Free & Fat Free
Pudding & Pie Filling
Chocolate Pudding Snacks
Chocolate Sugar Free & Fat Free Instant
Pudding & Pie Filling
Chocolate Sugar Free Cook & Serve
Pudding & Pie Filling
Chocolate Sugar Free Pudding Snacks
Chocolate Vanilla Swirls Fat Free
Pudding Snacks
Chocolate Vanilla Swirls Pudding
Snacks
Chocolate Vanilla Swirls Sugar Free
Pudding Snacks
Coconut Cream Cook & Serve Pudding
& Pie Filling
Coconut Cream Instant Pudding & Pie
Filling
Creamy Caramel Sugar Free Pudding
Snacks
Devil's Food & Chocolate Fat Free
Pudding Snacks
Devil's Food Fat Free Instant Pudding
& Pie Filling
Double Chocolate Sugar Free Pudding
Snacks
French Vanilla Instant Pudding & Pie
Filling
Lemon Cook & Serve Pudding & Pie
Filling
Lemon Instant Pudding & Pie Filling
Lemon Instant Sugar Free & Fat Free
Pudding & Pie Filling
Mixed Berry Smoothie Snacks
Oreo Pudding Snacks
Pistachio Instant Pudding & Pie Filling
Pistachio Instant Sugar Free & Fat Free
Pudding & Pie Filling
Pumpkin Spice Instant Pudding & Pie
Filling
Strawberries & Crème Swirled Pudding
Snacks - Crème Savers
Strawberry Banana Smoothie Snacks
Strawberry Cheesecake Snacks
Sundae Toppers Chocolate with
Chocolate Topping Pudding

Sundae Toppers Vanilla with Caramel
Topping Pudding Snacks
Sundae Toppers Vanilla with Chocolate
Topping Pudding
Tapioca Fat Free Cook & Serve Pudding
Tapioca Fat Free Pudding Snacks
Tapioca Pudding Snacks
Vanilla & Chocolate 100 Calorie Packs
Fat Free Pudding Snacks
Vanilla Caramel Sundaes 100 Calorie
Packs Fat Free Pudding Snacks
Vanilla Cook & Serve Pudding & Pie
Filling
Vanilla Cook & Serve Sugar Free
Pudding & Pie Filling
Vanilla Instant Pudding & Pie Filling
Vanilla Instant Sugar Free & Fat Free
Pudding & Pie Filling
Vanilla Pudding Snacks
Vanilla Sugar Free & Fat Free Instant
Pudding & Pie Filling
Vanilla Sugar Free Pudding Snacks
White Chocolate Fat Free Instant
Pudding & Pie Filling
White Chocolate Instant Sugar Free &
Fat Free Pudding & Pie Filling
X-Treme Chocolate Pudding Sticks

Junket
Junket (All BUT Hansen Island
Microwavable Fudge Mix)

Kozy Shack
Puddings (All)

Kroger ()
Pudding - Boxed
Pudding - Snack Cups

Laura Lynn (Ingle's)
Puddings RTE Dairy (All)

Lifeway
Lifeway (All)

Meijer
Pudding - Cook & Serve Butterscotch
Pudding - Cook & Serve Chocolate
Pudding - Cook & Serve Vanilla
Pudding & Pie Filling Instant -
Chocolate
Pudding & Pie Filling Instant - Coconut
Cream

Pudding & Pie Filling Instant - French Vanilla
Pudding & Pie Filling Instant - Pistachio
Pudding & Pie Filling Instant - Vanilla
Pudding Instant - Banana Cream
Pudding Instant - Butterscotch FF & SF
Pudding Instant - Chocolate FF & SF
Pudding Instant - Vanilla FF & SF
Pudding Premium - Chocolate Peanut Butter
Pudding Premium - French Vanilla
Pudding Premium - Orange Dream
Pudding Snack - Banana
Pudding Snack - Butterscotch
Pudding Snack - Chocolate
Pudding Snack - Chocolate Fat Free
Pudding Snack - Chocolate Fudge
Pudding Snack - Multi-Pack Chocolate & Vanilla
Pudding Snack - Tapioca
Pudding Snack - Vanilla

Mori-Nu
Mates Chocolate Pudding Mix
Mates Lemon Crème Pudding Mix
Mates Vanilla Pudding Mix

Publix ()
Chocolate Pudding
Fat Free Chocolate Pudding
Fat Free Chocolate-Vanilla Swirl Pudding
Rice Pudding
Sugar Free Chocolate-Vanilla Swirl Pudding
Tapioca Pudding

Safeway
Pudding - Instant
Pudding Cups

Stop & Shop
Butterscotch Pudding Mix
Chocolate Fudge Pudding Snack Cups
Chocolate Instant Pudding & Pie Filling
Chocolate Pudding Snack Cups
Instant Low Calorie Vanilla Pudding & Pie Mix
Refrigerated Chocolate Pudding
Refrigerated Chocolate/Vanilla Pudding

Refrigerated Fat Free Chocolate Pudding
Refrigerated Fat Free Chocolate/Vanilla Pudding
Rice Pudding
Sugar Free Chocolate Instant Pudding Mix
Tapioca Pudding Mix
Vanilla Pudding Snack Cups

Trader Joe's ()
Puddings - Chocolate
Puddings - Rice
Puddings - Tapioca

RICE CAKES

Giant
Rice Cakes - Plain Unsalted
Rice Cakes - Sour Cream & Onion

Kroger ()
Plain Rice Cakes
Salted Rice Cakes

Lundberg Family Farms
Eco-Farmed Rice Cakes - Brown Rice
Eco-Farmed Rice Cakes - Brown Rice (Salt Free)
Organic Rice Cakes - Brown Rice
Organic Rice Cakes - Brown Rice (Salt Free)
Organic Rice Cakes - Caramel Corn
Organic Rice Cakes - Cinnamon Toast
Organic Rice Cakes - Koku Seaweed
Organic Rice Cakes - Mochi Sweet
Organic Rice Cakes - Popcorn
Organic Rice Cakes - Sesame Tamari
Organic Rice Cakes - Sweet Green Tea with Lemon
Organic Rice Cakes - Tamari with Seaweed
Organic Rice Cakes - Wild Rice

Publix ()
Lightly Salted Rice Cakes
Mini Caramel Rice
Mini Cheddar Rice
Mini Ranch Rice
Unsalted Rice Cakes
White Cheddar Rice Cakes

Stop & Shop
Apple Cinnamon Rice Cakes
Rice Cakes - Caramel
Rice Cakes - Plain Salted & Unsalted
Rice Cakes - Sesame Unsalted
Rice Cakes - Sour Cream & Onion
Rice Cakes - White Cheddar

Trader Joe's ()
Lightly Salted Rice Cakes

TRAIL MIX

Bear Naked ()
High Sierra Blend Organic Trail Mix
Pacific Crest Organic Trail Mix

Enjoy Life Foods 👣 👣
Not Nuts! Beach Bash Trail Mix
Not Nuts! Mountain Mambo Trail Mix

Frito Lay ()
Original Trail Mix

Hy-Vee
Chocolate & Nut Trail Mix
Chocolate Nut Trail Mix
Raisin & Nut Trail Mix
Raisin Nut Trail Mix
Tropical Trail Mix

Planters 👣
Fruit & Nut Mix Trail Mix
Mixed Nuts & Raisins Trail Mix
Nut & Chocolate Mix Snack Packs Trail
   Mix
Nut & Chocolate Mix Trail Mix
Nuts, Seeds & Raisins Trail Mix

Safeway
Trail Mix with Candy Pieces

Trader Joe's ()
Antioxidant Nut and Berry Mix
Cranberry Trail Mix
Go Raw Trek Mix
Organic Trek Mix with Chocolate Chips
Rainbows End Trail Mix
Simply Almonds, Cashews &
   Cranberries Trek Mix
Simply The Best Trek Mix
Spicy Almonds, Cashews & Cranberries
   Trek Mix

Sweet, Savory & Tart Trek Mix
Tempting Trail Mix

MISCELLANEOUS

Corn Nuts 👣
Barbecue Crunchy Corn Snack
Chile Picante Crunchy Corn Snack
Nacho Cheese Crunchy Corn Snack
Original Crunchy Corn Snack
Ranch Crunchy Corn Snack
Salsa Jalisco Crunchy Corn Snack

Crunchies
100% Organic Peas
Corn Snack
Edamame
Grilled Edamame
Roasted Veggies
Salted Edamame
Tamari Edamame

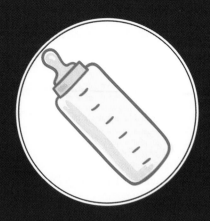

BABY FOOD & FORMULA

BABY FOOD

Beech-Nut

Good Evening Whole Grain Brown Rice Cereal

Rice Cereal

Stage 1 Fruits - Applesauce

Stage 1 Fruits - Chiquita Bananas

Stage 1 Fruits - Pears

Stage 1 Fruits - Prunes

Stage 1 Fruits Vegetables - Beginner Basics Assorted Fruit & Vegetable 18 Pk

Stage 1 Meats - Beef & Beef Broth

Stage 1 Meats - Chicken & Chicken Broth

Stage 1 Meats - Turkey & Turkey Broth

Stage 1 Meats - Veal & Veal Broth

Stage 1 Vegetables - Butternut Squash

Stage 1 Vegetables - Tender Golden Sweet Potatoes

Stage 1 Vegetables - Tender Sweet Carrots

Stage 1 Vegetables - Tender Sweet Peas

Stage 1 Vegetables - Tender Young Green Beans

Stage 2 Cereals - Rice Cereal & Apples with Cinnamon

Stage 2 Desserts - Dutch Apple Dessert

Stage 2 Desserts - Fruit Dessert

Stage 2 Desserts - Vanilla Custard Pudding with Apples

Stage 2 Dinners - Apples & Chicken

Stage 2 Dinners - Chicken & Rice Dinner

Stage 2 Dinners - Chicken Noodle Dinner

Stage 2 Dinners - Four Delicious Dinner Varieties 18 Pack

Stage 2 Dinners - Homestyle Chicken Soup

Stage 2 Dinners - Macaroni & Beef with Vegetables

Stage 2 Dinners - Pineapple Glazed Ham

Stage 2 Dinners - Sweet Potatoes & Chicken

Stage 2 Dinners - Turkey Rice Dinner

Stage 2 Dinners - Vegetables & Beef

Stage 2 Dinners - Vegetables & Chicken

Stage 2 Dinners - Vegetables & Ham

Stage 2 Dinners Good Evening - Creamy Chicken Noodle Dinner

Stage 2 Dinners Good Evening - Ginger Chicken & Veggies

Stage 2 Dinners Good Evening - Ham, Pineapple & Rice

Stage 2 Dinners Good Evening - Hearty Vegetable Stew

Stage 2 Dinners Good Evening - Sweet Potato & Turkey

Stage 2 Dinners Good Evening - Turkey Tetrazzini

Stage 2 Fruit Yogurts - Banana Apple Yogurt

Stage 2 Fruits - Apples & Bananas

Stage 2 Fruits - Apples & Blueberries

Stage 2 Fruits - Apples & Cherries

Stage 2 Fruits - Apples & Pears

Stage 2 Fruits - Apples, Mango & Kiwi

Stage 2 Fruits - Apples, Pears & Bananas

Stage 2 Fruits - Applesauce

Stage 2 Fruits - Applesauce 4 Pack

Stage 2 Fruits - Apricots with Pears & Apples

Stage 2 Fruits - Chiquita Bananas

Stage 2 Fruits - Chiquita Bananas & Strawberries

Stage 2 Fruits - Chiquita Bananas 4 Pack

Stage 2 Fruits - Chiquita Bananas with Pears & Apples

Stage 2 Fruits - Cinnamon Raisin Pears with Apples

Stage 2 Fruits - Four Delicious Fruit Varieties 18 Pack

Stage 2 Fruits - Peaches

Stage 2 Fruits - Peaches & Bananas

Stage 2 Fruits - Pears

Stage 2 Fruits - Pears & Pineapple

Stage 2 Fruits - Pears & Raspberries

Stage 2 Fruits - Pears 4 Pack

Stage 2 Fruits - Plums with Apples & Pears

Stage 2 Fruits - Prunes with Pears

Stage 2 Fruits Desserts Dha Plus - Dha Plus+ Apple Delight

Stage 2 Fruits Dha Plus - Dha Plus+ Banana Supreme

Stage 2 Fruits Hispanic Variety - Guava

Stage 2 Fruits Hispanic Variety - Mango

Stage 2 Fruits Hispanic Variety - Papaya

Stage 2 Fruits Vegetables - Sweet Potatoes & Apples

Stage 2 Vegetables - Butternut Squash

Stage 2 Vegetables - Carrots & Peas

Stage 2 Vegetables - Corn & Sweet Potatoes

Stage 2 Vegetables - Country Garden Vegetables

Stage 2 Vegetables - Four Delicious Vegetable Varieties 18 Pack

Stage 2 Vegetables - Mixed Vegetables

Stage 2 Vegetables - Sweet Corn Casserole

Stage 2 Vegetables - Tender Golden Sweet Potatoes

Stage 2 Vegetables - Tender Sweet Carrots

Stage 2 Vegetables - Tender Sweet Peas

Stage 2 Vegetables - Tender Young Green Beans

Stage 2 Vegetables Dha Plus - Dha Plus+ Carrots

Stage 2 Vegetables Dha Plus - Dha Plus+ Garden Vegetables

Stage 2 Vegetables Dha Plus - Dha Plus+ Sweet Potatoes

Stage 3 Cereals - Rice Cereal & Pears

Stage 3 Desserts - Banana Pudding

Stage 3 Desserts - Fruit Dessert

Stage 3 Dinners - Country Vegetables & Chicken

Stage 3 Dinners - Good Evening Country Vegetables with Beef

Stage 3 Dinners - Good Evening Vegetable Turkey Dinner

Stage 3 Dinners - Turkey Rice Dinner

Stage 3 Fruits - Apples & Bananas

Stage 3 Fruits - Apples & Cherries

Stage 3 Fruits - Applesauce

Stage 3 Fruits - Chiquita Bananas

Stage 3 Fruits - Peaches

Stage 3 Fruits - Pears

Stage 3 Vegetables - Carrots & Peas

Stage 3 Vegetables - Green Beans, Corn & Rice

Stage 3 Vegetables - Sweet Potatoes

Table Time - Apple Dices in White Grape Juice from Concentrate

Table Time - Carrot Dices

Table Time - Green Bean Dices

Table Time - Pear Dices in White Grape Juice From Concentrate

Table Time Dinners - Turkey Stew with Rice

Meijer

Little Fruit - Apple

Little Fruit - Strawberry/Banana

Little Veggies - Corn

BABY JUICE & OTHER DRINKS

Beech-Nut

Apple Juice

Dha Plus+ Yogurt Blends with Juice-

Mixed Berry

Dha Plus+ Yogurt Blends with Juice-
Tropical Fruit

Gentle Juice Variety Pack

Good Evening Veggie Delight Juice

Good Morning Chiquita Banana Juice
with Yogurt

Juice Blends Variety Pack

Mixed Fruit Juice

Pear Juice

White Grape Juice

Bright Beginnings

Pediatric Nutrition Drinks (All)

Hy-Vee

Mother's Choice Infant Water

Mother's Choice Infant Water with
Fluoride

Mother's Choice Pediatric Vanilla Drink

Mother's Choice Pediatric Vanilla with
Fiber Drink

Meijer

Bright Beginnings Soy Vanilla PND

Chocolate PND

Gluco-Burst - Arctic Cherry

Gluco-Burst - Chocolate Diabetic
Nutritional Drink

Strawberry PND

Van w/Fiber PND

Vanilla Pediatric Nutritional Drink

Vanilla Soy PND

PediaSure

PediaSure Products

FORMULA

Bright Beginnings

Infant Formulas (All)

EnfaCare

Pediatric Products (All)

Enfamil

Pediatric Products (All)

Meijer

Follow-On w/DHA

Gentle Protein w/DHA

Lactose Free w/DHA

Milk w/DHA

Regular Term Formula

Soy Term Formula

Soy w/DHA

Nestlé ()

Infant Formulas (All)

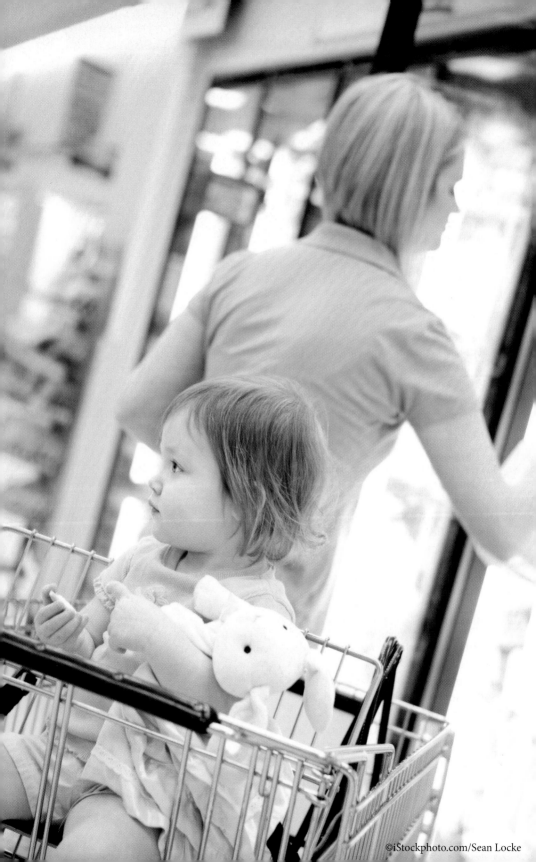

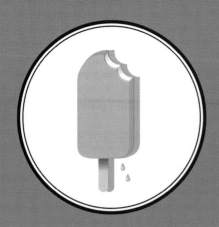

FROZEN FOODS

BEANS

Albertsons
Frozen Beans

Hy-Vee
Frozen Baby Lima Beans

Nature's Promise (Stop & Shop)
Organic Edamame in Pod

Publix ()
Spec. Butter Beans

Giant
Baby Lima Beans

Fordhook Lima Beans

Stop & Shop
Baby Lima Beans
Fordhook Lima Beans

COOKIE DOUGH

French Meadow Bakery
All Natural Gluten-Free Chocolate Chip
Cookie Dough

Gluten-Free Pantry, The
Buckwheat Raisin Cookie Dough

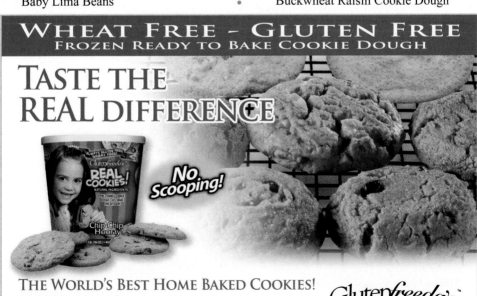
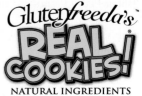

Chocolate Chunk Cookie Dough

Glutenfreeda Real Cookies! ႘ ႘

Chip Chip Hooray!
Chocolate Minty Python
Peanut Envy
Peanut, Paul & Mary
Snicker Poodles
Sugar Kookies

Trader Joe's ()

Gluten Free Peanut Butter Cookie
Dough

FROZEN YOGURT

Dreyer's

see Edy's (same parent company)

Edy's

Fat Free Yogurt - Vanilla
Slow Churned Yogurt Blends - Black
Cherry Vanilla Swirl
Slow Churned Yogurt Blends -
Cappuccino Chip
Slow Churned Yogurt Blends - Caramel
Praline Crunch
Slow Churned Yogurt Blends -
Chocolate Vanilla Swirl
Slow Churned Yogurt Blends - Peach
Slow Churned Yogurt Blends -
Strawberry
Slow Churned Yogurt Blends - Vanilla

Hood

Chocolate Almond Praline Frozen
Yogurt
Fat Free Double Raspberry Frozen
Yogurt

Lucerne (Safeway)

Fat Free Vanilla Frozen Yogurt

Publix ()

Black Cherry Premium Low Fat Frozen
Yogurt
Butter Pecan Premium Low Fat Frozen
Yogurt
Chocolate Premium Low Fat Frozen
Yogurt
Neapolitan Premium Low Fat Frozen
Yogurt
Peach Premium Low Fat Frozen Yogurt

Peanut Butter Cup Premium Low Fat
Frozen Yogurt
Strawberry Premium Low Fat Frozen
Yogurt
Vanilla Orange Premium Low Fat
Frozen Yogurt
Vanilla Premium Low Fat Frozen
Yogurt

Turkey Hill

Frozen Yogurt - Chocolate Cherry
Cordial
Frozen Yogurt - Chocolate
Marshmallow
Frozen Yogurt - Fudge Ripple
Frozen Yogurt - Neapolitan
Frozen Yogurt - Nutty Caramel Caribou
(Limited Edition)
Frozen Yogurt - Vanilla Bean
Frozen Yogurt Smoothie - Orange
Cream Swirl
Frozen Yogurt Smoothie - Peach Mango
Frozen Yogurt Smoothie - Pomegranate
Blueberry & Cream with Açai
Frozen Yogurt Smoothie - Raspberry
Lemonade

WholeSoy & Co. ႘

Soy Frozen Yogurt (All)

FRUIT

Albertsons

Frozen Fruit

Europe's Best

Fruits (All)

Giant

Berry Medley
Blackberries
Blueberries
Dark Sweet Cherries
Mango
Mixed Fruit
Peaches
Pineapple
Raspberries - in Syrup
Raspberries - Plain
Sliced Strawberries - Plain
Sliced Strawberries - with Artificial

Sweetener
Sliced Strawberries - with Sugar
Strawberries

Hy-Vee
Frozen Blueberries
Frozen Cherry Berry Blend
Frozen Red Raspberries
Frozen Sliced Strawberries
Frozen Whole Strawberries

Kroger ()
Plain Frozen Fruit

Meijer
Frozen Berry Medley
Frozen Blackberries
Frozen Blueberries
Frozen Dark Sweet Cherries
Frozen Mango Chunks
Frozen Mango Sliced
Frozen Mixed Fruit
Frozen Organic Blueberries
Frozen Organic Peaches
Frozen Organic Raspberries
Frozen Organic Strawberries
Frozen Pineapple Chunks
Frozen Raspberries
Frozen Raspberries - Individually Qk
   Frozen
Frozen Sliced Peaches
Frozen Strawberries - Individually Qk
   Frozen
Frozen Strawberries - Sliced
Frozen Tart Cherries
Frozen Triple Berry Blend
Frozen Tropical Fruit Blend

Publix ()
Blackberries
Blueberries
Cherries - Dark Sweet
Cranberries
Mixed Berries
Mixed Fruit
Peaches - Sliced
Raspberries
Strawberries - Sliced, Sweetened
Strawberries - Whole

Stop & Shop
Berry Medley

Blackberries
Blueberries
Dark Sweet Cherries
Mango
Mixed Fruit
Peaches
Pineapple
Raspberries
Raspberries in Syrup
Sliced Strawberries
Sliced Strawberries in Sugar
Sliced Strawberries with Artificial
   Sweetener
Strawberries

Wyman's
Wyman's (All)

ICE CREAM

Dreyer's
also see Edy's (same parent company)
Grand Ice Cream - Coffee
New and Exciting Fun Flavors - Mocha
   Almond Fudge

Edy's
Fat Free No Sugar Added - Chocolate
   Fudge
Fat Free No Sugar Added - Vanilla
   Chocolate
Grand Ice Cream - Chocolate
Grand Ice Cream - Chocolate Chip
Grand Ice Cream - Double Vanilla
Grand Ice Cream - French Vanilla
Grand Ice Cream - Mint Chocolate Chip
Grand Ice Cream - Neapolitan
Grand Ice Cream - Rocky Road
Grand Ice Cream - Strawberry
Grand Ice Cream - Vanilla
Grand Ice Cream - Vanilla Bean
Grand Ice Cream - Vanilla Chocolate
Grand Ice Cream - Vanilla Fudge Swirl
Grand Ice Cream Pints - Chocolate
Grand Ice Cream Pints - Mint Chocolate
   Chip
Grand Ice Cream Pints - Strawberry
Grand Ice Cream Pints - Vanilla
Limited Edition - Banana Nut

Limited Edition - Banana Split
Limited Edition - Eggnog
Limited Edition - Mango
Limited Edition - Peppermint
Limited Edition - Pineapple Coconut
Limited Edition - Pumpkin
Limited Edition - Root Beer Float
Loaded - Chocolate Peanut Butter Cup
Loaded - Nestle Butterfinger
New and Exciting Fun Flavors - Butter Pecan
New and Exciting Fun Flavors - Cherry Chocolate Chip
New and Exciting Fun Flavors - Dulce de Leche
New and Exciting Fun Flavors - Espresso Chip (Edy's Brand Only)
New and Exciting Fun Flavors - Peanut Butter Cup
New and Exciting Fun Flavors - Spumoni
New and Exciting Maxx Pints - Chocolate Peanut Butter Chunk
New and Exciting Maxx Pints - Nestle Butterfinger
Slow Churned Light - Butter Pecan
Slow Churned Light - Caramel Delight
Slow Churned Light - Chocolate
Slow Churned Light - Chocolate Chips
Slow Churned Light - Chocolate Fudge Chunk
Slow Churned Light - Coffee
Slow Churned Light - French Vanilla
Slow Churned Light - Fudge Tracks
Slow Churned Light - Mint Chocolate Chips
Slow Churned Light - Neapolitan
Slow Churned Light - Peanut Butter Cup
Slow Churned Light - Raspberry Chip Royale
Slow Churned Light - Rocky Road
Slow Churned Light - Strawberry
Slow Churned Light - Take The Cake
Slow Churned Light - Vanilla
Slow Churned Light - Vanilla Bean
Slow Churned Limited Edition - Eggnog
Slow Churned Limited Edition - Most Orange-inal (American Idol)
Slow Churned Limited Edition - One Split Wonder (American Idol)
Slow Churned Limited Edition - Peppermint
Slow Churned Limited Edition - Pumpkin
Slow Churned Limited Edition - Winning Idol Flavor
Slow Churned No Sugar Added - Butter Pecan
Slow Churned No Sugar Added - Coffee
Slow Churned No Sugar Added - French Vanilla
Slow Churned No Sugar Added - Fudge Tracks
Slow Churned No Sugar Added - Mint Chocolate Chip
Slow Churned No Sugar Added - Neapolitan
Slow Churned No Sugar Added - Triple Chocolate
Slow Churned No Sugar Added - Vanilla
Slow Churned No Sugar Added - Vanilla Bean

Giant

Andes Crème De Methe Ice Cream
Black Cherry Ice Cream
Black Raspberry Ice Cream
Butter Pecan Ice Cream
Butterscotch Ripple Ice Cream
Cherry Vanilla Ice Cream
Chocolate Ice Cream
Chocolate Marshmallow Ice Cream
Coffee Ice Cream
Light Butter Pecan Ice Cream
Light Vanilla Ice Cream
Mint Chocolate Chip Ice Cream
Moose Tracks Ice Cream
Natural Butter Pecan Ice Cream
Natural Chocolate Chip Ice Cream
Natural Chocolate Ice Cream
Natural Coffee Ice Cream
Natural French Vanilla Ice Cream
Natural Mint Chocolate Chip Ice Cream
Natural Mocha Almond Ice Cream

Natural Strawberry Ice Cream
Natural Vanilla Bean Ice Cream
Natural Vanilla Fudge Ripple Ice Cream
Peanut Butter Jumble Ice Cream
Strawberry Ice Cream
Toffee Crunch Ice Cream
Vanilla Fudge Ice Cream
Vanilla Ice Cream

Guaranteed Value (Stop & Shop)

Chocolate Ice Cream
Chocolate Marshmallow
Fudge Royal Ice Cream
Neapolitan Ice Cream
Vanilla Ice Cream
Vanilla Orange Ice Cream

Hood

Butterscotch Blast
Chippedy Chocolaty
Chocolate
Classic Trio
Creamy Coffee
Fudge Twister
Golden Vanilla
Holiday Eggnog (Seasonal)
Light Almond Praline Delight
Light Butter Pecan
Light Butter Toffee Crunch
Light Caribbean Coffee Royale
Light Creamy Vanilla
Light Raspberry Swirl
Maple Walnut
Natural Vanilla Bean
New England Creamery - Bear Creek Caramel
New England Creamery - Boston Vanilla Bean
New England Creamery - Cape Cod Fudge Shop
New England Creamery - Light Butter Pecan
New England Creamery - Light Chocolate Chip
New England Creamery - Light Coffee
New England Creamery - Light French Silk
New England Creamery - Light Main Blueberry & Sweet Cream
New England Creamery - Light Martha's Vineyard Black Raspberry
New England Creamery - Light Mint Chocolate Chip
New England Creamery - Light Under The Stars
New England Creamery - Light Vanilla
New England Creamery - Maine Blueberry & Sweet Cream
New England Creamery - Martha's Vineyard Black Raspberry
New England Creamery - Moosehead Lake Fudge
New England Creamery - Mystic Lighthouse Mint
New England Creamery - New England Homemade Vanilla
New England Creamery - New England Lighthouse Coffee
New England Creamery - North End Spumoni
New England Creamery - Vermont Maple Nut
Patchwork
Peppermint Stick (Seasonal)
Red Sox Ice Cream (All Flavors)
Strawberry

Hy-Vee

Butter Crunch Ice Cream
Cherry Nut Ice Cream
Cherry Nut Light Ice Cream
Chocolate Chip Ice Cream
Chocolate Chip Light Ice Cream
Chocolate Ice Cream
Chocolate Marshmallow Ice Cream
Chocolate/Vanilla Flavored Ice Cream
Dutch Chocolate Light Ice Cream
Fudge Marble Ice Cream
Mint Chip Ice Cream
Neapolitan Ice Cream
Neapolitan Light Ice Cream
New York Vanilla Ice Cream
Peanut Butter Fudge Ice Cream
Peppermint Ice Cream
Strawberry Ice Cream
Vanilla Flavored Ice Cream
Vanilla Light Ice Cream

It's Soy Delicious
- Almond Pecan
- Awesome Chocolate
- Black Leopard
- Carob Peppermint
- Chocolate Almond
- Chocolate Peanut Butter
- Espresso
- Green Tea
- Mango Raspberry
- Pistachio Almond
- Raspberry
- Tiger Chai
- Vanilla
- Vanilla Fudge

Louis Trauth Dairy
- Louis Trauth Dairy (All BUT Lowfat Buttermilk, Cookies N Cream Ice Cream, Chocolate Chip Cookie Dough Ice Cream, Ice Cream Sandwiches, and Sundae Nut Cones)

Lucerne (Safeway)
- Egg Nog Ice Cream

Meijer
- Awesome Strawberry Ice Cream
- Black Cherry Ice Cream
- Bordeaux Cherry Chocolate Ice Cream
- Butter Pecan Ice Cream
- Candy Bar Swirl Ice Cream
- Carb Conquest Chocolate
- Carb Conquest Vanilla
- Cherry Sherbert
- Chocolate Chip Ice Cream
- Chocolate Ice Cream
- Chocolate Peanut Butter Fudge Ice Cream
- Chocolate Thunder Ice Cream
- Combo Cream
- Cotton Candy Ice Cream
- Dulce De Leche Ice Cream
- Fat Free No Sugar Added Caramel Pecan Crunch
- Fat Free No Sugar Added Vanilla w/ Splenda
- Fudge Swirl Ice Cream
- Golden Vanilla Ice Cream
- Heavenly Hash Ice Cream
- Lemonberry Twist Sherbet
- Lime Sherbet
- Lite N.S. Added Butter Pecan w/ Splenda
- Lite Neapolitan Ice Cream
- Lite No Sugar Added Vanilla w/Splenda
- Mackinac Fudge Ice Cream
- Meijer Gold - Caramel Toffee Swirl
- Meijer Gold - Double Nut Chocolate
- Meijer Gold - Georgian Bay Butter Pecan
- Meijer Gold - Peanut Butter Fudge Swirl
- Meijer Gold - Peanut Butter Fudge Tracks
- Meijer Gold - Thunder Bay Cherry
- Meijer Gold - Victorian Vanilla
- Mint Chocolate Ice Cream
- Neapolitan Ice Cream
- Peppermint Ice Cream
- Praline Pecan Ice Cream
- Scooperman Ice Cream
- Tin Roof Ice Cream
- Vanilla Ice Cream

Midwest Country Fare (Hy-Vee)
- Chocolate Chip Ice Cream
- Chocolate Ice Cream
- Light Vanilla Ice Cream
- Neapolitan Ice Cream
- Vanilla Ice Cream

Nestlé Ice Cream
- Vanilla Almond No Sugar Added Slow Churned Light Ice Cream Bars

Organic So Delicious Dairy Free
- Butter Pecan
- Chocolate Peanut Butter
- Chocolate Velvet
- Creamy Lemon
- Creamy Orange
- Creamy Raspberry
- Creamy Vanilla
- Dulce De Leche
- Mint Marble Fudge
- Mocha Fudge
- Neapolitan
- Strawberry

Publix ( )

Banana Split Premium Ice Cream
Bear Claw Premium Ice Cream
Black Jack Cherry Premium Ice Cream
Buckeye's & Fudge Premium Limited
  Edition Ice Cream
Butter Pecan Premium Homemade Ice
  Cream
Butter Pecan Premium Ice Cream
Caramel Mountain Tracks Premium
  Limited Edition Ice Cream
Cherry Nut Premium Ice Cream
Chocolate Almond Premium Ice Cream
Chocolate Cherish Passion Premium Ice
  Cream
Chocolate Chip Premium Homemade
  Ice Cream
Chocolate Chip Premium Ice Cream
Chocolate Ice Cream
Chocolate Low Fat Ice Cream
Chocolate Marshmallow Swirl Ice
  Cream
Chocolate Peanut Butter Swirl Ice
  Cream
Chocolate Premium Ice Cream
Coffee Premium Ice Cream
Double Chocolate Chunk Premium
  Homemade Ice Cream
Dulce de Leche Premium Ice Cream
Egg Nog Premium Limited Edition Ice
  Cream
French Silk Duo Premium Limited
  Edition Ice Cream
French Vanilla Premium Ice Cream
Fudge Royal Ice Cream
Fudge Royal Low Fat Ice Cream
Heavenly Hash Premium Ice Cream
Maple Walnut Premium Limited Edition
  Ice Cream
Mint Chocolate Chip Premium Ice
  Cream
Monkey Business Premium Limited
  Edition Ice Cream
Neapolitan Ice Cream
Neapolitan Low Fat Ice Cream
Neapolitan Premium Ice Cream
Otter Paws Premium Ice Cream

Peanut Butter Goo Goo Premium Ice
  Cream
Peppermint Stick Premium Limited
  Edition Ice Cream
Rum Raisin Premium Limited Edition
  Ice Cream
Santa's White Christmas Premium Ice
  Cream
Strawberry Premium Homemade Ice
  Cream
Strawberry Premium Ice Cream
Vanilla Ice Cream
Vanilla Low Fat Ice Cream
Vanilla Premium Homemade Ice Cream
Vanilla Premium Ice Cream
Vanilla Strawberry Ice Cream

Purely Decadent Dairy Free

Cherry Nirvana
Chocolate Obsession
Coconut Craze
Cookie Dough (Gluten Free)
Mint Chocolate Chip
Mocha Almond Fudge
Peanut Butter Zig Zag
Pomegranate Chip
Praline Pecan
Purely Vanilla
Rocky Road
So Very Strawberry
Turtle Trails

Reed's

Reed's (All)

Rice Dream

Cocoa Marble Fudge
Neapolitan
Vanilla

Select Brand (Safeway)

Caramel Cashew Ice Cream
Chocolate Chunk Ice Cream
Coffee Ice Cream
Dutch Chocolate Ice Cream
Fat Free Caramel Swirl Ice Cream
Fat Free No Sugar Added Vanilla Ice
  Cream
Light Peppermint Ice Cream
Mocha Ice Cream
Mother Load Ice Cream

Ole' Vanilla Ice Cream
Pecan Praline Ice Cream

Soy Dream

Butter Pecan
Chocolate
French Vanilla
Green Tea
Mocha Fudge
Strawberry Swirl
Vanilla
Vanilla Fudge Swirl

Stop & Shop

Butterscotch Ripple Ice Cream
Chocolate Chip Ice Cream
Coffee Ice Cream
Country Club Ice Cream
Heavenly Hash Ice Cream
Natural Butter Pecan Ice Cream
Natural Chocolate Chip Ice Cream
Natural Chocolate Ice Cream
Natural Coffee Ice Cream
Natural French Vanilla Ice Cream
Natural Mint Chocolate Chip Ice Cream
Natural Mocha Almond Ice Cream
Natural Strawberry Ice Cream
Natural Vanilla Bean Ice Cream
Natural Vanilla Fudge Ripple Ice Cream
Neapolitan Ice Cream
Peppermint Stick Ice Cream
Strawberry Ice Cream
Vanilla Fudge Swirl Ice Cream
Vanilla Ice Cream

Tillamook

Ice Cream (All BUT Caramel Toffee
Crunch, Cookies and Cream, Cookie
Dough, German Chocolate Cake and
Marionberry Pie)

Trader Joe's ()

French Vanilla Ice Cream
Ice Cream - Chocolate
Soy Cream - Cherry Chocolate Chip
Soy Cream - Mango Vanilla
Soy Cream - Vanilla

Turkey Hill

All Natural Recipe - Coffee
All Natural Recipe - Mint Chocolate
Chip

All Natural Recipe - Neapolitan
All Natural Recipe - Nutty Neapolitan
All Natural Recipe - Vanilla Bean
Cool Moos - Chocolate
Creamy Commotions - Moose Tracks
Duetto - Chocolate and Coconut
(Limited Edition)
Duetto - Lemon
Duetto - Mango
Duetto - Raspberry
Duetto - Root Beer
Light Ice Cream - Banana Split
Light Ice Cream - Chocolate Chip
Light Ice Cream - Chocolate Nutty
Moose Tracks
Light Ice Cream - Moose Tracks
Light Ice Cream - Raspberry Chocolate
Chunk
Light Ice Cream - Vanilla Bean
No Sugar Added Ice Cream - Cherry
Fudge Ripple
No Sugar Added Ice Cream - Dutch
Chocolate
No Sugar Added Ice Cream - Peanut
Brittle
No Sugar Added Ice Cream - Vanilla
Bean
Premium Ice Cream - Banana Split
Premium Ice Cream - Black Cherry
Premium Ice Cream - Black Raspberry
Premium Ice Cream - Butter Pecan
Premium Ice Cream - Choco Mint Chip
Premium Ice Cream - Chocolate
Marshmallow
Premium Ice Cream - Chocolate Peanut
Butter Cup
Premium Ice Cream - Colombian
Coffee
Premium Ice Cream - Dutch Chocolate
Premium Ice Cream - Eagles
Touchdown Sundae
Premium Ice Cream - French Vanilla
Premium Ice Cream - Fudge Ripple
Premium Ice Cream - Jets Sundae Blitz
Premium Ice Cream - Neapolitan
Premium Ice Cream - Orange Cream
Swirl
Premium Ice Cream - Original Vanilla

Premium Ice Cream - Peanut Butter Ripple
Premium Ice Cream - Rocky Road
Premium Ice Cream - Rum Raisin
Premium Ice Cream - Strawberries & Cream
Premium Ice Cream - Vanilla & Chocolate
Premium Ice Cream - Vanilla Bean

JUICE & JUICE DRINKS

Giant
Frozen Concentrate 100% Grape Juice
Frozen Concentrate Cranberry Cocktail
Frozen Concentrate Grape Cocktail
Frozen Concentrate Lemonade
Frozen Concentrate Limeade
Frozen Concentrate Orange Juice
Frozen Concentrate Pink Lemonade
Frozen Concentrate White Grape Cocktail
Frozen Concentrate Wildberry Punch
Fruit Punch (Green, Red)

Hy-Vee
Apple Juice Frozen Concentrate
Fruit Punch Frozen Concentrate
Grape Juice Cocktail Frozen Concentrate
Lemonade Frozen Concentrate
Limeade Frozen Concentrate
Orange Juice Frozen Concentrate
Orange Juice with Added Calcium Frozen
Pineapple Juice From Concentrate
Pink Lemonade Frozen Concentrate

Langers
Juices (All)

Meijer
Frozen Apple Juice Concentrate
Frozen Fruit Punch Concentrate
Frozen Grape Juice Concentrate
Frozen Grapefruit Juice Concentrate
Frozen Lemonade Concentrate
Frozen Limeade Concentrate
Frozen O.J. Concentrate Pulp Free
Frozen O.J. Concentrate w/Calcium

Frozen Orange Juice Concentrate
Frozen Orange Juice Concentrate - High Pulp
Frozen Pink Lemonade Concentrate
White Grape Juice Cocktail Concentrate

Midwest Country Fare (Hy-Vee)
Orange Juice Frozen Concentrate

Old Orchard
Old Orchard Juices

Publix ()
Frozen Concentrated Orange Juice

Stop & Shop
Frozen Concentrate 100% Grape Juice
Frozen Concentrate Apple Juice
Frozen Concentrate Cranberry Cocktail
Frozen Concentrate Fruit Punch
Frozen Concentrate Grape Cocktail
Frozen Concentrate Lemonade
Frozen Concentrate Limeade
Frozen Concentrate Orange Juice
Frozen Concentrate Pink Lemonade
Frozen Concentrate White Grape Cocktail
Frozen Concentrate Wildberry Punch

Trader Joe's ()
Concentrates - Lemon
Concentrates - Orange

Welch's
Welch's (All)

MEAT

Applegate Farms
Applegate Farms (All BUT Chicken Nuggets, Chicken Pot Pie, & Chicken Strips)

Bell & Evans
Chicken Burgers

Bubba Burger
Bubba Burger (All)

Empire Kosher
Frozen Chicken
Frozen Ground Turkey
Frozen Whole Turkey & Turkey Breasts
Individually Quick Frozen Chicken Parts

Jennie-O ()

Frozen Ground Seasoned Turkey
Frozen Ground Turkey
Frozen Turkey Breast (Gravy packet NOT GF)
Frozen Turkey Burgers
Prime Young Turkey - Frozen (Gravy packet NOT GF)

Kroger ()

Frozen Plain Chicken Breast
Frozen Plain Chicken Thighs
Frozen Plain Chicken Wings
Frozen Plain Turkey Breast
Frozen Plain Turkey Thighs

Mama Lucia

Fully Cooked Sausage Meatballs Made with Beef

Manor House (Safeway)

Frozen Enhanced Turkey

Meijer

Breast Split Frzn
Breast Tenders Frzn
Frozen Duckling
Frozen Turkey Breast
Frozen Turkey Breast - Young

Perdue

Individually Frozen - Chicken Breasts
Individually Frozen - Chicken Tenderloins
Individually Frozen - Chicken Wings

Philly-Gourmet

All Beef Sandwich Steaks
Pure Beef Homestyle Patties

Pilgrim's Pride

Marinated Individually Quick Frozen - Boneless/Skinless Breasts
Marinated Individually Quick Frozen - Boneless/Skinless Thighs
Marinated Individually Quick Frozen - Drum
Marinated Individually Quick Frozen - Drummettes
Marinated Individually Quick Frozen - Split Breast
Marinated Individually Quick Frozen - Tenderloins
Marinated Individually Quick Frozen - Thighs
Marinated Individually Quick Frozen - Wing Sections

Publix ()

Frozen Boneless Skinless Chicken Breasts
Frozen Boneless Skinless Chicken Cutlets
Frozen Chicken Breast Tenderloins
Frozen Chicken Wingettes

Shelton's

Chicken Franks
Ground Turkey Chub
Ground Turkey Chub White
Smoked Chicken Franks
Smoked Turkey Franks
Spicy Chicken Dogs
Spicy Turkey Dogs
Turkey Breakfast Strips
Turkey Burgers
Turkey Franks
Uncured Chicken Bologna
Uncured Turkey Bologna

Trader Joe's ()

Chili Lime Chicken Burgers
Seasoned Rack of Lamb

Wellshire Farms

Frozen Beef Hamburgers
Frozen Turkey Burgers

NOVELTIES

Dibs

Bite Sized Ice Cream with Coating - Chocolate
Bite Sized Ice Cream with Coating - Mint
Bite Sized Ice Cream with Coating - Peanut Butter w/Peanut Butter Center
Bite Sized Ice Cream with Coating - Rocky Road
Bite Sized Ice Cream with Coating - Strawberry
Bite Sized Ice Cream with Coating - Vanilla
Vanilla Snack Bags

Dreyer's
Strawberry Fruit Bar

Edy's
Strawberry Fruit Bar

Eskimo Pie
Dark Chocolate Coated Vanilla
Dark Chocolate Coated Vanilla Bar
King Size Original Vanilla Bar
Vanilla & Chocolate

Gaga's SherBetter
To Go - Chocolate
To Go - Lemon
To Go - Orange
To Go - Raspberry

Giant
Chocolate Ice Cream Cups
Citrus Pops
Jr Pops
No Sugar Added Fudge Pops
Orange Cream Bars
Twin Pops
Vanilla Ice Cream Cup

Hood
Fudge Stix
Hendries Citrus Stix
Hendries Kids Karnival Stix
Hendries Kids Stix
Hendries Mix Stix
Hendries NSA Citrus 'N Berry
Hendries Pop Stix
Hoodsie Cups
Hoodsie Pops - 6 Flavor Assortment
   Twin Pops
Hoodsie Sundae Cups
Ice Cream Bar
Orange Cream Bar
Rocket

Hy-Vee
Assorted Twin Pops
Chocolate & Strawberry Sundae Cups
Fat Free No Sugar Added Fudge Bars
Fudge Bars
Galaxy Reduced Fat Ice Cream Bars
Pops - Cherry, Orange & Grape
Reduced Fat Galaxy Bars

Louis Trauth Dairy
Louis Trauth Dairy (All BUT Lowfat
   Buttermilk, Cookies N Cream Ice
   Cream, Chocolate Chip Cookie Dough
   Ice Cream, Ice Cream Sandwiches,
   and Sundae Nut Cones)

Lucerne (Safeway)
Fudge Ice Cream Bars
Orange Ice Cream Bars
Root Beer Float Ice Cream Bars
Toffee Brittle Ice Cream Bars
Vanilla Ice Cream Bars
Vanilla Sundae Ice Cream Bars
Vanilla Sundae Ice Cream Cups
Vanilla/Sherbet Ice Cream Bars

Meijer
Brr Bar
Dream Bars
Frozen Novelties - Gold Bar
Frozen Novelties - Toffee Bar
Fudge Bars
Ice Cream Bars
Juice Stix
No Sugar Added Fudge Bars
No Sugar Added Party Pops (Assorted)
Orange Glider
Party Pops - Orange/Cherry/Grape/L
Red White and Blue Pops
Toffee Bars
Twin Pops

Minute Maid
Juice Bars - Orange, Cherry, and Grape

Nestlé Ice Cream
Butterfinger Loaded Bar
Creamy Coconut Fruit Bar
Fruit Bar Variety Pack - Lime/
   Strawberry/Wildberry
Fruit Bars Mini Snack Size - Cherry/
   Grape/Tropical
Fruit Bars Mini Snack Size - Orange &
   Cream/Raps Cream/Lime Cream
Grape Fruit Bar
Itzakadoozie Ice Pop
Lemonade Fruit Bar
Lime Fruit Bar
No Sugar Added Fruit Bar Variety
   Pack - Black Cherry/Strawberry Kiwi/

Mixed Berry
No Sugar Added Fruit Bar Variety Pack
 - Raspberry/Strawberry/Tangerine
Orange & Cream Fruit Bar
Push-Up Orange
Push-Up Rainbow
Rainbow Push-Ups
Shrek Push-Up Variety Pack
Shrek Puss in Boots Push-Up Variety
 Pack
Shrek Sludge Fudge Bar
Shrek Swamp Pops Ice Pops
Strawberry Fruit Bar
Strawberry-Banana Smoothies Fruit &
 Yogurt Bars
Tangerine Fruit Bar
Vanilla Milk Chocolate Slow Churned
 Light Ice Cream Bars
Variety Pack Push-Ups - Cherry,
 Orange, Berry

Organic So Delicious Dairy Free ☼
Creamy Fudge Bar
Creamy Vanilla Bar
Vanilla & Almonds Bar

Publix ()
Banana Pops
Cream Pops
Fudge Bar
Fudge Sundae Cups
Ice Cream Bar
Ice Cream Squares
No Sugar Added Fudge Pops
No Sugar Added Ice Cream Bars
No Sugar Added Ice Cream Squares
No Sugar Added Ice Pop
Orange, Cherry and Grape Junior Ice
 Pops
Red White and Blue Junior Ice Pops
Toffee Bar
Twin Pops
Vanilla Cups

Purely Decadent Dairy Free ☼
Purely Vanilla Bar
Vanilla Almond Bar

Safeway
Assorted Ice Pops
Basic Red Vanilla Ice Cream

Kreme Koolers

Select Brand (Safeway)
Caramel Caribou Ice Cream Bars
Fruit Bars (All Flavors)

Skinny Cow, The
Low Fat Fudge Bars
Skinny Mini Fudge Bars
Vanilla and Caramel Skinny Dippers
Vanilla and Mint Skinny Dippers

So Delicious Dairy Free ☼
Creamy Orange Bar
Creamy Raspberry Bar
Kidz - Assorted Fruit Pops
Kidz - Fudge Pops

Sweet Nothings ☼
Fudge Bar
Mango Raspberry Bar

Trader Joe's ()
Blissful Ice Cream Bar
Dark Chocolate Dipped Strawberries
Fruit Floes
Gone Bananas Chocolate Dipped
 Bananas
Mango Passion Exotique
Strawberries N' Crème
Truffle Bites

Welch's
Welch's (All)

PIZZA & CRUSTS

Amy's Kitchen
Rice Crust Cheese Pizza
Rice Crust Spinach Pizza
Single Serve Non-Dairy Rice Crust
 Cheese Pizza

Chebe ☼ ☼
Pizza Crusts

Ener-G
Rice Pizza Shells
Yeast Free Rice Pizza Shells

Foods By George
Pizza
Pizza Crusts

Gluten-Free & Fabulous
Cheese Pizza

Pepperoni Pizza
Pizza Crust

Glutino 🍴
Pizza - 3 Cheese with Brown Rice Crust
Pizza - Duo Cheese
Pizza - Spinach / Feta
Pizza - Spinach Soy Cheese with Brown Rice Crust

Ian's Natural Foods 🍴 🍴 ()
Wheat Free Gluten Free French Bread Pizza

Mariposa Baking Company 🍴
Pizza Crust

POTATOES

Alexia Foods ()
Potato Products (All)

Dr. Praeger's
Potato Littles
Sweet Potato Littles
Sweet Potato Pancakes

Giant
Crinkle Cut French Fries
Crispy Fries
Extra Crispy Crinkle Cut Fries
Hash O' Brien
Puffs with Onions
Shoestring Fries
Shredded Hash Browns
Southwestern Style Hash Browns
Steak Fries
Straight Cut French Fries

Hy-Vee
Frozen Country Style Hash Brown Potatoes
Frozen Crinkle Cut Fries
Frozen Criss Cut Potatoes
Frozen Steak Fries
Hash Brown Potatoes

Ian's Natural Foods 🍴 🍴 ()
Alphatots

Ingles Markets
Frozen Potatoes (All BUT Seasoned Fries)

Kroger ()
Plain Frozen Potatoes - Salted

McCain Foods ()
5 Minute Shoestring French Fries
Classic Cut French Fries
Crinkle Cut French Fries
HomeStyle BabyCakes
Mash-Bites Potatoes
Premium Golden Crisp Crinkle Cut Fry
Premium Golden Crisp Fast Food Fries Shoestring Cut
Premium Golden Crisp Straight Cut French Fry
Roasters - All American
Roasters - French Onion
Roasters - Grilled Garlic & Onion
Shoestring French Fries
Smiles Fun Shaped Potatoes
Steak Fries
Straight Cut French Fries
Tasti Tater Shaped Potatoes

Meijer
Frozen French Fries
Frozen French Fries Crinkle Cut
Frozen French Fries Quickie Crinkles
Frozen French Fries Shoestring
Frozen French Fries Steak Cut
Frozen Hashbrowns
Frozen Hashbrowns - Shredded
Frozen Hashbrowns - Southern Style
Frozen Hashbrowns - Western Style
Frozen Potatoes - Crinkle Cut Fries
Frozen Potatoes - French Fried Crinkle Cut
Frozen Potatoes - Tater Tots
Frozen Potatoes - Tater Treats

Ore-Ida ()
Cottage Fries
Country Style Hashbrowns
Crunch Time Classics Crinkle Cut
Crunch Time Classics Straight Cut
Deep Fries Crinkle Cuts
Extra Crispy Fast Food Fries
French Fries
Golden Crinkles
Golden Fries
Golden Patties

Hash Browns
Pixie Crinkles
Potato Wedges with Skins
Potatoes O'Brien
Shoestrings
Snackin' Fries
Southern Style Hash Browns
Steak Fries
Tater Tots (All Varieties)

Publix ()

Crinkle Cut Fries
Golden Fries
Shoestring Fries
Southern Style Hash Browns
Steak Fries
Tater Bites
Tater Puffs

Safeway

Crinkle Cut Potatoes
Crispy Fries
French Fried Potatoes
Hash Browns - Country Style
Hash Browns - Shredded
Hash Browns - Southern Style
O'Brien Potatoes
Potato Sticks
Restaurant Style Crinkle Cut Potatoes
Shoestring Potatoes
Steak Cut Potatoes
Twice Baked Potatoes

Select Brand (Safeway)

Roasted Rosemary Wedges

Simply Potatoes

Simply Potatoes (All Varieties)

Stop & Shop

Butter Twice Baked Potatoes
Cheddar Cheese Twice Baked Potatoes
Crinkle Cut French Fries
Crispy Fries
Extra Crispy Crinkle Cut Fries
Frozen Natural Wedges
Puffs with Onions
Shoestring Fries
Shredded Hash Browns
Sour Cream & Chive Twice Baked
  Potatoes
Southwestern Style Hash Browns

Steak Fries
Straight Cut French Fries

Trader Joe's ()

Crinkle Wedge Potatoes
Organic Frozen French Fries
Pacific Northwest Crinkle Wedge
  Potatoes

PREPARED MEALS & SIDES

Amy's Kitchen

Asian Noodle Stir-Fry
Baked Ziti Bowl
Baked Ziti Kids Meal
Black Bean Enchilada Whole Meal
Black Bean Tamale Verde Whole Meal
Black Bean Vegetable Enchilada
Black Bean Vegetable Enchiladas -
  Light in Sodium
Brown Rice & Vegetables Bowl
Brown Rice & Vegetables Bowl - Light
  in Sodium
Brown Rice, Black-Eyed Peas & Veggie
  Bowl
Cheese Enchilada
Cheese Enchilada Whole Meal
Cheese Tamale Verde Whole Meal
Cream of Rice Hot Cereal Bowl
Garden Vegetable Lasagna
Indian Mattar Paneer
Indian Mattar Paneer - Light in Sodium
Indian Mattar Tofu
Indian Palak Paneer
Indian Paneer Tikka
Indian Vegetable Korma
Mexican Casserole Bowl
Mexican Casserole Bowl - Light in
  Sodium
Mexican Tamale Pie
Rice Mac & Cheese
Santa Fe Enchilada Bowl
Shepherd's Pie
Shepherd's Pie - Light in Sodium
Teriyaki Bowl
Thai Stir-Fry
Tofu Rancheros
Tofu Scramble

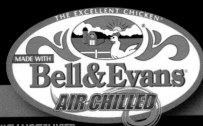
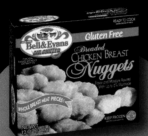
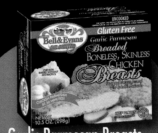
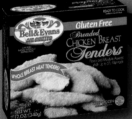
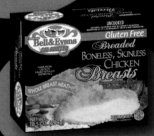
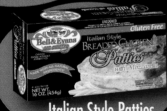
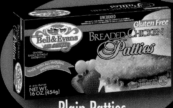

Tortilla Casserole & Black Beans Bowl

Bell & Evans
BBQ Wings
Buffalo Style Wings
Gluten Free Breaded Breasts
Gluten Free Breaded Patties
Gluten Free Garlic Parmesan Breaded Breasts
Gluten Free Italian Style Breaded Patties
Gluten Free Nuggets
Gluten Free Tenders
Grilled BBQ Breasts
Grilled Breasts
Grilled Buffalo Style Breasts

Cedarlane Natural Foods
Five Layer Mexican Dip
Three Layer Enchilada Pie

Coleman Natural
Buffalo Wings

Contessa
Jambalaya
Paella
Ragin' Cajun Shrimp
Seafood Veracruz
Shrimp on the Bar-B
Shrimp Santa Fe
Shrimp Scampi
Thai Style Coconut Chicken
Thai Style Curry Chicken
Whiskey Jack Shrimp

Delimex ()
3-Cheese Taquitos
Beef Deli Bulk Pack Tamales
Beef Tamales (Costco)
Beef Tamales (Sam's Club)
Beef Tamales (Trader Joe's)
Beef Taquitos
Beef Taquitos (Costco)
Beef Taquitos (Sam's Club)
Beef Tamales
Beef Taquitos
Cheese Deli Bulk Pack Tamales
Chicken & Cheese Tamales
Chicken & Cheese Tamales (Trader Joe's)
Chicken Deli Bulk Pack Tamales

Chicken Taquitos
Chicken Taquitos (Costco)
Schwan's Beef Tamales
Schwan's Beef w/Salsa Taquitos
Smart & Final Beef Taquitos
Taquitos - Mini Beef Snacker Tray with Salsa

Dr. Praeger's
Broccoli Little
Potato Crusted Fillet Fish Sticks (Ensure GF version, as a non-GF option exists)
Potato Crusted Fish Fillets (Ensure GF version, as a non-GF option exists)
Potato Crusted Fishies (Ensure GF version, as a non-GF option exists)
Spinach Littles

El Monterey ()
Chicken Corn Taquitos
Shredded Steak Corn Taquitos

Empire Kosher
Fully Cooked Barbecue Chicken (Fresh Or Frozen)
Fully Cooked Barbecue Turkey (Fresh Or Frozen)

Giant
Wings - Buffalo
Wings - Honey BBQ

Gluten Free Café ☃
Asian Noodles
Fettuccini Alfredo
Lemon Basil Chicken
Pasta Primavera

Glutino ☃
Chicken Alfredo
Chicken Pad Thai
Chicken Pomodoro
Chicken Ranchero
Macaroni & Cheese
Penne Alfredo
Penne Mushroom

Goya ()
Classic Entrees - Ground Beef, Potatoes in Seasoned Sauce with Rice
Classic Entrees - Pigeon Peas & Rice
Classic Entrees - Rice with Chicken

Homestyle Meals
   Frozen Fully Cooked Baby Back Ribs

Ian's Natural Foods ☃ ☃ ()
   Lightly Battered Fish - Wheat & Gluten
      Free Recipe
   Wheat Free Gluten Free Recipe Chicken
      Finger Meal
   Wheat Free Gluten Free Recipe Chicken
      Nuggets
   Wheat Free Gluten Free Recipe Chicken
      Patties
   Wheat Free Gluten Free Recipe Fish
      Sticks
   Wheat Free Gluten Free Recipe Mac &
      Meat Sauce
   Wheat Free Gluten Free Recipe Mac &
      NO Cheese
   Wheat Free Gluten Free Recipe Popcorn
      Turkey Corn Dogs

Murray's Chicken
   Gluten-Free Chicken Nuggets

Organic Bistro ☃ ()
   Chicken Citron

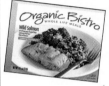
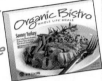
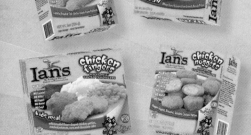
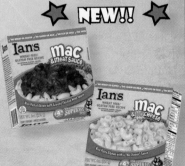
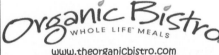

Ginger Chicken
Jamaican Jerk Shrimp Cake
Pasta Puttanesca
Savory Turkey
Sockeye Salmon Cake
Spiced Chicken Morocco
Wild Salmon

Rice Expressions
Rice Products (All)

Rosina
Italian Sausage Meatballs

S'Better Farms
Chicken Ballontine
Chicken Fingers
Chicken Siciliano
Chicken Szechwan
Party Wings

Select Brand (Safeway)
Gourmet Club Eating Right - Chicken
Lettuce Wraps
Gourmet Club Eating Right - Ginger
Chicken

Simply Enjoy (Giant)
Butter Chicken
Pad Thai with Chicken
Tikka Masala

Simply Enjoy (Stop & Shop)
Butter Chicken
Pad Thai with Chicken
Tikka Masala

South Beach Living
Caprese Style Chicken Frozen Entrée
Savory Beef Frozen Entree

Starfish
Gluten Free Battered Cod
Gluten Free Battered Haddock

Stop & Shop
Buffalo Style Wings
Honey BBQ Wings
Spinach, Artichoke & Cheese Dip

Tabatchnick Fine Foods
Black Bean
Broccoli Cheese
Cabbage
Corn Chowder
Cream of Broccoli
Cream of Mushroom

Cream of Spinach
Creamed Spinach
Lentil
New England Potato
Pea
Potato
Rock Island
Salmon Chowder
Southwest Bean
Tomato Rice
Vegetarian Chili
Wild Rice
Yankee Bean

Trader Joe's ()
Bacon Wrapped Scallops
Biryani
Chicken Biryani
Chicken Chile Verde
Chicken Enchiladas in Salsa Verde
Chicken Gorgonzola
Chicken Masala
Chicken Tandoori Rice Bowl
Chicken Taquitos
Chicken Wings
Eggplant Parmesan - Grilled Not Fried
Enchilada - Organic Black Bean and
Corn
Flame Grilled Buffalo Patties
Handcrafted Green Chile and Cheese
Tamales
Handmade Green Chili and Cheese
Tamales
Marinated Ahi Tuna Steaks
Marinated Wild White King Salmon
Fillets
Organic Rice (All)
Peruvian Style Chimichurri Rice
Premium Salmon Patties
Quinoa Pilaf with Shrimp and
Vegetables
Salmon Burger
Seasoned Mahi Mahi Fillets
Shepherds Pie (Beef)
Shrimp Scampi
Shrimp Stir-Fry
Southwest Style Turkey Burger
Stuffed Poblano Peppers

Tamales - Beef
Tamales - Cheese
Tamales - Chicken
Taquitos - Black Bean
Taquitos - Chicken
Thai Style Lemongrass Chicken w/Rice
Ultimate Seafood Kabobs

Wellshire Kids

Frozen Dino Shaped Chicken Bites
Uncured Beef Corn Dogs
Uncured Chicken Corn Dogs

SAUSAGE

Jones Dairy Farm

All Natural Golden Brown Fully
Cooked & Browned Sausage Patties
All Natural Golden Brown Light Fully
Cooked & Browned Sausage & Rice
Links
All Natural Golden Brown Made From
Beef Fully Cooked & Browned
Sausage Links
All Natural Golden Brown Mild Fully
Cooked & Browned Sausage Links
All Natural Golden Brown Spicy Fully
Cooked & Browned Sausage Links

Shelton's

Turkey Breakfast Sausage
Turkey Italian Sausage
Turkey Sausage Patties

Wellshire Farms

Frozen Chicken Apple Patties
Frozen Chicken Apple Sausage Links
Frozen Country Sage Sausage Links
Frozen Country Sage Sausage Patties
Frozen Original Breakfast Sausage
Links
Frozen Original Breakfast Sausage
Patties
Frozen Sunrise Maple Sausage Links
Frozen Sunrise Maple Sausage Patties
Frozen Turkey Maple Patties
Frozen Turkey Maple Sausage Links

SHERBET & SORBET

Alpine Ice Natural Frozen Desserts

Bolder Berry
Green Tea Verbena
Hibiscus Rose
Mango Passion
Plum Lucky

Dreyer's

see Edy's (same parent company)

Edy's

Berry Rainbow Sherbet
Orange Cream Sherbet
Swiss Orange Sherbet
Tropical Rainbow Sherbet

Gaga's SherBetter

SherBetter - Chocolate
SherBetter - Lemon
SherBetter - Orange
SherBetter - Rainbow
SherBetter - Raspberry

Giant

Lemon Lime Sherbet
Orange Sherbet
Pineapple Sherbet
Rainbow Sherbet
Raspberry Sherbet

Guaranteed Value (Stop & Shop)

Rainbow Sherbet

Hood

New England Creamery - Black
Raspberry Sherbet
New England Creamery - Orange
Sherbet
New England Creamery - Rainbow
Sherbet
New England Creamery - Wildberry
Sherbet
Sherbet (All)

Hy-Vee

Lime Sherbet
Orange Blossom Ice Cream & Sherbet
Orange Sherbet
Pineapple Sherbet
Rainbow Sherbet
Raspberry Sherbet

Meijer
Orange Sherbet
Pineapple Sherbet
Rainbow Sherbet
Raspberry Sherbet

Publix ( )
Cool Lime Sherbet
Exotic Fruit Medley Sherbet
No Sugar Added Sunny Orange Sherbet
Peach Mango Passion Sherbet
Rainbow Dream Sherbet
Raspberry Blush Sherbet
Sunny Orange Sherbet
Tropic Pineapple Sherbet
Tropical Swirl Sherbet

Safeway
Chocolate Sorbet
Raspberry Sorbet

Trader Joe's ( )
Mango Tangerine Sorbet
Sorbet (All)

Turkey Hill
Sherbet - Fruit Rainbow
Sherbet - Orange Grove
Venice Premium Ice - Lemon & Cherry
Venice Premium Ice - Mango

VEGETABLES

Albertsons
Frozen Broccoli
Frozen Carrots
Frozen Cauliflower
Frozen Green Beans
Frozen Peas
Frozen Spinach
Frozen Squash
Frozen Turnip Greens
Frozen Vegetable Blends (All BUT
  Sweet Onion Rounds)

Europe's Best
Vegetables (All)

Giant
Broccoli - Chopped
Broccoli - Cuts
Broccoli - Florets
Broccoli, Cauliflower, Pepper Mix

Broccoli, Corn and Red Peppers
Cauliflower
Chopped Green Pepper
Collard Greens
Corn - Cut
Corn - On The Cob
Corn - Supersweet On The Cob
Country Blend
Green Beans - Cut
Green Beans - French
Green Beans - Whole
Green Beans and Wax Beans
Japanese Stir Fry Blend
Kale - Chopped
Kale - Leaf
Latino Blend
Mixed Vegetables
Mustard Greens - Chopped
Mustard Greens - Leaf
Peas and Diced Carrots
Petite Peas - No Salt Added
Petite Peas - Regular
Ranchero Blend
Soup Mix Vegetables
Spinach - Chopped
Spinach - Leaf
Spinach - Whole Leaf
Stir Fry Vegetables
Succotash
Sugar Snap Peas
Sweet Peas
Turnip Greens
Whole Okra
Zucchini

Grand Selections (Hy-Vee)
Frozen Caribbean Blend Vegetables
Frozen Normandy Blend Vegetables
Frozen Petite Green Peas
Frozen Petite Whole Carrots
Frozen Riviera Blend Vegetables
Frozen Sugar Snap Peas
Frozen Super Sweet Cut Corn
Frozen White Shoepeg Corn
Frozen Whole Green Beans

Hy-Vee
California Blend
Corn On The Cob

Cream Style Golden Corn
Frozen Broccoli Cuts
Frozen Broccoli Florets
Frozen Brussels Sprouts
Frozen California Mix
Frozen Cauliflower Florets
Frozen Chopped Broccoli
Frozen Chopped Spinach
Frozen Crinkle Cut Carrots
Frozen Cut Golden Corn
Frozen Cut Green Beans
Frozen French Cut Green Beans
Frozen Italian Blend
Frozen Leaf Spinach
Frozen Mixed Vegetables
Frozen Oriental Vegetables
Frozen Sweet Peas
Frozen Winter Mix
Mini Corn On The Cob
Whole Kernel Golden Corn

Ingles Markets
Frozen Vegetables (All BUT Breaded Okra, Hushpuppies & Onion Rings)

Kroger ()
Plain Frozen Vegetables

Meijer
Frozen Beans - Green Cut
Frozen Beans - Green French Cut
Frozen Beans - Green Italian Cut
Frozen Broccoli Chopped
Frozen Broccoli Cuts
Frozen Broccoli Spears
Frozen Brussels Sprouts
Frozen Carrots Crinkle Cut
Frozen Carrots Whole Baby
Frozen Cauliflower Florets
Frozen Chinese Pea Pods
Frozen Collards Chopped
Frozen Corn - Whole Kernel
Frozen Corn - Whole Kernel Golden
Frozen Corn Cob Mini Ear
Frozen Corn On Cob
Frozen Edamame (Soybeans)
Frozen Mixed Vegetables
Frozen Okra - Chopped
Frozen Okra - Whole
Frozen Onions - Chopped

Frozen Organic Green Peas
Frozen Organic Mixed Vegetables
Frozen Peas - Green
Frozen Peas - Green Petite
Frozen Peas & Carrots
Frozen Peppers - Green, Chopped
Frozen Spinach - Chopped
Frozen Spinach - Leaf
Frozen Squash - Cooked
Frozen Vegetables - California Style
Frozen Vegetables - Fiesta
Frozen Vegetables - Florentine
Frozen Vegetables - Italian
Frozen Vegetables - Mexican
Frozen Vegetables - Oriental
Frozen Vegetables - Parisian Style
Frozen Vegetables - Stew Mix
Frozen Vegetables - Stir Fry

Midwest Country Fare (Hy-Vee)
Frozen Broccoli Cuts
Frozen Brussels Sprouts
Frozen California Blend
Frozen Cauliflower
Frozen Chopped Broccoli
Frozen Cut Corn
Frozen Cut Green Beans
Frozen Green Peas
Frozen Mixed Vegetables

Nature's Promise (Stop & Shop)
Organic Asparagus Spears
Organic Broccoli Mini Spears
Organic Corn - Corn On The Cob
Organic Corn - Cut Corn
Organic Cut Leaf Spinach
Organic Mixed Vegetables
Organic Peas
Organic Whole & Cut Green Beans

Publix ()
Alpine Blend
Broccoli - Chopped
Broccoli - Cuts
Broccoli - Spears
Brussels Sprouts
California Blend
Carrots - Crinkle Cut
Carrots - Whole Baby
Cauliflower

Collard Greens, Chopped
Corn - Cut
Corn On The Cob
Del Oro Blend
Field Peas w/Snap
Green Beans - Cut
Green Beans - French Cut
Green Peppers - Diced
Gumbo Mix
Italian Blend
Japanese Blend
Mixed Vegetables
Okra - Cut
Okra - Whole Baby
Onions - Diced
Oriental Blend
Peas
Peas - Blackeye
Peas - Butter
Peas - Crowder
Peas - Green
Peas - Petite
Peas - Purple Hull
Peas and Carrots
Rhubarb
Roma Blend
Soup Mix w/Tomatoes
Spinach - Chopped
Spinach - Cut Leaf
Spinach - Leaf
Squash - Cooked
Squash - Yellow Sliced
Succotash
Turnip Greens - Chopped
Turnip Greens w/Diced Turnips

Raley's ()
Whole Asparagus Spears

Seapoint Farms
Seapoint Farms
Seapoint Farms

Stop & Shop
Asparagus - Spears, Tips & Cuts
Broccoli - Chopped, Cuts & Spears
Broccoli and Cauliflower
Brussels Sprouts
Cauliflower
Chopped Green Pepper

Collard Greens
Cooked Squash
Corn - Cut
Corn - On The Cob
Corn - Supersweet Corn On The Cob
Corn and Butter
Corn and Peas
Country Blend
Cut Wax Beans
Green Beans - Cut, French, with Garlic,
    Italian & Whole
Green Beans and Wax Beans
Japanese Stir Fry Blend
Kale
Latino Blend
Mixed Vegetables
Mustard Greens
Peas and Diced Carrots
Ranchero Blend
Rutabagas
Spinach - Chopped
Spinach - Leaf
Stew Vegetables
Sweet Peas
Whole Okra
Zucchini

VEGGIE BURGERS

Amy's Kitchen
Bistro Burger
Dr. Praeger's
Gluten Free California Veggie Burger
Nature's Promise (Giant)
Garlic and Cheese Veggie Burger
Soy Vegetable Burger
Vegan Soy Vegetable Burger
Nature's Promise (Stop & Shop)
Garlic & Cheese Veggie Burger
Soy Vegetable Burger
Vegan Soy Vegetable Burger
Organic Sunshine Burgers
Organic Sunshine Burgers (All)
Sol Cuisine
Organic Falafel with Sauce
Original
Spicy Bean

Vegetable

Trader Joe's ()
Tofu Veggie Burger

Turtle Island Foods
SuperBurgers

WAFFLES & FRENCH TOAST

Glutino ☡
Cinnamon French Toast

Ian's Natural Foods ☡ ☡ ()
Wheat Free Gluten Free French Toast
Sticks

LifeStream () ☡
Buckwheat Wildberry Waffles
Mesa Sunrise Waffles

Trader Joe's ()
Gluten Free Homestyle Pancakes
Wheat Free Toaster Waffles

Van's All Natural
Wheat-Free/Gluten-Free Apple
Cinnamon Waffles
Wheat-Free/Gluten-Free Blueberry
Waffles
Wheat-Free/Gluten-Free Buckwheat
Waffles
Wheat-Free/Gluten-Free Flax Waffles
Wheat-Free/Gluten-Free Mini Waffles
Wheat-Free/Gluten-Free Original
Waffles

MISCELLANEOUS

Chebe ☡ ☡
Bread Sticks
Frozen Rolls
Sandwich Buns
Tomato-Basil Breadsticks

Giant
Spinach, Artichoke & Cheese Dip

Goya ()
Frozen Recaito
Frozen Sofrito

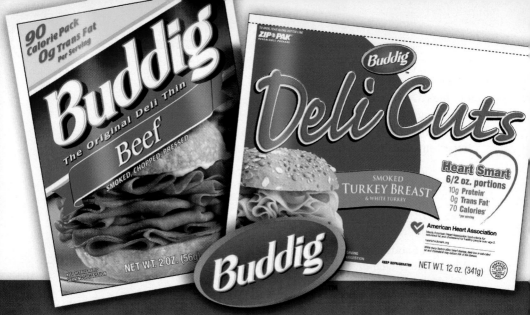

Free of Gluten. Full of Flavor.

Go gluten free with Buddig and Old Wisconsin.® Buddig Original and Deli Cuts are great-tasting, naturally high in protein and low in fat. Deli Cuts have recently been certified by the American Heart Association® to display their heart-check mark, making them an even better way to help you control your diet. Old Wisconsin products offer a wide range of hardwood-smoked beef and turkey meat snacks to fit your lifestyle. Enjoy naturally gluten free lunchmeat and snacks with the Buddig and Old Wisconsin family of products.*

Visit *buddig.com* and *oldwisconsin.com* to learn more or visit your local grocery retailer.

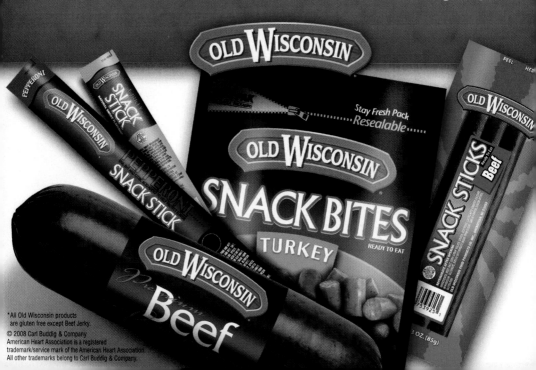

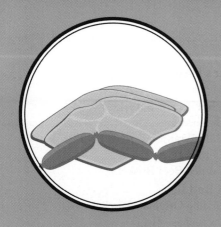

©istockphoto.com/Mei-Yan Irene Chan

MEAT

BACON

Applegate Farms
Applegate Farms (All BUT Chicken Nuggets, Chicken Pot Pie, & Chicken Strips)

Bar-S
Bar-S (All BUT Chuck Wagon Brand Franks & Bar-S Corn Dogs)

Beelers
Bacons (All)

Butcher's Cut (Safeway)
Bacon (All Varieties, must have EST 13331)

Cloverdale Foods
Bacon (All)

Coleman Natural
Bacon

Columbus Salame
Pancetta

Ejays So. Smokehouse
Canadian Style Bacon
Mesquite Smoked Jalapeno Pork Bacon
Mesquite Smoked Pork Bacon

Garrett County Farms
Bacon

Giant
Sliced Bacon - Regular
Sliced Bacon - Thick Sliced

Hormel ()
Bacon Bits & Pieces
Black Label - Bacon
Canadian Style Bacon
Fully Cooked Bacon
Microwave Bacon

Natural Choice - Canadian Bacon
Natural Choice - Uncured Bacon
Natural Choice - Uncured Lower Sodium Bacon
Old Smokehouse - Bacon
Pillow Pack - Canadian Bacon

Hormel Red Label ()
Bacon

Hormel Value Brand ()
Sliced Bacon

Hy-Vee
Hickory Smoked Fully Cooked Bacon

Jennie-O ()
Extra Lean Turkey Bacon
Turkey Bacon

Jones Dairy Farm
Farm Fresh & Tender Sliced Canadian Bacon
Slab Bacon
Sliced Bacon - Regular
Sliced Bacon - Thick

Kroger ()
Bacon - Plain

Laura Lynn (Ingle's)
Bacon
Bacon Chips

Meijer
Bacon
Bacon - Lower Sodium

Oscar Mayer ᏰᎧ
America's Favorite Bacon - Lower Sodium
America's Favorite Bacon - Natural Smoked Uncured

America's Favorite Bacon - Naturally
  Hardwood Smoked
Bacon - Hearty Thick Cut
Bacon - Ready To Serve
Canadian Bacon - Ready To Serve
Center Cut Bacon
Hearty Thick Cut Ready To Serve
  Bacon
Real Bacon Bits

Publix ()
Bacon (All Varieties)

Range Brand ()
Bacon

Stop & Shop
Center Cut Sliced Bacon
Lower Sodium Bacon
Maple Flavored Bacon
Regular Sliced Bacon

Trader Joe's ()
Turkey Bacon
Uncured Bacon

Vac Pac Meats (Safeway)
Pancetta Italian Bacon

Wellshire Farms
Classic Sliced Dry Rubbed Bacon
Classic Sliced Turkey Bacon
Dry Rubbed Center Cut Bacon
Range Sliced Dry Rubbed Bacon
Range Sliced Peppered Bacon
Sliced Applewood Smoked Maple
  Bacon
Sliced Beef Bacon
Sliced Canadian Style Bacon
Sliced Pancetta Bacon
Sliced Peppered Turkey Bacon

BEEF

Albertsons
Wafer Sliced Lunchmeat (Albertson's
  Brand Only)

Applegate Farms
Applegate Farms (All BUT Chicken
  Nuggets, Chicken Pot Pie, & Chicken
  Strips)

Boar's Head
Meats (All)

Butcher's Cut (Safeway)
Beef Burgers
Bulk Wrapped Corned Beef Brisket
Corned Beef
Corned Beef Brisket

Carl Buddig 🦴
Buddig Original "Big Pak" Deli
  Pouches - Beef
Buddig Original "Big Pak" Deli
  Pouches - Corned Beef
Buddig Original Deli Pouches - Beef
Buddig Original Deli Pouches - Corned
  Beef
Buddig Original Deli Pouches -
  Pastrami
Buddig Original in Resealable
  Containers - Beef
Buddig Original in Resealable
  Containers - Corned Beef
Buddig Original Value Pack Deli
  Pouches - Beef
Buddig Original Value Pack Deli
  Pouches - Corned Beef

Coleman Natural
Fresh Meat Products

Columbus Salame
Choice Pastrami
Choice Roast Beef
Corned Beef Choice
Italian Roast Beef

Fast Classics
Bacon Cheeseburger
Beef Burger

Fast Fixin'
Philly Beef

Homestyle Meals
Shredded Beef in BBQ Sauce

Hormel ()
Always Tender - Flavored Fresh Beef
  Peppercorn
Always Tender - Non-Flavored Fresh
  Beef
Deli Sliced Cooked Corned Beef
Deli Sliced Cooked Pastrami
Deli Sliced Seasoned Roast Beef

Natural Choice - Roast Beef
Pillow Pack - Dried Beef
Refrigerated Entrées - Beef Roast Au
Jus

Hy-Vee
Luncheon Meat
Quarter Pounders
Thin Sliced Beef
Thin Sliced Corned Beef
Thin Sliced Pastrami

Isaly's
Deli Meats (All)

Land O' Frost
Lunchmeats (All BUT Taste Escapes
Lemon Pepper Chicken)

Meijer
Beef Slice Chipped Meats
Corned Beef Sliced Chipped Meat
Pastrami Sliced Chipped Meat

Oscar Mayer 🖎
Roast Beef - Slow Roasted Shaved Deli
Fresh Meats

Primo Taglio (Safeway)
Cooked Corned Beef
Pastrami Coated with Spices
Seasoned Roast Beef (Coated with
Seasonings)

Publix ()
Beef Pot Roast with Home-Style Gravy
(Fully Cooked)
Corned Beef (Sliced Lunch Meats)
Peppered Beef (Sliced Lunch Meats)

Publix GreenWise Market ()
Sirloin for Kabobs
Sirloin for Stir Fry
Top Round for Stir Fry

Safeway
Corned Beef (Deli Counter)

Smith's
Ham
Roast Beef

Thumman's
All Natural Black Angus Cooked
Corned Beef Round
All Natural Black Angus Pastrami
Round

Bottom Roast Beef
Cajun Style Beef Top Round London
Broil
Cap Corned Beef
Capless Roast Beef
Cooked Brisket
Cooked Corned Beef Round - Capless
Corned Beef Bottom
First Cut Corned Beef - Coed
First Cut Corned Beef Brisket - Raw
First Cut Pastrami
Fresh Cooked Brisket
Hamberger and Beef Patties
Italian Style Roast Beef - Capless
Pastrami
Pastrami Bottom
Raw Corned Beef Brisket
Ripple Roast Beef

Trader Joe's ()
Fully Cooked & Seasoned Prime Rib of
Beef

Vac Pac Meats (Safeway)
Cooked Corned Beef
Mortadella - Pistachio Nuts and Black
Pepper Added
Pastrami Coated with Seasonings -
Caramel Color Added
Roast Beef - Coated with Garlic,
Dextrose and Spices

Wellshire Farms
Sliced Beef Pastrami Round
Sliced Corned Beef Round
Sliced Top Round Roast Beef

BOLOGNA

Applegate Farms
Applegate Farms (All BUT Chicken
Nuggets, Chicken Pot Pie, & Chicken
Strips)
Bar-S
Bar-S (All BUT Chuck Wagon Brand
Franks & Bar-S Corn Dogs)
Boar's Head
Meats (All)
Cloverdale Foods
Deli Meats (All)

ALWAYS READ LABELS

Empire Kosher
Chicken Bologna - Slices
Turkey Bologna - Slices
Turkey Bologna Roll

Hy-Vee
Beef Bologna
Bologna
Garlic Bologna
German Brand Bologna
Thick Bologna
Thin Bologna
Turkey Bologna

Louis Rich And Oscar Mayer ⌒
50% Less Fat Turkey Bologna
Turkey Bologna

Old Wisconsin ☗ ()
Ring Bologna

Oscar Mayer ⌒
98% Fat Free Bologna
Beef Bologna
Bologna
Cheese Bologna
Light Beef Bologna
Light Bologna

Perdue
Deli Turkey Bologna

Plainville Farms
Plainville Farms (All BUT gravy and
dressing)

Publix ()
Beef Bologna (Sliced Lunch Meats)
German Bologna (Sliced Lunch Meats)

Seltzer's
Lebanon Bolognas (All)

Smith's
Bologna

Thumman's
Angle Cut Bologna
Beef Bologna
Chub Bologna
Garlic Bologna
Ham Bologna
Jumbo Bologna
Long Bologna
Lower Sodium Bologna
Old Fashioned Bologna

Red Bologna
Ring Bologna
Thick Bologna

Wellshire Farms
Sliced Old Fashioned Deli Style Beef
Bologna
Sliced Turkey Bologna

CHICKEN

Albertsons
Wafer Sliced Lunchmeat (Albertson's
Brand Only)

Applegate Farms
Applegate Farms (All BUT Chicken
Nuggets, Chicken Pot Pie, & Chicken
Strips)

Boar's Head
Meats (All)

Butcher's Cut (Safeway)
Boneless Skinless Chicken Breast
Young Chicken Thighs

Carl Buddig ☗
Buddig Deli Cuts - Rotisserie Chicken
Buddig Original "Big Pak" Deli
Pouches - Chicken
Buddig Original Deli Pouches - Chicken
Buddig Original in Resealable
Containers - Chicken
Buddig Original Value Pack Deli
Pouches - Chicken

Empire Kosher
Filled Chicken Breasts with Broccoli
Filling
Filled Chicken Breasts with Mixed
Vegetable Filling
Fresh Chill Pack Chicken & Turkey
Fresh Rotisserie Chicken
Fully Cooked Barbecue Chicken (Fresh
Or Frozen)
Ground Chicken

Fast Classics
Buffalo Wings
Fire Roasted Chicken Breast
Honey BBQ Chicken Wings
Tomato Basil Chicken Breast

Fast Fixin'

Breakaway Chicken SteakEze
Grilled Chicken Breast
Grilled Chicken Breast - Fajita
Grilled Chicken Breast-Mesquite
Restaurant Style - Buffalo Wings
Restaurant Style - Italian Chicken Slices
Restaurant Style - Southwestern
  Chicken Slices

FreeBird

Grilled Breast Filets
Grilled Strips
Party Wings - BBQ Style
Party Wings - Buffalo
Party Wings - Rotisserie-Style

Homestyle Meals

Shredded Chicken in BBQ Sauce

Hormel ()

Always Tender - Italian Flavored Fresh
  Chicken
Always Tender - Lemon-Pepper
  Flavored Fresh Chicken
Always Tender - Roast Flavored Fresh
  Chicken
Natural Choice - Grilled Chicken Strips
Natural Choice - Oven Roasted Chicken
  Strips

Hy-Vee

Boneless Skinless Chicken Thighs For
  Fajitas
Buffalo Style Flavored Chicken Wings
Herb Garlic Flavored Chicken Breasts
  with Rib Meat
Lemon Butter Flavored Chicken Breasts
  with Rib Meat
Thin Sliced Chicken

Jennie-O ()

Turkey Store - Buffalo Style Deli
  Chicken Breast
Turkey Store - Mesquite Smoked Deli
  Chicken Breast
Turkey Store - Oven Roasted Deli
  Chicken Breast

Land O' Frost

Lunchmeats (All BUT Taste Escapes
  Lemon Pepper Chicken)

Louis Rich And Oscar Mayer ⟨⟩

White Chicken Oven Roasted

Meijer

Chicken Slice Chipped Meat

Oscar Mayer ⟨⟩

Chicken Breast Oven Roasted Deli
  Fresh Meats
Chicken Breast Oven Roasted Thin
  Sliced Deli Fresh Meats
Chicken Breast Rotisserie Style Shaved
  Deli Fresh Meats
Honey Roasted Chicken Breast Cuts
Oven Roasted Chicken Breast Cuts

Perdue

Buffalo Chicken Wings Hot N Spicy
  Seasoned
Carving - Chicken Breast, Oven
  Roasted
Ground Breast of Chicken
Ground Chicken
Ground Chicken Burgers
Perfect Portions - Boneless Skinless
  Chicken Breasts
Perfect Portions - Boneless Skinless
  Chicken Breasts, Italian Style
Rotisserie Chicken - Barbecue
Rotisserie Chicken - Italian
Rotisserie Chicken - Lemon Pepper
Rotisserie Chicken - Oven Roasted
Rotisserie Chicken - Toasted Garlic
Rotisserie Chicken - Tuscany Herb
  Roasted
Rotisserie Oven Stuffer Roaster
Rotisserie Oven Stuffer Roaster Breast
Short Cuts - Carved Chicken Breast
  Grilled Italian Style
Short Cuts - Carved Chicken Breast
  Grilled Lemon Pepper
Short Cuts - Carved Chicken Breast
  Grilled Southwestern Style
Short Cuts - Carved Chicken Breast
  Honey Roasted
Short Cuts - Carved Chicken Breast
  Original Roasted
Sliced Chicken Breast - Oil Fried

Pilgrim's Pride

Buffalo Wings - Fully Cooked

Chicken - Marinated (Chill Pack in A Tray)

Marinated Italian Chicken Breasts (Chill Pack in Tray)

Marinated Lemon-Pepper Chicken Breasts (Chill Pack in Tray)

Primo Taglio (Safeway)

Chicken Breast (Oven Roasted) Browned in Hot Cottonseed Oil

Publix ()

Apple Wood Smoked Rotisserie Chicken - Deli

Barbecue Flavored with Barbecue Seasoning and Sauce Rotisserie Chicken (Deli)

Barbecue Flavored with Barbecue Seasoning Rotisserie Chicken (Deli)

Fully Cooked Whole, Smoked Chicken

Lemon Pepper Flavored with Lemon & Herb Seasoning Rotisserie Chicken (Deli)

Original Roasted Rotisserie Chicken (Deli)

Safeway

Deli Roasted Chicken (Deli Counter)

Thumman's

All Natural Oven Roasted Gourmet Chicken Breast

All Natural Oven Roasted Hickory Smoked Chicken Breast

Oven Roasted Chicken Breast - Barbaque Style

Oven Roasted Chicken Breast - Buffalo Style

Oven Roasted Premium Chicken Breast - Browned in Oil

Trader Joe's ()

BBQ Shredded Chicken

Fully Cooked & Seasoned Roasted Chicken

Grilled Balsamic & Rosemary Chicken Breast

Grilled Chicken Strips

Grilled Lemon Pepper Chicken Breast

Just Chicken - Plain

Ukrop's

Kitchen Entrees - Grilled Chicken Breast

Kitchen Entrees - Grilled Chicken Breast with Honey BBQ Sauce

Kitchen Entrees - Grilled Chicken Breast with Lemon Sauce

Kitchen Entrees - Parmesan Chicken Tenders

Kitchen Entrees - Rotisserie Chicken

Kitchen Entrees - Sliced Grilled Breast of Chicken

Wellshire Farms

Sliced Oven Roasted Chicken Breast

Wellshire Kids

Refrigerated Dino Shaped Chicken Bites

HAM & PROSCIUTTO

Albertsons

Wafer Sliced Lunchmeat (Albertson's Brand Only)

Applegate Farms

Applegate Farms (All BUT Chicken Nuggets, Chicken Pot Pie, & Chicken Strips)

Bar-S

Bar-S (All BUT Chuck Wagon Brand Franks & Bar-S Corn Dogs)

Beelers

Hams (All)

Boar's Head

Meats (All)

Butcher's Cut (Safeway)

Cooked Ham - 95% Fat Free

Shank Cut Ham

Spiral Sliced Ham (Glaze packet is NOT GF)

Carl Buddig 𝕭

Buddig Deli Cuts - Brown-Sugar Ham

Buddig Deli Cuts - Honey Ham

Buddig Deli Cuts - Smoked Ham

Buddig Original "Big Pak" Deli Pouches - Ham

Buddig Original "Big Pak" Deli Pouches - Honey Ham

Buddig Original Deli Pouches - Ham
Buddig Original Deli Pouches - Honey
  Ham
Buddig Original in Resealable
  Containers - Ham
Buddig Original in Resealable
  Containers - Honey Ham
Buddig Original Value Pack Deli
  Pouches - Ham
Buddig Original Value Pack Deli
  Pouches - Honey Ham

Cloverdale Foods
Ham (All)

Columbus Salame
Applewood Smoked Ham
Brown Sugar Ham
Ham Black Forest
Honey Ham
Italian Style Ham
Maple Syrup Honey Ham
Proscuitto

Ejays So. Smokehouse
Black Forest Ham Steak

Giant
Cooked Ham - 97% Fat Free

Hormel ()
Black Label - Chopped Ham
Cure 81 - Bone-In Ham
Cure 81 - Boneless Ham
Cure 81 - Old Fashioned Spiral Ham
Deli Sliced Black Forest Ham
Deli Sliced Cooked Ham
Deli Sliced Double Smoked Ham
Deli Sliced Honey Ham
Deli Sliced Prosciutto Ham
Diced Ham
Julienne Ham
Luncheon Meat
Natural Choice - Cooked Deli Ham
Natural Choice - Honey Deli Ham
Natural Choice - Smoked Deli Ham
Refrigerated Entrées - Glazed Ham with
  Maple & Brown Sugar

Hy-Vee
96% Sliced Cooked Ham
Brown Sugar Spiral Sliced Ham
Chopped Ham

Cooked Ham
Deli Thin Slices - Honey Ham
Deli Thin Slices - Smoked Ham
Honey & Spice Spiral Sliced Ham
Thin Sliced Ham with Natural Juices
Thin Sliced Honey Ham with Natural
  Juices

Isaly's
Deli Meats (All)

Jones Dairy Farm
Country Carved Honey & Brown Sugar
  Cured Ham Slices
Farm Fresh & Tender Ham Slices
Farm Fresh & Tender Ham Steak
Farm Fresh & Tender Hams

Land O' Frost
Lunchmeats (All BUT Taste Escapes
  Lemon Pepper Chicken)

Meijer
Double Smoked Ham
Ham Sliced Chipped Meats
Honey Ham - 97% Fat Free
Honey Roasted Ham
Sliced Cooked Ham - 97% Fat Free

Oscar Mayer ✑
Baked Ham
Boiled Ham
Chopped Ham
Chopped Honey Ham
Chopped with Smoke Flavor Ham
Ham - Brown Sugar Shaved Deli Fresh
  Meats
Ham - Brown Sugar Thin Sliced Deli
  Fresh Meats
Ham - Cooked 96% Fat Free Deli Fresh
  Meats
Ham - Cooked Deli Fresh Meats
Ham - Honey 96% Fat Free
Ham - Honey Deli Fresh Meats
Ham - Honey Shaved Deli Fresh Meats
Ham - Smoked 96% Fat Free
Ham - Smoked 97% Fat Free Thin
  Sliced Deli Fresh Meats
Ham - Smoked Deli Fresh Meats
Ham - Smoked Shaved Deli Fresh
  Meats
Ham - Virginia Brand Shaved Deli

Fresh Meats
Honey Ham
Natural Smoked Ham

Perdue

Deli Turkey Ham - Hickory Smoked

Plainville Farms

Plainville Farms (All BUT gravy and dressing)

Primo Taglio (Safeway)

Maple Ham (Old Fashioned) with Natural Juices

Prosciutto Dry Cured Ham

Publix ()

Cooked Ham (Sliced Lunch Meats)

Extra Thin Sliced Honey Ham (Sliced Lunch Meats)

Hickory Smoked Ham - Semi-Boneless, Fully Cooked

Honey Cured Bone-In Ham - Brown Sugar Glazed

Honey Cured Bone-In Ham with Brown Sugar Glaze Mix Packet

Honey Cured Boneless Ham with Brown Sugar Glaze

Honey Kut Ham (Sliced Lunch Meats)

Low Salt Ham (Sliced Lunch Meats)

Spiral Sliced Ham

Sweet Ham (Sliced Lunch Meats)

Tavern Ham (Sliced Lunch Meats)

Virginia Brand Ham (Sliced Lunch Meats)

Stop & Shop

Cooked Ham - 97% Fat Free

Cooked Ham with Natural Juices - 98% Fat Free

Danish Brand Ham with Natural Juices - 97% Fat Free

Thumman's

All Natural Black Forest Brand Ham

Black Forest Brand Ham

Bone and Tied Ham

Bone in Smoked Short Shank Virginia Ham

Boneless Fully Cooked Smoked Virginia Ham

Brown Sugar Coated Cooked Ham

Chef's Slice Ham

Easy Slice Spiral Cut Ham

Flat Smoked Ham

Honey Cured Baked Baby Ham

Honey Cured Baked Ham

Jersey Made Hot Ham

Jersey Made Oblong Ham

Jersey Made Ready to Eat Flat Ham

Jersey Made Ripple Ham

Jersey Made Ripple Smoked Ham

Jersey Made Ripple Virgina Ham

Natural Casing Hot Ham

Our Ham-O-Collo Cooked Hot Ham

Our Hot Ham

Oven Roasted Fresh Ham - Homestyle

Ready To Eat Hot Ham

Ripple Hot Ham

Ripple Proscuittini

Ripple Roast Pork

Round Proscuitto

Short Cut Deluxe Cooked Ham - Baby

Short Cut Deluxe Cooked Ham - Baby

Short Cut Deluxe Cooked Ham - Lower Sodium

Short Cut Deluxe Cooked Ham - Prague Shaped

Short Cut Deluxe Cooked Ham - Small Round Shape

Short Cut Deluxe Cooked Ham - Square Shape

Short Cut Deluxe Cooked Ham - Tear Drop Shape

Small Round Smoked Ham

Wally Oblong Box Ham

Wally Oblong Ham

Wally Pear Shape Ham

Wally Pear Shape Ham Box

Wally Square Ham

Trader Joe's ()

Prosciutto Di Italia

Spiral Ham with Glaze Pack

Ukrop's

Kitchen Entrees - Spiral Sliced Ham

Vac Pac Meats (Safeway)

Black Forest Ham with Natural Juices - Coated with Caramel Color

Old Fashioned Maple Ham with Natural Juices

Prosciutto Dry Cured Ham

Wellshire Farms
Black Forest Boneless Ham Nugget
Black Forest Deli Ham
Old Fashioned Boneless Half Ham
Old Fashioned Boneless Whole Ham
Salt Cured Ham Café Slices
Semi Boneless Half Ham
Sliced Black Forest Ham
Sliced Ham Capicola
Sliced Tavern Ham
Sliced Virginia Brand Ham
Sunday Breakfast Ham
Virginia Brand Boneless Ham Steak
Virginia Brand Buffet Ham

HOT DOGS & FRANKS

Applegate Farms
Applegate Farms (All BUT Chicken
Nuggets, Chicken Pot Pie, & Chicken
Strips)
Bar-S
Bar-S (All BUT Chuck Wagon Brand
Franks & Bar-S Corn Dogs)
Boar's Head
Meats (All)
Butcher's Cut (Safeway)
Jumbo Franks (includes Chicken &
Pork)
Jumbo Turkey Franks
Cloverdale Foods
Franks (All)
Coleman Natural
Hot Dogs
Empire Kosher
Chicken Franks
Turkey Franks
Hormel ()
Wranglers Franks
Jennie-O ()
Turkey Franks
Johnsonville
Johnsonville (All BUT Beer 'n
Bratwurst and Cooked Beer Brats)

Louis Rich And Oscar Mayer 🖉
Bun Length Turkey Franks
Cheese Dogs Turkey Franks
Turkey Franks
Oscar Mayer 🖉
98% Fat Free Weiners
Bun-Length Beef Franks
Hot and Spicy XXL Hot Dogs
Jumbo Beef Franks
Light Beef Franks
Light Weiners
Little Smokies
Little Smokies Cheese
Little Wieners
Premium Beef XXL Hot Dogs
Regular Beef Franks
Regular Weiners
Smoked XXL Hot Dogs
Smokies Sausage
The Cheesiest Cheese Dogs
Turkey Franks
Turkey Hot Dogs
XXL Deli Style Beef Franks
Publix ()
Beef Franks
Beef Hot Dogs
Meat Franks
Meat Hot Dogs
Sabrett
All Beef Frankfurters (Skinless and
Natural Casing)
Safeway
Jumbo Beef Franks
Select Brand (Safeway)
Beef Franks
Smith's
Wieners
Thumman's
4-1 Franks
All Beef Loose Franks
All Beef Package Franks
All Natural Pork and Beef Frankfurters
Cocktail Franks
Loose Franks
Natural Casing Franks
PushCart Natural Casing Franks
Pushcart Skinless Franks

Wellshire Farms
Cheese Frank
Chicken Hot Dogs
NY Style Big Beef Franks
Old Fashioned Beef Frank
Original Deli Frank
Premium Beef Frank
Turkey Franks

MEAT ALTERNATIVES

Lightlife
Tofu Pups
Sol Cuisine
Organic Sol Ground (Veggie Ground)
Organic Tofu Ribz

PEPPERONI

Hormel ()
Pepperoni
Pillow Pack - Turkey Pepperoni
Hy-Vee
Pepperoni
Primo Naturale
Dried Pepperoni
Sliced Dried Pepperoni
Wellshire Farms
Sliced Beef Pepperoni

PORK

Boar's Head
Meats (All)
Byron's Pork BBQ
Byron's Pork BBQ (Sold at Sam's Club)
Columbus Salame
Capicolla Hot
Capicolla Mild
Coppa
Fire Roast Pork Roast
Fire Roasted Pork
Fast Fixin'
Ribz For Sandwiches
Homestyle Meals
Pork Baby Back Ribs with BBQ Sauce

Shredded Pork in BBQ Sauce
Hormel ()
Always Tender - Adobo Pork Cubes
Flavored Fresh Pork
Always Tender - Citrus Flavored Fresh
Pork
Always Tender - Fajita Pork Strips
Flavored Fresh Pork
Always Tender - Lemon-Garlic
Flavored Fresh Pork
Always Tender - Mesquite Flavored
Fresh Pork
Always Tender - Mojo Criollo Flavored
Fresh Pork
Always Tender - Non-Flavored Fresh
Pork
Always Tender - Onion-Garlic Flavored
Fresh Pork
Always Tender - Original Flavored
Fresh Pork
Always Tender - Raspberry Chipotle
Flavored Fresh Pork
Always Tender - Sun-Dried Tomato
Flavored Fresh Pork
Refrigerated Entrées - Pork Roast Au
Jus
Publix ()
Pork Loin in Teriyaki Sauce (Fully
Cooked)
Spanish Style Pork (Sliced Lunch
Meats)
Select Brand (Safeway)
St. Louis Style Smoke House Signature
Ribs
Trader Joe's ()
Baby Back Pork Ribs
BBQ Shredded Pork
Pork in Barbecue Sauce
Ukrop's
Kitchen Entrees - Herb Roasted Pork
Loin
Kitchen Entrees - Southern Style Pork
BBQ
Kitchen Entrees - Virginia Pork BBQ

Salami

Columbus Salame
All Natural Herb Salame
All Natural Hot Fennel Salame
All Natural Italian Dry Salame
All Natural Pepper Salame
All Natural Sopressata
Cacciatore
Crespone
Felino
Finocchiona
Genoa Salame
Habanero Hot Salame
Herb Salame
Hot Fennel Salame
Italian Dry Salame
Lite Salame
Low Sodium Salame
Pepper Salame
Salame Cotto
Salame Secchi
Sopressata

Empire Kosher
Turkey Salami - Slices
Turkey Salami Roll

Hormel ()
Hard Salami (Snack Size)
Homeland - Hard Salami
Italian Dry Salami (Snack Size)
Pillow Pack - Hard Salami
Pillow Pack - Pepperoni

Hy-Vee
Cooked Salami

Louis Rich And Oscar Mayer ⬿
50% Less Fat Turkey Cotto Salami
Turkey Cotto Salami

Old Wisconsin 🍴 ()
Beer Salami

Oscar Mayer ⬿
Hard Salami Sausage
Salami - Beef Deli Thin Deli Fresh
Meats

Perdue
Deli Turkey Salami

Primo Naturale
Chub Hard Salami

Chub Salami with Black Pepper
Chub Salami with Herbs
Chub Salami with Wine
Sliced Coppa Salami
Sliced Hard Salami
Sliced Original Salami with Wine
Sliced Premium Genoa Salami
Sliced Salami with Black Pepper
Sliced Salami with Herbs

Primo Taglio (Safeway)
Cervelat Salami
Genoa Salami
Salami (Peppered) Coated with Gelatin
& Black Pepper
Sopressata

Publix ()
Hard Salami - Reduced Fat (Sliced
Lunch Meats)

Safeway
Genoa Salami (Deli Counter)
Hard Salami (Deli Counter)

Thumman's
Cooked Salami

Vac Pac Meats (Safeway)
Genoa Salami
Peppered Salami - Coated with Black
Pepper and Gelatin
Sopressata

Wellshire Farms
Sliced Cooked Salami
Sliced Old Fashioned Deli Style Beef
Salami

Sausage

Applegate Farms
Applegate Farms (All BUT Chicken
Nuggets, Chicken Pot Pie, & Chicken
Strips)

Bar-S
Bar-S (All BUT Chuck Wagon Brand
Franks & Bar-S Corn Dogs)

Beelers
Sausages (All)

Bilinski's
Bilinski's (All)

Boar's Head
Meats (All)
Butcher's Cut (Safeway)
Bratwurst
Italian Sausage - Regular & Mild
Polska Kielbasa
Smoked Sausage
Canino's Sausage Company 🏅 🏅
Bratwurst
Breakfast Sausage
German Brand Sausage
Hot Italian
Hot! Chorizo
Mild Italian
Polish Sausage
Spicy Cajun Style Sausage
Sweet Italian Sausage
Cloverdale Foods
Sausage (All)
Columbus Salame
Mortadella
Mortadella w/Pistachio
Di Lusso ()
Beef Summer Sausage
Ejays So. Smokehouse
Smoke Jalapeno Sausage
Smoked Kielbasa
Empire Kosher
Chicken Sausage Mushroom & Garlic
Chicken Sausage Sun Dried Tomato
    Basil
Chicken Sausage Sweet Apple &
    Cinnamon
Farmington (Save-A-Lot)
Farmington Pork Sausage, Mild
Global Gourmet
Andouille Chicken Sausage
Apple Oven Roasted Chicken Sausage
Artichoke and Calamata Olive Chicken
    Sausage
Chipotle Pepper Chicken Sausage
Feta Cheese & Fresh Spinach Chicken
    Sausage
Fontina Cheese & Roasted Garlic
    Chicken Sausage
Spicy Italian Chicken Sausage

Sun Dried Tomato Chicken Sausage
Hormel ()
Crumbled Sausage
Little Sizzlers - Sausage Links & Patties
Smokies
Summer Sausage (Snack Size)
Hy-Vee
Bratwurst
Bratwurst - Grill Pack
Sausage Links
Sausage Patties
Jennie-O ()
Breakfast Lover's - Turkey Sausage
Extra Lean Smoked Kielbasa Turkey
    Sausage
Extra Lean Smoked Turkey Sausage
Turkey Store - Cheddar Turkey
    Bratwurst Fresh Dinner Sausage
Turkey Store - Hot Italian Fresh Dinner
    Sausage
Turkey Store - Lean Turkey Bratwurst
    Fresh Dinner Sausage
Turkey Store - Maple Links Fresh
    Breakfast Sausage
Turkey Store - Mild Links Fresh
    Breakfast Sausage
Turkey Store - Mild Patties Fresh
    Breakfast Sausage
Turkey Store - Sweet Italian Fresh
    Dinner Sausage
Johnsonville
Johnsonville (All BUT Beer 'n
    Bratwurst and Cooked Beer Brats)
Jones Dairy Farm
All Natural Hearty Pork Sausages
All Natural Light Pork Sausage & Rice
    Links
All Natural Little Pork Sausages
All Natural Original Pork Sausage Roll
All Natural Pork Sausage Patties
Chub Braunschweiger Liverwurst - 20%
    Bacon
Chub Braunschweiger Liverwurst -
    Light
Chub Braunschweiger Liverwurst -
    Original
Chub Braunschweiger Liverwurst - with

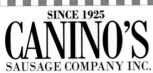

SINCE 1925

CANINO'S
SAUSAGE COMPANY INC.

— QUICK FACTS —

- **GLUTEN FREE,**
  Soy FREE & Dairy FREE
- Contains NO MSG, Nitrates, Preservatives, or Artificial Colors
- Contains ALL NATURAL ingredients
- ALL PRODUCTS made with ONLY the finest ground pork
- LESS FAT than the USDA recommended amount
- Colorado Company since 1925

Onion
Chunk Braunschweiger - Light
Chunk Braunschweiger - Original
Sliced Braunschweiger

Nature's Promise (Giant)
Italian Spicy Pork Sausage
Mild Italian Chicken Sausage
Red Pepper and Provolone Pork Sausage
Spiced Apple Chicken Sausage
Spinach and Feta Chicken Sausage
Sun Dried Tomato and Basil Chicken Sausage

Nature's Promise (Stop & Shop)
Italian Spicy Pork Sausage
Mild Italian Chicken Sausage
Red Pepper & Provolone Pork Sausage
Spiced Apple Chicken Sausage
Spinach & Feta Chicken Sausage
Sun Dried Tomato & Basil Chicken Sausage

Old Wisconsin
Beef Stick Summer Sausage - Beef
Beef Stick Summer Sausage - Original

Braunschweiger
Braunschweiger - Onion & Parsley
Grilling Sausages - Festival Bratwurst
Grilling Sausages - Natural Casing Wieners
Grilling Sausages - Polish Kielbasa
Grilling Sausages - Smoked Sausage with Cheddar
Hand-tied Summer Sausage - Beef
Hand-tied Summer Sausage - Beef Garlic
Hand-tied Summer Sausage - Garlic
Hand-tied Summer Sausage - Original
Liver Sausage
Party Summer Sausage
Summer Sausage - Beef
Summer Sausage - Beef Garlic
Summer Sausage - Garlic
Summer Sausage - Original
XX Summer Sausage

Oscar Mayer
Beef Summer Sausage
Summer Sausage

Perdue
Seasoned Fresh Lean Turkey Sausage - Hot Italian
Seasoned Fresh Lean Turkey Sausage - Sweet Italian

Plainville Farms
Plainville Farms (All BUT gravy and dressing)

Premio
Bratwurst
Cheese and Basil
Hot
Luganiga
Mild
Pepper, Onion and Mushroom
Sweet
Sweet Basil
Tomato, Garlic and Rosemary

Primo Italian (Save-A-Lot) ()
Primo Italian Mild & Hot Sausage ()

Primo Naturale
Dried Hot Chorizo
Sliced Dried Chorizo
Sliced Hot Chorizo

Sliced Sopressata
Sopressata
Stick Dried Chorizo
Sweet Abruzzi Sausage

Primo Taglio (Safeway)
Mortadella - Black Pepper Added

Publix ()
Fresh Bratwurst
Fresh Chorizo
Fresh Italian - Hot
Fresh Italian - Mild
Fresh Turkey Italian - Hot
Fresh Turkey Italian - Mild

Select Brand (Safeway)
Beef Hot Link Sausage
Beef Smoked Sausage
Cajun Style Link Sausage
Chicken Andouille Sausage
Chicken Apple Sausage
Italian Pork Sausage
Italian Sausage
Polish Sausage
Turkey Chicken Parmesan Basil
Sausage
Turkey Chicken Sun Dried Tomato
Sausage

Smith's
Sausages

Thumman's
Bratwurst
Braunschweiger - Chub Yellow Casing
Liverwurst
Braunschweiger - Fresh Liverwurst
Braunschweiger - White Casing
Liverwurst
Braunschweiger - Yellow Casing
Liverwurst
Chub Smoked Liverwurst
Hog Casing Sausage
Italian Hot Sausage
Italian Sausage Hot Package
Italian Sausage Sweet Package
Italian Sweet Sausage
Kielbasi Loaf
Kielbasi Loose
Knockwurst
Liverwurst Cap

Loose Knockwurst
Mama Kielbasa
Pre-Cooked Bratwurst
Pre-Cooked Sausage
Sausage Patties
Sheep Casing Sausage

Trader Joe's ()
Sausage (All)

Villa Roma
Sausage Products (All)

Wellshire Farms
Aged Cheddar Bratwurst
Mild Italian Style Turkey Dinner Link
Sausage
Morning Maple Turkey Breakfast Link
Sausage
Original Bratwurst
Polska Kielbasa
Pork Andouille Sausage
Pork Chorizo Sausage
Pork Linguica Sausage
Pork Liverwurst
Pork Sausage with Green Peppers &
Onions
Pork Sausage with Jalapeno & Aged
Cheddar
Roasted Garlic & Parsley Turkey
Dinner Link Sausage
Smoked Bratwurst
Smoked Pork Kielbasa Links
Spicy Hot Style Bratwurst
Turkey Andouille Sausage
Turkey Dinner Sausage Links -
Jalapeno Herb
Turkey Kielbasa
Turkey Liverwurst

SEAFOOD

Captains Choice (Safeway)
Cod Fillets
Cooked Tail On Shrimp

SeaPak ()
Shrimp Scampi

Trader Joe's ()
Crabmeat (Deli)
Smoked Salmon (Deli)

TOFU & TEMPEH

Eden Foods
Dried Tofu

Giant
Tofu - Extra Firm
Tofu - Firm

Lightlife
Garden Veggie Tempeh
Organic Flax Tempeh
Organic Soy Tempeh
Organic Wild Rice Tempeh

Mori-Nu
Chinese Spice Seasoned Tofu
Japanese Miso Seasoned Tofu
Organic Silken Tofu
Silken Extra Firm Tofu
Silken Firm Tofu
Silken Lite Extra Firm Tofu
Silken Lite Firm Tofu
Silken Soft Tofu

Sol Cuisine
Organic Herb Tofu
Organic Sesame Ginger Tofu
Organic Tofu

Stop & Shop
Tofu - Extra Firm
Tofu - Firm

Sunergia Soyfoods
More Than Tofu Organic Garlic Shitake
More Than Tofu Organic Indian Masala
More Than Tofu Organic Italian Herb
More Than Tofu Organic Jalapeno
Spinach
More Than Tofu Organic Peanut Ginger
More Than Tofu Organic Pesto
More Than Tofu Organic Savory
Portabella
More Than Tofu Organic Spicy Indian
More Than Tofu Organic Spicy Thai

Trader Joe's ()
Tofu - Extra Firm
Tofu - Organic Firm

Turtle Island Foods
Organic Five Grain Tempeh
Spicy Veggie Tempeh

TURKEY

Albertsons
Wafer Sliced Lunchmeat (Albertson's
Brand Only)

Applegate Farms
Applegate Farms (All BUT Chicken
Nuggets, Chicken Pot Pie, & Chicken
Strips)

Bar-S
Bar-S (All BUT Chuck Wagon Brand
Franks & Bar-S Corn Dogs)

Boar's Head
Meats (All)

Butcher's Cut (Safeway)
Ground Turkey
Oven Roasted Turkey Breast - 98% Fat
Free & Regular

Carl Buddig 🍴
Buddig Deli Cuts - Honey-Roasted
Turkey
Buddig Deli Cuts - Oven-Roasted
Turkey
Buddig Deli Cuts - Smoked Turkey
Buddig Original "Big Pak" Deli
Pouches - Honey-Roasted Turkey
Buddig Original "Big Pak" Deli
Pouches - Oven-Roasted Turkey
Buddig Original "Big Pak" Deli
Pouches - Turkey
Buddig Original Deli Pouches - Honey-
Roasted Turkey
Buddig Original Deli Pouches - Oven-
Roasted Turkey
Buddig Original Deli Pouches - Turkey
Buddig Original in Resealable
Containers - Honey-Roasted Turkey
Buddig Original in Resealable
Containers - Turkey
Buddig Original Value Pack Deli
Pouches - Honey-Roasted Turkey
Buddig Original Value Pack Deli
Pouches - Oven-Roasted Turkey
Buddig Original Value Pack Deli
Pouches - Turkey

Columbus Salame
Herb Roasted Turkey

Herb Turkey Breast
Holiday Carving Turkey
Honey Turkey Breast
Maple Honey Turkey Breast
Pepper Turkey
Reduced Sodium Turkey
Smoked Turkey Breast
Turkey Fire Roasted

Empire Kosher

Fresh Chill Pack Chicken & Turkey
Fresh Ground Turkey
Fully Cooked Barbecue Turkey (Fresh
  Or Frozen)
Preferred - Signature Edition Smoked
  Turkey Breast, Skinless
Preferred - Signature Edition Turkey
  Breast Pastrami, Skinless
Preferred - Signature Edition Turkey
  Pastrami, Skinless
Premiere - Signature Edition All Natural
  Turkey Breast Skinless
Premiere - Signature Edition All Natural
  Turkey Breast with Skin
Signature Edition - Oven Prepared
  Turkey Breast
Signature Edition - Smoked Turkey
  Breast
Smoked Turkey Breast - Slices
Turkey Breast - Slices
Turkey Burgers
Turkey Pastrami - Slices
White Turkey Roll

Giant

Honey Turkey Breast - 97% Fat Free
Oven Roasted Turkey Breast - 97% Fat
  Free
Smoked Turkey Breast

Hormel ()

Deli Sliced Oven Roasted Turkey Breast
Deli Sliced Smoked Turkey Breast
Julienne Turkey
Natural Choice - Honey Deli Turkey
Natural Choice - Oven Roasted Deli
  Turkey
Natural Choice - Smoked Deli Turkey

Hy-Vee

Deli Thin Slices - Honey Roasted
  Turkey Breast
Deli Thin Slices - Oven Roasted Turkey
  Breast
Thin Sliced Honey Turkey
Thin Sliced Turkey
Turkey

Isaly's

Deli Meats (All)

Jennie-O ()

Apple Cinnamon Turkey Breast
Cajun-Style Refrigerated Qtr Turkey
  Breasts
Cracked Pepper Refrigerated Qtr
  Turkey Breasts
Festive Tender Cured Turkey
Garlic Peppered Turkey Breast
Grand Champion - Hickory Smoked
  Turkey Breast
Grand Champion - Homestyle Pan
  Roasted Turkey Breast
Grand Champion - Honey Cured Turkey
  Breast
Grand Champion - Mesquite Smoked
  Turkey Breast
Grand Champion - Oven Roasted
  Turkey Breast
Grand Champion - Tender Browned
  Turkey Breast
Hickory Smoked Refrigerated Qtr
  Turkey Breasts
Honey Cured Refrigerated Qtr Turkey
  Breasts
Honey Maple Turkey Breast
Hot Red Peppered Turkey Breast
Italian Style Turkey Breast
Maple Spiced Turkey Breast
Mesquite Smoked Turkey Breast
Natural Choice - Oven Roasted Turkey
  Breast
Natural Choice - Peppered Turkey
  Breast
Natural Choice - Tender Browned
  Turkey Breast
Oven Roasted Refrigerated Qtr Turkey
  Breasts

Oven Roasted Turkey Breast
Pan Roasts with Gravy - White
Pan Roasts with Gravy - White/Dark Combo
Peppered Turkey Breast
Prime Young Turkey - Fresh (Gravy packet NOT GF)
Refrigerated Dark Turkey Pastrami
Refrigerated Honey Cured Turkey Ham
Refrigerated Turkey Ham
Smoked Peppered Turkey Breast
Smoked Turkey Breast
Smoked Turkey Wings & Drumsticks
Sun-Dried Tomato Refrigerated Qtr Turkey Breasts
Tender Browned Turkey Breast
Tomato Basil Turkey Breast
Turkey Store - Cracked Pepper Hickory Smoked Turkey Breast
Turkey Store - Extra Lean Fresh Ground Turkey
Turkey Store - Fresh Lean Turkey Patties
Turkey Store - Garlic & Herb Oven Ready Turkey
Turkey Store - Garlic Pesto Hickory Smoked Turkey Breast
Turkey Store - Homestyle Oven Ready Turkey
Turkey Store - Honey Cured Hickory Smoked Turkey Breast
Turkey Store - Honey Cured Smoked Turkey Breast
Turkey Store - Honey Mesquite Turkey Breast
Turkey Store - Italian Fresh Ground Turkey
Turkey Store - Lean Fresh Ground Turkey
Turkey Store - Lemon-Garlic Flavored Tenderloins
Turkey Store - Oven Ready Turkey Breast (Gravy packet NOT GF)
Turkey Store - Oven Roasted Turkey Breast
Turkey Store - Seasoned Pepper Flavored Tenderloins
Turkey Store - Sun Dried Tomato

Hickory Smoked Turkey Breast
Turkey Store - Tequila Lime Flavored Tenderloins
Turkey Store Fresh Tray - Breast Slices
Turkey Store Fresh Tray - Breast Strips
Turkey Store Fresh Tray - Tenderloins
Turkey Store So Easy - BBQ Glazed Breast Filets
Turkey Store So Easy - Broccoli & Cheese Stuffed Breasts
Turkey Store So Easy - Honey Glazed Breast Filets
Turkey Store So Easy - Pepper Cheese & Rice Stuffed Breasts
Turkey Store So Easy - Slow Roasted Turkey Breast
Turkey Store So Easy - Swiss Cheese & Ham Stuffed Breasts

Land O' Frost
Lunchmeats (All BUT Taste Escapes Lemon Pepper Chicken)

Louis Rich And Oscar Mayer ✍
Smoked Chopped 50% Less Fat Turkey Ham
Turkey Breast Hickory Smoked 98% Fat Free
Turkey Breast Oven Roasted
Turkey Ham
Turkey Smoked White 95% Fat Free
Turkey White Smoked

Meijer
Fresh Hen Turkey
Fresh Tom Turkey
Fresh Turkey Breast
Hen Turkey
Hickory Smoked Turkey Breast
Honey Roasted Turkey Breast
Meijer Gold - Hen Turkey
Meijer Gold - Tom Turkey
Tom Turkey
Turkey Basted w/Timer
Turkey Breast Fresh
Turkey Breast Zipper 97% Fat Free
Turkey Fresh Natural
Turkey Sliced Chipped Meat

Norbest
Turkey Products (All)

Norwestern ()
- Deli Turkey - Hickory Smoked
- Deli Turkey - Oven Roasted
- Deli Turkey - Turkey Pastrami

Oscar Mayer ⌒
- Honey Smoked Lean White Turkey
- Oven Roasted White Turkey
- Smoked White Turkey
- Turkey- Oven Roasted 98% Fat Free Deli Fresh Meats
- Turkey - Smoked 97% Fat Free Deli Fresh Meats
- Turkey Breast - Honey Smoked Shaved Deli Fresh Meats
- Turkey Breast - Honey Smoked Thin Sliced Deli Fresh Meats
- Turkey Breast - Mesquite Shaved Deli Fresh Meats
- Turkey Breast - Mesquite Thin Sliced Deli Fresh Meats
- Turkey Breast - Oven Roasted Deli Fresh Meats
- Turkey Breast - Oven Roasted Shaved Deli Fresh Meats
- Turkey Breast - Oven Roasted Thin Sliced Deli Fresh Meats
- Turkey Breast - Smoked Deli Fresh Meats
- Turkey Breast - Smoked Shaved Deli Fresh Meats
- Turkey Breast - Smoked Thin Sliced Deli Fresh Meats
- Turkey Variety Pack
- Variety Pack - Turkey Breast - Honey Roasted/Oven Roasted/Hickory Smoked

Perdue
- Carving - Turkey Breast, Hickory Smoked
- Carving - Turkey Breast, Honey Smoked
- Carving - Turkey Breast, Mesquite Smoked
- Carving - Turkey Breast, Oven Roasted
- Carving - Turkey Ham, Honey Smoked
- Carving - Whole Turkey
- Carving Classics - Pan Roasted Turkey Breast, Cracked Pepper
- Carving Classics - Turkey Breast Pan Roasted
- Carving Classics - Turkey Breast Pan Roasted, Honey Smoked
- Deli Dark Turkey Pastrami - Hickory Smoked
- Deli Pick Ups - Sliced Turkey Breast, Golden Browned
- Deli Pick Ups - Sliced Turkey Breast, Honey Smoked
- Deli Pick Ups - Sliced Turkey Breast, Mesquite Smoked
- Deli Pick Ups - Sliced Turkey Breast, Oven Roasted
- Deli Pick Ups - Sliced Turkey Breast, Smoked
- Deli Pick Ups - Sliced Turkey Ham, Honey Smoked
- Deli Turkey Breast - Oil Browned
- Fresh Ground Breast of Turkey
- Fresh Lean Ground Turkey
- Ground Turkey Burgers
- Healthsense - Turkey Breast, Oven Roasted (Fat Free, Reduced Sodium)
- Rotisserie Turkey Breast
- Short Cuts - Carved Turkey Breast Oven Roasted
- Slicing - Turkey Ham
- Tender & Tasty Products
- Whole Turkeys Seasoned with Broth

Plainville Farms
- Plainville Farms (All BUT gravy and dressing)

Primo Taglio (Safeway)
- Dinner Roast Turkey Breast
- Honey Maple Turkey Breast
- Mesquite Smoked Turkey Breast with Natural Mesquite Smoke Flavoring Added
- Natural Hickory Smoked Peppered Turkey Breast with Natural Smoke Flavoring
- Natural Hickory Smoked Turkey Breast with Natural Smoke Flavoring
- Pan Roasted Turkey Breast Browned in Hot Cottonseed Oil

Salsa Seasoned Cooked and Cured
Turkey Breast

Publix ()

Extra Thin Sliced Oven Roasted Turkey
Breast (Sliced Lunch Meats)

Extra Thin Sliced Smoked Turkey
Breast (Sliced Lunch Meats)

Fresh Young Turkey - Whole

Fresh Young Turkey Breast

Fully Cooked Smoked Turkey (Whole)

Fully Cooked Smoked Turkey Breast

Fully Cooked Turkey Breast (Deli)

Fully Cooked Turkey, Whole (Deli)

Ground Turkey

Ground Turkey Breast

Smoked Turkey (Sliced Lunch Meats)

Turkey Breast (Sliced Lunch Meats)

Safeway

Roasted Turkey Breast (Deli Counter)

Stop & Shop

Oven Roasted Turkey Breast - Fat Free

Smoked Turkey Breast

Thumman's

All Natural Oven Roasted Gourmet
Turkey Breast

All Natural Oven Roasted Hickory
Smoked Turkey Breast

Golden Roasted Filet of Turkey - Cajun
Style

Golden Roasted Filet of Turkey -
Craked Pepper and Paprika Coated

Golden Roasted Filet of Turkey - Honey
and Molasses Coated

Golden Roasted Filet of Turkey - Italian
Style

Golden Roasted Filet of Turkey -
Lemon Pepper Coated

Golden Roasted Filet of Turkey - Lower
Sodium

Golden Roasted Filet of Turkey -
Pastrami Seasoning

Golden Roasted Filet of Turkey -
Rotisserie Flavor

Golden Roasted Filet of Turkey - Santa
Fe Style

Golden Roasted Gourmet Turkey

Golden Roasted Skinless Filet of Turkey

- Hickory Smoked

Oven Roasted Premium Turkey Breast

Petite Filet of Turkey - Hickory Smoked
(Skinless and with Skin)

Premimum White Filet of Turkey -
Skinless

Premium White Filet of Turkey

Trader Joe's ()

Mesquite Smoked Turkey Breast Sliced
(East Coast)

Vac Pac Meats (Safeway)

Cracked Pepper Turkey Breast with
Natural Smoke Flavoring

Hickory Smoked Turkey Breast with
Natural Smoke Flavoring

Oven Roasted Turkey Breast

Wellshire Farms

All Natural Pan Roasted Turkey Breast

All Natural Smoked Turkey Breast

Sliced Oven Roasted Turkey Breast

Sliced Smoked Turkey Breast

Sliced Turkey Ham

Turkey Breast Oven Roasted

Turkey Ham Buffet Half Ham

Turkey Ham Steak

MISCELLANEOUS

Albertsons

Wafer Sliced Lunchmeat (Albertson's
Brand Only)

Columbus Salame

Head Cheese

Head Cheese Hot

Hy-Vee

Ham & Cheese Loaf

Old Fashioned Loaf

Pickle Loaf

Spiced Luncheon Loaf

Nature's Promise (Giant)

Deli Meats (All Varieties)

Old Wisconsin ☸ ()

Pate - Black Pepper

Pate - Braunschweiger Spreadable

Pate - Onion & Parsley

Oscar Mayer ᵔ

Variety Pack - Bologna/Turkey/Ham

Variety Pack - Fat Free Ham & Turkey
Variety Pack - Ham/Turkey
Variety Pack - Ham/Turkey/Canadian
  Style Bacon
Variety Pack - Salami/Bologna/Ham

Publix ()

Olive Loaf (Sliced Lunch Meats)
Pickle & Pimento Loaf (Sliced Lunch
  Meats)

Thumman's

Blood and Tongue Loaf
Head Cheese
Luncheon Loaf
Old Fashion Head Cheese
Olive Loaf
Pickle and Pimento Loaf
Pizza Topping

Index of Advertisers

CARL BUDDIG

www.buddig.com 888.633.5684

EREWHON

www.usmillsllc.com 800.422.1125

Since 1966 Erewhon® has provided great tasting, gluten-free cereals that are organic. Visit our website for our Crispy Rice Snacks recipe that the whole family will enjoy.

FOOD FOR LIFE

www.foodforlife.com 800.797.5090

With over 30 years producing gluten-free products, Food For Life maintains very strict standards in the production of our gluten-free product line for the protection of our customers.

GLUTENFREEDA REAL COOKIES!

www.glutenfreedafoods.com 360.755.1300

IAN'S NATURAL FOODS

www.iansnaturalfoods.com 800.543.6637

Ian's manufactures both frozen and dry foods, all of which are independently tested, assuring our foods average less than 2.5 parts per million gluten.

MARY'S GONE CRACKERS

www.marysgonecrackers.com 888.258.1250

5 flavors of crackers and 3 flavors of Sticks & Twigs, manufactured in dedicated g-f, nut-free, dairy-free, kosher and organic facility. 2008 Outstanding Cracker award winner (NASFT).

BARD'S TALE BEER

www.bardsbeer.com 877.440.2337

CHEBE BREAD PRODUCTS

www.chebe.com 800.217.9510

Our facility is 100% gluten-free. Many of our products are free of allergens, such as soy, corn, lactose, yeast, tree nuts and peanuts.

CHERRYBROOK KITCHEN

www.cherrybrookkitchen.com. 866.458.8225

Cherrybrook Kitchen makes great-tasting baking mixes and snacks that are wheat-free/gluten-free, as well as peanut-free, dairy-free, egg-free and nut-free.

ENDANGERED SPECIES CHOCOLATE

www.chocolatebar.com. 800.293.0160

Endangered Species Chocolate uses ethically-traded, shade-grown cacao to make all-natural and organic chocolate bars. All milk and dark chocolate products are Certified Gluten-Free by the Gluten-Free Certification Organization.

GLUTINO

www.glutenfree.com 800.291.8386

PAMELA'S PRODUCTS

www.pamelasproducts.com 707.462.6605

Since 1988, Pamela's Products has set the standard in great tasting gluten-free foods. We offer award-winning cookies and baking mixes.

R.W. GARCIA

www.rwgarcia.com. 408.287.4616

WHOLESOME SWEETENERS

www.OrganicSugars.biz. 800.680.1896

Wholesome Sweeteners award-winning Fair Trade Certified, Organic & Natural Sugars, Syrups, Agave Nectars and Honeys are all gluten free.

CANINO'S SAUSAGE COMPANY

www.caninosausage.com 800.538.0148

MARIPOSA BAKING COMPANY

www.mariposabaking.com.............................510.595.0955

Mariposa handcrafts delights in our 100% dedicated GF bakery. We've Been Nibbled! Our products were selected as outstanding by The Nibble.

ORGANIC BISTRO

www.theorganicbistro.com 480.664.8729

Organic Bistro Whole Life Meals are easy to prepare frozen meals made with 100% Gluten-Free, organic and premium natural ingredients. Each recipe is developed by a registered dietician, naturopathic physician and chef for optimal nutrition and taste.

RED STAR YEAST

www.redstaryeast.com 800.445.4746

Red Star Yeast, making gluten-free yeast for over 125 years! Go to our website for more Gluten Free recipes - www.redstaryeast.com

WOODCHUCK DRAFT CIDER

www.woodchuck.com..................................802.388.0700

Woodchuck Draft Cider was born in Vermont in 1991. Made by people who care about purity, taste and authenticity, Woodchuck offers a handcrafted quality with a unique taste.

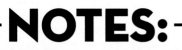

NOTES:

THE GLUTEN-FREE DIET:
AN EASY REFERENCE INGREDIENTS TABLE

✓	Gluten-Free
✗	NOT Gluten-Free
?	Maybe - depends on manufacturer

Need a refresher on the gluten-free diet? These grains are safe: rice, soy, corn, potatoes, tapioca, buckwheat, arrowroot, amaranth, millet, quinoa, sorghum and teff. When plain, you can also eat: fruits, vegetables, milk, meat, eggs, beans, oil, wine, and distilled alcohols like vodka and gin.

As for what's off limits, "no wheat, rye, barley and oats*" in practice means, no (wheat) flour, pasta, croutons, bread, cookies, and "hidden" gluten sources like soy sauce, beer, and licorice. (But don't despair, there ARE specialty GF versions of these products in this guide!) Beyond these basics, even the most experienced shopper can stumped by mysterious ingredients like "guar gum."

We hope this ingredient list will make label-reading easier than ever, for both new and experienced GF shoppers!

Ingredient		Ingredient		Ingredient	
Agar-Agar	✓	Durum	✗	Mono and Diglycerides	✓
Alcohol, Distilled	✓	Einkorn	✗	Monosodium Glutamate (MSG)	✓
Algin	✓	Farina	✗	Mustard Flour	?
Annatto	✓	Flax	✓	Natural Colors	✓
Arabic Gum	✓	Fructose	✓	Natural Flavors	✓
Artificial Colors	✓	Fumaric Acid	✓	Polysorbates	✓
Artificial Flavoring	✓	Gelatin	✓	Psyllium	✓
Ascorbic Acid	✓	Glucose	✓	Rennet	✓
Aspartame	✓	Glucose Syrup	✓	Rice Malt	✓
Baking Powder	?	Glutamic Acid	✓	Rice Syrup	?
Beer	✗	Glutinous Rice	✓	Rum	✓
Beta Carotene	✓	Glycerides	✓	Saccharin	✓
BHA	✓	Glycol	✓	Seitan	✗
BHT	✓	Graham Flour	✗	Semolina	✗
Bulgur	✗	Guar Gum	✓	Silicon Dioxide	✓
Calcium Disodium EDTA	✓	Gum Arabic	✓	Sodium Benzoate	✓
Caprylic Acid	✓	Hydrolyzed Corn Protein	✓	Sodium Nitrate	✓
Caramel Color	✓	Hydrolyzed Soy Protein	✓	Sodium Nitrite	✓
Carboxymethylcellulose	✓	Hydrolyzed Wheat Protein	✗	Sodium Sulphite	✓
Carnauba Wax	✓	Inulin	✓	Sorbate	✓
Carob Bean	✓	Invert Sugar	✓	Sorbic Acid	✓
Carrageenan	✓	Kamut	✗	Sorbitol	✓
Casein	✓	Lactic Acid	✓	Soy Sauce	✗
Cellulose Gum	✓	Lactose	✓	Spelt	✗
Citric Acid	✓	Lecithin	✓	Starch (on labels, this refers to cornstarch)	✓
Corn Gluten	✓	Malic Acid	✓	Stevia	✓
Corn Syrup	✓	Malt (e.g., malt extract, malt flavoring, malt vinegar)	✗	Sucralose	✓
Corn Syrup Solids	✓			Sucrose	✓
Cornstarch	✓	Maltitol	✓	Sulfites	✓
Couscous	✗	Maltodextrin	✓	Tabbouleh	✗
Cream of Tartar	✓	Maltose	✓	Tartaric Acid	✓
Dextrimaltose	✗	Mannitol	✓	Triticale	✗
Dextrins	?	Matzo (matzoh)	✗	Vanilla Extract	✓
Dextrose	✓	Molasses	✓	Vanilla Flavoring	✓
				Vanillin	✓
				Vinegar (All EXCEPT malt)	✓
				Vodka	✓
				Wheat Bran	✗
				Wheat Germ	✗
				Whey	✓
				Wine	✓
				Xanthan Gum	✓
				Xylitol	✓
				Yeast (All EXCEPT brewer's yeast)	✓

*See page 12 for a profile on "gluten-free" oats

This ingredient table was created in collaboration with Shelley Case, B.Sc., RD, registered dietitian and autho of Gluten-Free Diet: A Comprehensive Resource Guide. She is a member of the medical advisory board of the Celiac Disease Foundation and Gluten Intolerance Group. For more in-depth information about th gluten-free diet, ingredients, labeling laws and healthy eating, please visit www.glutenfreediet.ca.